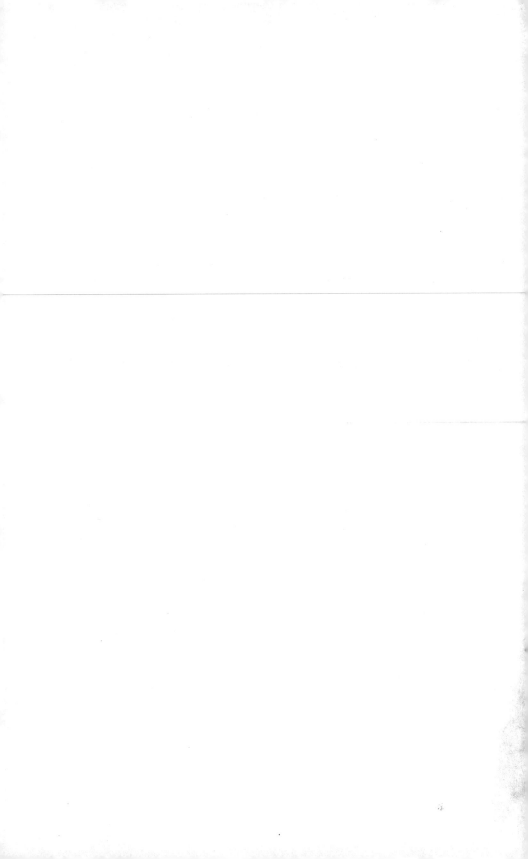

Drug Addiction
and its Treatment

Drug Addiction and its Treatment

Michael Gossop
Head of Research
National Addiction Centre
Institute of Psychiatry
Maudsley Hospital
London

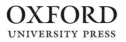

OXFORD
UNIVERSITY PRESS

OXFORD
UNIVERSITY PRESS

Great Clarendon Street, Oxford OX2 6DP

Oxford University Press is a department of the University of Oxford.
It furthers the University's objective of excellence in research, scholarship,
and education by publishing worldwide in

Oxford New York

Auckland Bangkok Buenos Aires Cape Town Chennai
Dar es Salaam Delhi Hong Kong Istanbul Karachi Kolkata
Kuala Lumpur Madrid Melbourne Mexico City Mumbai Nairobi
São Paulo Shanghai Taipei Tokyo Toronto

Oxford is a registered trade mark of Oxford University Press
in the UK and in certain other countries

Published in the United States
by Oxford University Press Inc., New York

© Oxford University Press, 2003

The moral rights of the author have been asserted
Database right Oxford University Press (maker)

First published 2003
Reprinted 2004

A catalogue record for this book is available from the British Library

Library of Congress Cataloging in Publication Data
(Data available)

ISBN 0 19 852608 3 (Pbk)

10 9 8 7 6 5 4 3 2

Typeset by Newgen Imaging Systems (P) Ltd., Chennai, India
Printed in Great Britain
on acid-free paper by
Biddles Ltd, King's Lynn, Norfolk

Preface

This book represents an attempt to discuss the nature of the most important and most widely used treatments for drug addiction, and to bring together the increasing evidence about their impact and effectiveness. It is intended to help bridge the gap that continues to exist between clinicians and academic researchers. My aim has been to present an up-to-date summary of the range of drug problems and of the treatments and interventions that are available to help tackle these problems. Within this framework, I have tried to discuss the research evidence in a way which is relevant to the everyday clinical concerns of those who are actually involved in the process of treatment.

It is clear that the largest body of research evidence about addiction treatments and their effectiveness is derived from work conducted in the United States. This is, necessarily, reflected in the content of this book. Where appropriate, I have sought to include research material from other countries, and I have specifically sought to refer to addiction treatment research conducted in the UK.

It is, perhaps, necessary to say something about the words that we use to talk about drug addiction. For those whose taste runs to such matters, these offer endless opportunities for terminological discussions. For example, the very word addiction is itself strongly disliked by many because of its excess meaning. Are addiction and dependence synonymous? Should *addiction* be seen as a composite disorder which also includes other problems? Should we avoid the word altogether talk and restrict discussion to its specific components? My own view is that the word is not without its merits precisely because it does still capture something of the compulsion to use drugs and of the entanglement within continued drug taking that are at the heart of what we mean by this problem.

From a different perspective, others have argued that the term *addict* is pejorative, and at least one scientific journal refuses to accept articles containing the word on the grounds that it is likely to perpetuate negative stereotypes.

Abuse and *misuse* also create consternation. Even *treatment* has been challenged in this context. There has also been debate about whether it is appropriate to refer to those who receive treatment as *patients* (since they are neither passive, nor are they necessarily receiving treatment within a medical setting).

My own preferences for certain terms will no doubt become clear to the reader, but I have no particular commitment to any of these terms. When more precise and more useful terms become available they will be adopted. But first and foremost, I have tried to avoid getting bogged down in terminological issues. That is not to say that I think such questions are unimportant. Many of them are both important and interesting, and would probably form the basis of an interesting chapter in their own right. However, my primary concern has been to address the issues of addiction and its treatment rather than to become enmeshed in a discussion of the language that we use to talk about them.

During the period of more than 30 years that I have worked in this field, there has been important progress. Without question, we now have a greatly improved understanding of addiction and its treatment. Some new treatments have emerged, and many of the existing treatments have been refined, while some of the traditional generalised treatment efforts have not proved their worth and have withered and faded. However, there has not been (nor, in my opinion, is there likely to be) any radical "discovery" to transform the nature of addiction treatment by providing a fully effective and universally applicable treatment intervention. Perhaps for this reason, many of those who have not kept up with developments in the field, are disappointed that there is not a single and specific treatment for addiction, and cling to the misapprehension that drug addiction is an untreatable condition. I hope that the evidence presented in this book will help to correct this mistakenly pessimistic view. Nonetheless, our understanding of the addictions and of its treatment is still rudimentary, and the provision of effective clinical services is often less than optimal. Without question, there remains enormous scope for many further improvements.

London
September 2003

Michael Gossop

Contents

Abbreviations

5-HIAA	hydroxy-indole acetic acid-5	MAP	Maudsley Addiction Profile
5-HT	5-hydroxatryptamine (serotonin)	MDMA	3,4-methylamphetamine (Ecstasy)
AA	Alcoholics Anonymous	MET	motivational enhancement therapy
ACMD	Advisory Council on the Misuse of Drugs (UK)	MI	motivational interviewing
ASAM	American Society of Addiction Medicine	MMM	methadone medical maintenance
ASI	Addiction Severity Index	MMT	methadone maintenance treatment
CA	Cocaine Anonymous	MRT	methadone reduction treatment
CBT	cognitive behavioural therapy		
CNS	central nervous system	NA	Narcotics Anonymous
CS	conditioned stimuli	NIDA	National Institute on Drug Abuse (US)
CURB	Campaign for the Use and Restriction of Barbiturates (UK)	NDATUS	National Drug and Alcoholism Treatment Unit Survey (US)
DA	dopamine	NTORS	National Treatment Outcome Research Study (UK)
DARP	Drug Abuse Reporting Programme (US)	OTI	Opiate Treatment Index
DATOS	Drug Abuse Treatment Outcome Study (US)	PET	positron emission tomography
DAWN	Drug and Alcohol Women's Network (UK)	RP	relapse prevention
DSM	*Diagnostic and statistical manual of mental disorders*	SAMHSA	Substance Abuse and Mental Health Services Administration (US)
ECA	Epidemiological Catchment Area (study; US)	SDS	Severity of Dependence Scale
GABA	gamma-aminobutyric acid	SOWS	Short Opiate Withdrawal Scale
HBV	hepatitis B virus	SSRIs	serotonin reuptake inhibitors
HCV	hepatitis C virus	TCAs	tricyclic antidepressants
HIV	human immunodeficiency virus	TCs	therapeutic communities
		THC	tetrahydrocannabinol
ISDD	Institute for the Study of Drug Dependence (UK)	TOPS	Treatment Outcome Prospective Study (US)
LAAM	leva-alpha acetyl methadol	TSF	twelve-step facilitation (programme)
LSD	lysergic acid diethylamide		
MAOIs	monoamine oxidase inhibitors	VSA	volatile substance abuse

Chapter 1

A background to addiction and its treatment

What this book means by drug addiction is most often manifested, psychologically and behaviourally, in feelings of compulsion to use drugs and difficulty in resisting those urges. Addiction is a learned behavioural problem, a habit disorder. It differs fundamentally from the mere use of illegal drugs in that an addiction represents an altered relationship between the user and their drug(s). The precise psychological and neurophysiological foundations upon which this altered relationship is based have yet to be fully identified.

There are undoubtedly problems with precisely defining and delineating the disorder. Terms such as drug use, misuse, abuse, and addiction have created difficulties for many years. One partial solution to some of the terminological difficulties has been to talk about specific types of drug-related problems and about problem drug users. The Advisory Council on the Misuse of Drugs (ACMD) offered a broad definition of a problem drug user as anyone who experiences social, psychological, physical, or legal problems related to intoxication, and/or regular excessive consumption, and/or dependence as a consequence of their use of drugs (ACMD 1982).

Not all drug-related behaviours are seen as problems by drug users. Not all drug-related behaviours are defined as problems by those working in treatment services. The specification of different types of problem is an essential part of assessing treatment effectiveness and treatment need. The problems that may be caused by or that are associated with drug misuse include drug dependence, adverse effects upon physical and psychological health, and impairment of social functioning (interpersonal relationships, educational or occupational performance, and illegal activity).

The term addiction, and more particularly the term 'addict', is also sometimes thought to carry a social stigma that undermines attempts to provide more humane and effective treatments for people with addictive disorders. These terms ('addict' and 'addiction') are used throughout this book. There is no reason why they should be regarded as stigmatizing. They also have the not inconsiderable merit that they capture one of the most fundamental characteristics of the disorder, the feeling of entrapment and of loss of freedom of choice to control the behaviour. Although some people are able to escape their addiction to drugs without medical or other treatment interventions, most addicts struggle for months, and sometimes for years to overcome the ties of addiction.

Modern patterns of addiction

Drug addiction is a cause of great personal distress to users and their families. It is also a major public health problem. In the UK serious concern about such problems was first voiced during the 1960s. In one sense, the 'modern era' of drug addiction can be thought of as beginning in the 1960s. This was a time when many countries witnessed a sudden increase in the use of many drugs. The use of illicit drugs was not new, though previously this had tended to be confined to certain special groups (e.g. 'medical' addicts such as doctors and nurses or iatrogenic addicts whose addiction was a consequence of previous medical treatment). From the mid-1960s, a wider range of illegal drugs began to be used by many young people. Most worryingly, the drugs that were widely being used now included heroin. Since that time, the prevalence of drug misuse and drug problems has increased greatly.

The time-scale for the development of drug problems was similar in many other countries. For various reasons, including geography and political climate, some countries initially appeared to be relatively unaffected by the development of these 'new' drug problems. Almost every country in the world is now confronted by the need to find a satisfactory and effective response to the many problems that are associated with the abuse of illegal drugs. These countries stretch across the globe from Ireland to Russia, from Finland to South Africa, from Colombia to Australia, from the USA to China.

The costs of drug abuse in the UK cannot be calculated precisely but they are known to be massive. Every year the problems associated with drug abuse and its consequences cost the country many billions of pounds. The costs include expenditure on prevention, treatment, and rehabilitation programmes. Costs are also incurred for welfare and social services, and for policing, inter-diction, and processing offenders within the criminal justice system. There are further human and social costs associated with impaired health, damaged relationships, and lowered productivity, as well as the distress caused to others by drug-related crime.

Few social problems are as complicated or as mutable as drug misuse. With regard to the question of which drugs cause problems, it is probably safest to assume that any substance that affects the psychological state of the user can also cause problems. The prevalence of specific types of drug taking in society is not directly related to the extent to which those drugs create problems either for society or for the individual. Although cannabis is widely used, it seldom leads to problems requiring clinical intervention. However, the drugs that lead to dependence are especially problematic, both at the societal level, and for the individual user. The extent to which different drugs are associated with different risks of dependence has long been seen as a central question with regard to the abuse of drugs. This issue has considerable contemporary relevance in the UK as well as in many other countries because of the increasing concern about the availability and abuse of heroin, crack cocaine, and other drugs that produce severe dependence in many of the people who use them.

Alcohol is one of our most familiar and domestic drugs. However, this book is about drug addiction and is not primarily about drinking problems or alcohol addiction *per se*. The reason for introducing alcohol as a drug is that it plays an important part in the repertoire of the multiple drug user, and as such it will appear throughout the book as one drug among many. There is no doubt that alcohol is a 'real' drug in the same sense that heroin is a drug. Alcohol is one of the more powerful, addictive, and destructive drugs and is used on a large scale. It acts on the nervous system like an anaesthetic and, in large enough amounts, it is a poison that can kill. In sufficiently large doses alcohol is capable of killing any living organism, though cases in which alcohol poisoning leads to respiratory depression and to death are comparatively rare. In smaller amounts alcohol acts as a depressant drug. As such, it produces sufficient impairment of judgement and skills to lead to countless road traffic accidents, acts of aggression, and other assorted but more minor misjudgements that may nonetheless be regretted the morning after.

As a central nervous system depressant, alcohol acts in ways that are similar to those associated with the benzodiazepine tranquillizers and the barbiturate sedatives. As the blood alcohol level rises, brain functions change and deteriorate. The first consistent changes in mood and behaviour occur at about 50 mg per cent, at which level most people tend to feel carefree and relaxed. Complex skills such as driving may be affected at 30 mg per cent and are seriously affected at 80 mg per cent. By 100 mg per cent, movements become clumsy and emotional behaviour is impaired, and these effects become more marked as blood alcohol levels increase further. By 300 mg per cent confusion, inability to stand or to walk, and unconsciousness are evident, and the fatal concentration lies between 500 and 800 mg per cent (Royal College of Psychiatrists 1986). Addiction to alcohol is also an extremely serious problem. In some respects, it could be regarded as more serious than addiction to the illegal drugs. Certainly it affects many more people and causes great harm.

During the 1970s, and increasingly since that time, there has been a broad consensus that 'the addictions' can be regarded as a category of disorders characterized by the compulsive and dependent use of many different substances and behaviours. It has been suggested that this category of addictions may include not just drug dependence, alcoholism, and cigarette smoking (and other forms of nicotine dependence), but also a range of other behaviours that do not involve the consumption of psychoactive substances, such as gambling, some types of eating disorders, compulsive sexual behaviour, and even compulsive exercising.

Tailoring treatment to the addiction and to the addict

This broad view of the addictions has been useful in many respects. This book does not attempt a comparative evaluation of the nature of addiction to all of these different 'addictions'. It is perhaps time to ask whether this acceptance of the commonalities of different types of addictive behaviour should be questioned. What are the limits of the 'commonalities' view? It is possible that different addictions may share certain common features. For some purposes it may be sensible to regard them as having enough in common to justify membership of the category of 'addictions'. However, common membership of a category should not be confused with being identical. Elephants and monkeys are both animals. Apples and grapes are both fruit. But elephants are not monkeys. And apples are not grapes.

Despite some similarities, giving up heroin is not the same as giving up cigarettes. The cigarette smoker does not also have to learn a new social identity with new social roles after giving up: for many heroin addicts, drug taking is a central part of their lifestyle in which the use of heroin was a focal point, giving meaning and purpose to their daily lives. Giving up drinking is not the same as giving up injecting drugs intravenously. When a compulsive gambler gives up gambling, he or she may be preoccupied with thoughts about it, and have strong urges to return to the behaviour. But, however much these responses have similarities with the withdrawal syndromes that occur after discontinuation of drug use, they are not the same. Dependent heroin users will experience more than just psychological urges to return to heroin use. They will also have physical pain. During withdrawal, the dependent benzodiazepine or barbiturate user may have seizures. Even if all of these withdrawal reactions are seen as being distributed along a single continuum and differing only in terms of severity, this does not alter the fact that they differ in terms of their clinical significance and in the need for different clinical management.

One thesis of this book is that addiction treatment interventions should be appropriately responsive to the needs of individual drug misusers. The term 'addiction' can mislead us if it is taken to imply that the wide range of different presenting problems can be subsumed within some relatively fixed and unitary construct. In this respect, the term obscures more than it reveals. The need for responsiveness to individual differences requires attention to specifics. These include issues such as whether or not an addiction involves the use of a psychoactive substance, whether the substance is taken orally, by smoking, or intravenously, whether discontinuation will lead to a clinical withdrawal syndrome requiring medical treatment in its own right, and whether the addiction is integrated within the user's personality and social lifestyle or whether it is seen as an isolated item of problem behaviour.

Many drug addicts have social and/or psychological problems that precede their drug dependence. These may include social behavioural problems from an early age, educational failure, literacy problems, family disintegration, lack of legitimate job skills, or psychiatric disorders. Such problems tend not to resolve themselves simply because the individual gives up drugs and, unless specific services are made available to deal with them, these problems may continue to cause difficulties for the individual and for their chances of recovery. For many drug addicts, recovery is not only a matter of giving up drug-seeking behaviour but also involves tackling the social and behavioural problems that may have preceded the addiction and that have often been worsened by it. The treatment of drug addiction problems, therefore, may include interventions that extend beyond the focal point of drug consumption, and that tackle the personal and social impairments that may affect those who enter treatment.

The assessment of treatment need has been defined in terms of the ability to benefit from health care (Stevens and Raftery 1994). In this respect, the need for treatment or health care is more specific than the need for health. The need for treatment has a neutral or pragmatic meaning and has specific relevance to the provision of health care, whereas the need for health has a moral meaning. Need for treatment, in this context, should be interpreted with regard to the potential of specific types of treatment interventions to remedy drug-related problems. In the evaluation of the effectiveness of treatments for addiction problems, the elimination or reduction of drug use usually serves as a primary outcome measure. A more comprehensive assessment of the impact of treatment may also use secondary outcome measures to measure changes in health and social functioning.

The therapeutic landscape

The history of addiction treatment has often been characterized by fads and fashions. Some of the treatments that have been used have been, at best ineffective and at worst harmful and occasionally even dangerous. It is a sad reflection upon this field that practices and procedures for the treatment of addiction can so easily be introduced and applied without (or even contrary to) evidence. This is illustrated by the extraordinary range of interventions that have been used to help detoxify heroin addicts. Several of these treatments have been more dangerous than the untreated withdrawal syndrome (Kleber 1981). Interventions have included the administration of hyoscine, strychnine, and nitroglycerine, as well as belladonna treatments involving the administration of scopolamine (causing hallucinations and agitation and requiring physical restraint by 'a strong nurse'). Other extreme forms of treatment have included electroconvulsive therapy, and insulin-induced hypoglycaemia.

The risks of such treatments are indicated by reports that, in a hospital where 130 patients were given the hyoscine treatment, there were six deaths in a year. This should be judged in the context that, although the heroin withdrawal syndrome causes considerable discomfort, it is of relatively short duration and is not medically serious, much less life-threatening. The use of sodium thiocyanate was found to lead to delirium and psychosis, often lasting as long as 2 months.

Some of these treatments may now appear reassuringly old-fashioned and little more than historical curiosities. Other treatments from the past have more modern counterparts. Bromide sleep treatment was used in the early decades of the twentieth century, as was 'artificial hibernation' with up to 72 hours of sodium pentothal-induced narcosis. This also led to deaths. Kleber refers to the deaths of 2 out of 10 patients treated in this way. In recent years there has been an enthusiasm for accelerated heroin detoxification under anaesthesia. Such treatments tend most often to have been provided by privately operated (for profit) organizations.

For many years, the traditional view of drug addiction was extremely pessimistic about outcome. The received wisdom suggested that people who become dependent upon drugs seldom gave up, and that treatment had little effect. An editorial in the first edition of the *International Journal of the Addictions* stated that there is no relationship between treatment and outcome and that, regardless of the type of treatment provided, 'the great majority of addicts simply resume drug use' (Einstein 1966). Similarly, an early review of treatment evaluation studies noted that 'the treatment of heroin addiction has been singularly unsuccessful' (Callahan 1980). This traditional view tended to see addiction in terms of an inevitable and progressive deterioration, and some natural history formulations have been more concerned to account for the deterioration of the addict than to allow for the possibilities of recovery.

The notion that addiction involves a progressive and irreversible deterioration is a view that has considerable resonance with popular conceptions of addiction. In its crudest form it can be found in the 'dope fiend' myth of inevitable social, moral, and physical decline. This view has been with us since at least the end of the nineteenth century, and it is a testimony to its staying power that a variation on this theme surfaced in a UK government anti-heroin campaign, which under the slogan 'heroin screws you up' depicted rapid decline in health and loss of control over intake. A market research evaluation of the campaign showed that this led to an increased belief among young people that death was an inevitable consequence of heroin use.

Prior to the 1970s, there was virtually no formal understanding of the addictions, and little was known about how addiction could be effectively managed or treated. During the late 1960s or early 1970s, many countries established systems of addiction treatment services. Prior to that, treatment was provided by very small numbers of 'specialist' doctors, or in other types of services (mental hospitals, prisons). Differences in the governing ideas behind British and American addiction policies were articulated in the 1916 Harrison Act in the USA and the 1926 Rolleston Report in the UK. The USA tended to pursue a policy that was reliant solely on control measures. The UK took a more medicalized view of the disorder and its management. These differences are still reflected in the contrast between the British acceptance of harm-reduction measures that can be utilized to limit the damage to the continuing drug misuser, and the US goals of 'zero tolerance', 'user accountability', and a 'drug-free America' (Kleber 1993).

When the UK drug clinics were first established (after 1968), they were almost all run by psychiatrists. Diagnoses were assigned to drug-addicted patients on an *ad hoc* basis after an informal clinical interview. The diagnoses were often unreliable and provided almost no useful information about aetiology, course, or treatment needs. The consequences of this were less damaging than they might have been since the treatment options available at that time were so limited. Out-patient treatment involved unsystematic forms of prescribing (it would be misleading to describe this as representing any planned or systematic programme of maintenance). In-patient treatment usually took the form of loosely organized therapeutic communities with various 'eclectic' treatment interventions applied according to the clinical preferences of the staff. Behaviour therapy and biological psychiatry were still developing disciplines. Social and cognitive learning theories and had yet to make an impact upon the field.

The history of medicine suggests that the origins of treatment for any problem tend to follow the identification of severe cases and, during its early stages of development, treatment consists of applying whatever remedies are available when the problem is first recognized. The responsibility for the treatment of newly identified problems may initially fall upon those whose interests are regarded as most closely related to the new problem but, over time, additional personnel may enter the field.

The therapeutic landscape of addiction treatment has changed dramatically since the 1960s, and especially during the past 2 decades. Many promising treatment interventions and procedures and new therapeutic agents have been developed. Different forms of psychological treatments have been developed and have been provided in a systematic manner. There are a range of pharmacological options where once there were very few. There is increasing evidence about the effectiveness of many of these treatment options. There is a clearer understanding of the importance of the social environment, behavioural functioning, cognitive processes, and the use of active coping strategies during recovery. Nonetheless, the treatment and management of drug addiction continues to be characterized by new developments, changing perspectives, and by controversies of one kind or another. The need to develop and strengthen interventions that are effective in reducing the extent of drug problems and in helping users to give up drug taking remains a matter of importance.

Treatment is now provided by a wider range of personnel with differing backgrounds, and in a wider range of settings. Early treatments for drug addiction often assumed the need for intensive and specialized treatment. And, whereas it remains true that many of the most severely addicted drug users require intensive and specialized treatments to maximize their chances of recovery, there has been increasing recognition of the valuable role that can be played by other treatment options. An effective response to drug misuse and drug addiction cannot be regarded as the sole responsibility of specialized treatment services. Other services will necessarily come into contact with people with drug problems, and the responsibility for tackling these problems should be spread more widely.

Many different parties have an involvement or a strong interest in drug treatment services. These include: the *individual patients* entering treatment; the *clinical programmes* that offer different types of services; *family members* or others who are personally involved with those receiving treatment; third-party *treatment puchasers and funders* (national, regional, and local); and various types of *regulatory agencies* who oversee, evaluate, or enforce legal or clinical standards. There are also other concerned individuals and agencies that have personal or professional relationships with drug users in treatment. All of these groups tend to have different expectations about treatment and about what should count as a successful treatment outcome.

The people who seek treatment for addiction problems give a variety of reasons for doing so. In most cases, there are several underlying issues. These usually involve an awareness of some sort of problem that needs to be tackled. This may be a psychological or physical health problem (hopelessness and depression, a serious infection), or some sort of acute social problem (an impending court case, the prospect of imprisonment, threats from a partner). A starting point for recovery generally involves the individual coming to recognize that they have suffered (and often caused) significant personal and social harm.

It is not unusual for drug misusers to be ambivalent about treatment, and their commitment to change may fluctuate greatly across time. Conflict and ambivalence lie at the root of giving up an addiction. Individuals who were desperate for treatment prior to admission may be resistant to treatment and deny their presenting problems after admission. Ambivalence is common during the first days and weeks of treatment, and presents a challenge to clinicians. Ambivalence is different to denial. The ambivalence of the user toward treatment has several sources. It is always useful for treatment personnel to remember that, whereas they see only too clearly the presenting problems, for the user drugs are something that have, for many years, been a focal point for their lives and a source of repeated and intense positive reinforcement. Many drug addicts are seduced into mistaking the satisfaction of drug wants and needs for the satisfaction of most (and sometimes, all) other wants and needs.

Also, in contrast to the easily obtained hit from a drug, most addiction treatment programmes, especially if implemented according to best clinical practice, are rigorous and demanding. They impose controls and require behavioural and psychological change. The difficulties of beginning and remaining committed to this sort of extensive change should not be underestimated: it would be a major challenge for the most stable and socially integrated individual. For those who are ambivalent about treatment, the demands of treatment may lead them to drop out of the programme before it is completed.

The beliefs, attitudes, intentions, and wishes of the drug misuser are of great importance in the treatment process. As in the rehabilitation of other chronic illnesses such as multiple sclerosis or stroke, the treatment and rehabilitation of people with drug addiction problems is, in many respects, more similar to education than to medical treatment with drugs or surgery (D.L. McLellan 1997).

The processes of recovery are not always gradual and incremental but often reflect sudden changes in beliefs and behaviours. Recovery may also be highly idiosyncratic. Treatment is not an impersonal process offered by neutral agents. For the patient it can be an important life event, and the relationship between the patient and therapist can have great emotional and psychological significance. It is surprising, therefore, that addiction research has paid so little attention to the role of therapist characteristics and skills, and their influence upon outcome.

Assessing the effectiveness of treatment

Although the title of this book refers to the treatment of addiction, the problems associated with addiction generally extend beyond the dependence syndrome, and include other behaviours and disorders. Also, each drug user may experience different problems, which may range from the acute to the chronic, and from the mild to the extremely severe. Drug misuse and drug addiction problems are diverse and are manifested by people with different backgrounds and characteristics. There are also many different types of treatment approaches and interventions.

The effectiveness of treatment is a complicated matter to understand and assess. The question 'Does addiction treatment work?' is far too simple. Treatment involves a variety of different practices and procedures that are used with different populations and that are designed to achieve different goals. At the simplest level, treatment is required to tackle both the initiation of change and the maintenance of change. It is one thing to give up drugs. It is another to stay off drugs. Drug addiction treatments include a broad range of interventions that vary in content, duration, intensity, goal, setting, provider, and target population. Research data are increasingly becoming available on the effectiveness of this broad spectrum of treatments.

An important conclusion to be reached from a study of the treatment research literature is that no single type of treatment can be expected to be effective for everyone who has a drug addiction problem. Drug users are a diverse and heterogeneous group, and these individual differences may be relevant to the selection of an appropriate and effective treatment. Different individuals prefer and may benefit from different kinds of treatment. A range of promising alternatives are available, each of which may be optimal for different types of individuals.

Different treatment settings may be appropriate for different people. In-patient hospital care may be most appropriate for those with coexisting acute medical or severe psychiatric problems. Residential care in a non-medical setting may be most appropriate for people who are socially unstable but who do not have coexisting acute medical or severe psychiatric problems. Out-patient care may be indicated for socially stable individuals who do not have coexisting acute medical or severe psychiatric problems. The differences in problems and in the individuals with these problems must be taken into account before an informed decision can be made about what type of treatment is likely to be most appropriate. However, despite the widespread acceptance of these principles, current treatment provision at the programme level still tends to operate in a way that is more reflective of the view that 'one size fits all', with patients being expected to adjust to the programme being provided.

The pathways leading to recovery tend to be complicated, and the variety of possible outcomes is extremely great. People who are treated for drug addiction problems achieve a continuum of outcomes with respect to their drug-taking behaviour and their drug-related problems. Different types of drug consumption and drug problems may increase or decrease following treatment, and the outcomes for different people will follow different time courses. After treatment, some people may show initial improvement with subsequent deterioration. Others may initially show little change but then gradually achieve a range of possibly substantial improvements. Others may oscillate between outcomes, with periods of abstinence alternating with periods of drug use.

There is no single, universally applicable criterion for the assessment of outcome. Treatment response is not a simple matter of success or failure. As with many other treatments, the assessment of outcome involves degrees of improvement, and these may have different meanings for different individual cases. Although there is a general acceptance of such goals as improved health, or reduction or elimination of drug consumption, it is also necessary to be aware of the need for flexible goals that can be adapted to individual circumstances.

More specifically, drug use outcomes after treatment may include: abstinence from all forms of substance use maintained for a lifetime; abstinence followed by a temporary lapse, followed by abstinence regained; reductions in (but not abstinence from) illicit drug use; reductions in use of some illicit drugs but continued or increased use of others; substitution of heavy drinking for drug taking; no change in drug use behaviours but reductions in drug-related problems; and deterioration in drug use and in drug-related problems.

The question 'Does addiction treatment work?' also places too much weight on treatment. It does not put the processes of treatment into an appropriate perspective. Many factors contribute to outcome, and treatment is only one of these. Outcome is also influenced (often powerfully) by the psychological, social, and other characteristics of the individual, the nature and severity of the problem itself, and by a wide variety of posttreatment experiences and events. It is influenced by complex interactions between all of these factors. The probability of a positive outcome for a homeless heroin injector with a severe mental illness and HIV/AIDS is likely to be lower than that for a socially stable person with a dependence on prescribed psychoactive drugs taken orally. The probable differences in outcomes would remain even if each of these individuals received an individually tailored treatment intervention.

It is not uncommon for some drug-addicted individuals to lack the basic social behavioural skills and supports that they need to complete, and sometimes even to start the recovery process. Such individuals often require intensive and prolonged help to cope with the psychological, social, economic, and practical challenges of recovery. Patients who leave drug addiction programmes with continuing psychological or social adjustment have been found to be less likely to achieve or maintain satisfactory outcomes. Treatment of other life problems associated with drug misuse can improve outcome. After many years, or even decades, of living a life that has been built upon getting high, buying, selling, talking, and thinking drugs, it is not surprising that giving up and staying off drugs should prove to be an extremely difficult task.

Chapter 2

Drug use and multiple drug use

Over time there are variations in the emphasis given to different substances as 'main' problem drugs. Sometimes greater attention is given to heroin use. At other times, arguments are made for the primacy of problems associated with crack cocaine, amphetamines, tranquillizers, or other drugs. This chapter discusses the drugs that are most frequently linked to addiction problems. Although the drugs are discussed one at a time, they are seldom used in isolation. Drug users who seek treatment rarely confine their drug taking to just one substance. Almost always, they use several different drugs, and sometimes they use a wide range of drugs as part of a broad repertoire of multiple drug taking. It is commonplace to use shorthand terms such as 'heroin addict' or 'cocaine user' but these terms can be misleading. A 'heroin addict' is extremely unlikely to be only a user of heroin.

Multiple drug use may involve the concurrent or sequential use of different substances. There may also be different reasons for multiple drug use. These include the following.

- *Drug enhancement.* Several drugs may be used at the same time to enhance the combined psychoactive effects. The combined use of opiates and benzodiazepines, for example, may be intended to increase the overall level of sedation.

- *Modification of effect.* Different drugs may be combined to counteract the adverse or unwanted effects of one or more drugs. Cocaine and heroin may be used together so that either the heroin takes away some of the unpleasant overstimulation and anxiety caused by the cocaine, or so that the stimulant offsets the sedation of the heroin.

- *Substitution.* The user may take a different drug as a substitute for their preferred drug if this is not available. Some heroin users may take alcohol in this way when heroin is not available. Substitute drugs may also sometimes be used to self-medicate withdrawal symptoms. Some heroin users take benzodiazepines for this purpose.

- *Social reasons.* For some drug misusers, multiple drug use may be influenced by the social setting and the behaviour of other drug misusers.

Sometimes this may be reflected in a generalized pattern of multiple drug abuse where a wide range of substances are taken in what appears to be an indiscriminate manner. This tends not to be linked to physical dependence.

The drugs that are used are not a random selection of the available substances. Certain drugs regularly appear as the most frequently used, and as the main causes of problems. In the UK and in many other countries throughout the world, heroin is the drug that is most frequently mentioned by users in treatment. Other drugs are also often mentioned as 'secondary' drugs. Such drugs may or may not be seen as being problems by the users themselves, but they are usually an important part of the clinical picture, and the use of these drugs can complicate treatment in various ways.

Too narrow a focus upon specific drugs and their effects can be misleading. Addiction cannot be understood solely in terms of the intrinsic properties of drugs. The addiction liability of a drug is the product of complex interactions between the neurochemical effects of the drug, the ways in which the drug is used, the purposes for which it is taken, the psychology of the user, and the social circumstances within which the drug taking occurs.

Heroin and other opiates

Opium is extracted from the poppy. It is one of the oldest medications known to man, and was used by Hippocrates. The main active ingredient of opium is the alkaloid, morphine, which was first derived from opium in 1803. Heroin (diacetylmorphine) was first synthesized at St Mary's Hospital, London, and was introduced into medicine in 1898. At first, heroin was believed to be safe and non-addictive, and was even used to treat morphine addiction. A number of other drugs, including methadone, have similar pharmacological and behavioural effects, though methadone is a synthetic compound and is not derived from opium. Methadone is longer acting than heroin or morphine, and is more effective when given orally. Methadone was synthesized during the 1940s, and became an important treatment option after 1964 when Vince Dole and Marie Nyswander set up the first methadone maintenance clinic in New York City.

The different opiates differ in their relative strength and duration of action, but they have broadly the same effects. Each produces an initial stimulation of the central nervous system, followed by a more marked depressant effect. Opiates produce analgesia, reduced feelings of apprehension, and a suppression of the cough reflex, and it is for these reasons that they are prescribed in medicine. Their main use is to relieve pain. Interestingly, the use of heroin within general medicine as a drug to treat severe and intractable pain is not regarded as controversial within Britain. Heroin is carried by general practitioners (GPs) and is used to treat patients who have had heart attacks. Heroin is used to treat people who are in severe pain as a result of serious illnesses such as cancer. In this role, almost all British doctors see the drug as a useful adjunct to their pharmacopoeia.

Opiates also produce changes in the psychological state of the user. These effects are often described as drowsiness and feelings of tranquillity. When taken by routes such as intravenous injection, these drugs lead to a sharp and rapid increase in opioid levels in the brain, which is usually experienced as an intense feeling of euphoria, often described as a 'rush'. This euphoric effect is greatly sought after by opiate misusers, and is often one of the more powerful reasons given for repeated use of the drug.

The opiates act through several mechanisms, including stimulation of at least three types of opiate receptors in the brain, the mu (μ), kappa (κ), and delta (δ) receptors. Mu receptors are diffusely distributed throughout the limbic system. The delta receptor is also located in the limbic system but in areas that do not overlap with the mu receptor distribution. The kappa receptor is distributed in the nucleus accumbens, the ventral tegmental area, the hypothalamus, and regions of the thalamus (Mansour *et al.* 1994). The action of the drug on these systems (and especially upon the mu receptors) is largely responsible for the reinforcing properties of opiates (Katz 1989).

Heroin is often seen as the archetypal drug of addiction. Black-market heroin in Britain has been available in different forms at different times. During the 1960s, most UK heroin was available as pharmaceutical diamorphine hydrochloride (usually tablets), which was obtained from chemist burglaries or through the diversion of heroin prescribed to addict patients. Currently, pharmaceutical heroin is only prescribed to a very small number of addict patients, and is rarely available on the streets. Where it is available, it is in the form of freeze-dried ampoules.

The first imported black-market heroin was from South-east Asia. This was available during the late 1960s and early 1970s, and was known as 'Chinese heroin'. During the 1970s, and following the Iranian revolution, the black market in heroin was dominated by the large-scale importation of a brown form of heroin, and south-west Asian heroin began to flood the British market between 1978 and 1979 (Lewis 1994). Street prices for heroin fell by as much as 25 per cent between 1980 and 1983 with no decrease in purity. By 1982, the area around northern Pakistan and Afghanistan had established its place as the major supplier for the UK market, and south-west Asian heroin continues to be the form of heroin that is most widely available in the UK.

The chemical nature of heroin is determined by the type of manufacturing process used, and this is often associated with the country of origin. Iranian and Pakistani heroin is characterized by a crude separation of morphine prior to acetylation. Samples are likely to consist of heroin in base form. Between 1978 and 1982, all but one of the Iranian heroin seizures made by UK Customs were of heroin base (O'Neil *et al.* 1984). A number of these samples additionally contained caffeine, which has been found to increase the efficiency of the delivery process (Strang *et al.* 1997*c*).

As a base form of heroin, south-west Asian heroin is suited to 'chasing the dragon' and not to injecting, and its arrival in the UK was an important factor leading to the spread of heroin chasing. Purity levels are directly related to illicit manufacturing processes and importation channels, and the purity of this form of black-market heroin has remained generally within the 20–50 per cent range (Strang *et al.* 1997*c*). Purity levels can change rapidly. For instance, in the USA where heroin was of very low purity for many years, the purity of heroin in New York City and Philadelphia increased from around 35 to over 75 per cent within a period of about 2 years during the late 1990s (Kreek 2000).

There is an important relationship between the different forms in which a drug is available and the route by which it is likely to be used. Chinese heroin is almost always available in its salt form (diamorphine hydrochloride). The salt form of heroin is soluble and can be injected or taken intranasally by 'snorting'. Attempts to smoke it will destroy almost all of the active form of the drug. In contrast, base forms of heroin are suited to smoking but not to intranasal or to intravenous use. It is possible, however, to convert the base form of heroin into a salt that can be dissolved and injected by the addition of an acid (many British heroin users add lemon juice or citric acid).

It is often stated that all drugs of abuse can be regarded as positive reinforcers. This is correct. However, it fails to give sufficient weight to the observation that drug abusers have clear, and often subtle preferences for different drugs and for different forms of the same drugs (Gossop and Connell 1975). Heroin users usually have preferences for one or another type of heroin and, in certain respects, drug abusers, and even drug addicts, can be seen as consumers in a marketplace with a variety of choices (Strang and King 1996). Conversely, not all drugs are attractive to all drug users. For example, the rate of alcohol abstainers among heroin addicts is much higher than would be expected (Gossop *et al.* 2000*b*).

Where methadone can be obtained on the black market, it is widely used by opiate addicts. At one time during the 1970s, methadone was so widely available as a street drug in London that, among the opiate addicts seeking treatment, almost as many were primarily dependent upon methadone as upon heroin. Gossop and Connell (1975) reported that 39 per cent of a clinical sample of drug addicts stated that methadone was their preferred drug compared to 46 per cent who preferred heroin (with 15 per cent preferring methylamphetamine). Where methadone is available in the form of ampoules (i.e. as an injectable drug), it is seen by some opiate users as being a more attractive option than heroin. Metrebian *et al.* (1998) found that more than a third (36 per cent) of opiate-dependent patients receiving prescribed opiates preferred injectable methadone to injectable heroin.

Among opiate addicts in treatment, almost half (49 per cent) were found to have used non-prescribed methadone during the 3 months prior to admission to treatment, with more than a quarter of them (29 per cent) being regular users of non-prescribed methadone (Gossop *et al.* 1998*b*). Best *et al.* (1997) found several relationships between the ways in which opiate addicts used methadone and heroin. For example, use of prescribed take-home methadone during the early part of the day was associated with reduced levels of illicit heroin use. Those who took methadone later in the day were more likely to use illicit heroin. Best *et al.* suggested that this might indicate an intention by opiate users to avoid any methadone blockade of the euphoric effects of heroin by taking the heroin for the 'high' and saving the methadone to avoid withdrawal.

Central nervous system stimulants: amphetamines and cocaine

Amphetamine was discovered in 1887, and first marketed in 1932 as an over-the-counter benzedrine (amphetamine sulphate) inhaler to treat nasal congestion. Amphetamine tablets became available in 1935, and at about this time the first reports appeared describing the potential dangers of addiction to amphetamine medications.

The amphetamines are a class of drugs containing a large number of psychoactive substances. Their overall effect is to increase the amount of available dopamine and noradrenaline (also called norepinephrine) in the central nervous system (CNS). Depending upon their chemical structure, amphetamines can produce stimulation, hallucinogenic effects, appetite-suppressant effects, or a mixture of these effects. Amphetamines can be taken by mouth, by snorting, smoking, and by injection.

Amphetamines can be obtained by diversion from legitimate medical channels. They are also illegally manufactured. Amphetamines are relatively easy to manufacture, and home laboratories have been able to prepare large quantities of the drug, usually in the form of amphetamine sulphate. This is one of the most common illegal preparations, and it is cheaply and widely available throughout the UK.

A stronger form of the drug, methylamphetamine, is also occasionally available. Methamphetamine is the crystalline hydrochloride salt, sometimes called 'ice'. The drug can be heated and inhaled from a pipe similar to those used to smoke crack cocaine (Cho 1990). The euphoric effect of methamphetamine is said to last much longer than that of crack cocaine and, depending upon the dosage, can last from 7 to 24 hours, (Perez-Reyes *et al.* 1991). The crash after methamphetamine use is regarded by users as being more intense and longer lasting than that for e̶i̶t̶h̶e̶r̶ ...

The use of amphet... ...widesp... ... an countries. In Sweden a... ...is the m... ...n. Concerns about the w... ...in Australia (Hando *et a*... ...nt who report ampheta... ...in recent years (Darke *et*... ...a-mines have been trie... ...y 1 per cent, and Klee (... ...d only to cannabis in po... ...n within some wester... ...A (Rawson *et al.* 2002).

Amphetamines ma... ...d energy, hyperactivity, ...l effects are usually dose... ...ied by uncontrollable... ...d vision, increased hear... ...rates and body temperature, loss of appetite, and impaired speech. Other physical side-effects may include dizziness, tremor, headache, flushed skin, chest pain with palpitations, vomiting, and abdominal cramps.

Amphetamine users may have problems with anxiety, tension, and irrational fears. The likelihood of such problems increases with repeated doses or unusually high doses of the drug. Williamson *et al.* (1997) investigated adverse effects associated with the use of three different stimulants (amphetamines, MDMA/Ecstasy, and cocaine) among a non-clinical sample of drug users. Amphetamines were associated with the greatest number of adverse effects. These effects were also rated as more severe than those of Ecstasy and cocaine. More than one-third of the amphetamine users described 'severe' sleep disturbances, and between 10 and 20 per cent of users reported severe problems with paranoia, depression, anxiety, and irritability. Polydrug users (who used opiates, opioids, and benzodiazepines as well as stimulants) were more likely to report adverse effects associated with their stimulant drug use than the drug users who were using stimulants only.

injecting stimulants produces a sudden euphoric sensation (a 'rush' or 'flash'). Stimulant use often occurs in binges during which users may smoke or inject themselves repeatedly and at frequent intervals over periods varying from several hours to several days. Often the user remains awake and does not eat, and they may use alcohol and other drugs to counter the overstimulation associated with the high doses of stimulants. Binges often continue until the user is exhausted, the toxic effects become too great, or supplies run out.

Benzodiazepines

Benzodiazepines have been widely used to treat psychological disorders since the 1950s. The commercial success of the benzodiazepines was partly due to their acting as a safer alternative to the barbiturates. Benzodiazepines are more effective in reducing anxiety, have fewer and less severe side-effects, and are much safer than barbiturates in overdoses. They are also attractive to many drug users, though it is only comparatively recently that attention turned to their misuse as 'street' drugs. Prescott (1983), for example, suggested that 'In contrast to the enormous general consumption of benzodiazepines, their abuse "for kicks" by young drug takers is distinctly uncommon . . . . They are not "fun drugs".' Others also argued that benzodiazepines were likely to have little appeal for illicit drug abusers (Marks 1985a; Woods 1987). However, Petursson and Lader (1984) reported that drug addicts who took large doses of diazepam, either on its own or with opiates, experienced a pleasant relaxed sensation that was recognized as a drug 'high'.

Benzodiazepines are only infrequently used as the main drug of dependence, but are often used as part of a pattern of multiple drug use (and multiple dependence). Benzodiazepines have been widely misused by polydrug users in many countries since the early 1980s. Among heroin addicts treated at the Maudsley Hospital in London, the percentage who were regular users of benzodiazepines doubled between 1988 and 1991. In 1991, about one-third were regular users of benzodiazepines, and about half of the regular users were physically dependent and required detoxification treatment for a benzodiazepine withdrawal syndrome (Davison and Gossop 1996).

More than a third (37 per cent) of amphetamine users in Sydney were found to have used benzodiazepines, and problems of polydrug use, psychopathology, general health, and social functioning were all worse among drug users who took benzodiazepines (Darke et al. 1994). A study in Baltimore found that benzodiazepines were widely abused by opiate addicts in methadone mainten-ance treatments and that these drugs were rated as producing a satisfactory drug 'high' (Iguchi et al. 1993).

In a survey of patterns of benzodiazepine use by drug addicts attending treatment services in seven cities across Britain, Strang *et al.* (1994*a*) found that the use of benzodiazepines was extremely common. The most worrying practice involved the injection of benzodiazepines, and the benzodiazepine most likely to be injected was temazepam. Temazepam capsules originally contained the drug in liquid form. This was popular among intravenous users since it was easily injected. The manufacturers replaced the original preparation with a hard gel formulation in 1989 to discourage abusers of this drug from attempting to inject it (Drake and Ballard 1988). However, a substantial proportion of drug users continued to inject temazepam by heating the hard capsules in an oven or microwave and injecting the sticky solution through a wide-bore needle.

Ruben and Morrison (1992) reported that 70 per cent of the patients attending their treatment services in the north-west of England were injecting temazepam capsules. Although, from a public health perspective, the altered formulation could be seen as having the advantage of reducing the numbers of people injecting temazepam, it also puts those who do continue to inject at increased risk of harm (Strang *et al.* 1992*b*). Such risks include the possible 'blocking' of peripheral veins in the arms and legs, skin abscesses, and the development of deep vein thrombosis. Problems can be exacerbated if large quantities of temazepam are abused.

More recent evidence suggests that the prevalence of benzodiazepine injecting has fallen. A study of drug-dependent patients attending three drug treatment clinics in London found that, although all benzodiazepine abusers had previously used temazepam, less than one-quarter of the sample reported current use of temazepam (Gossop *et al.* 1997*a*). Only 5 per cent of the sample were currently injecting temazepam and, of those who were injecting temazepam, most described this form of use as infrequent and opportunistic rather than as a regular activity. Where temazepam was used, the doses taken varied widely but were often extremely high. The average amount used was 95 mg per day though some of the drug takers reported using massive amounts. Two of this sample reported using amounts of about 1000 mg (50 or more 20 mg capsules) in a day. Extremely high-dose abuse of temazepam was also reported by Seivewright and Dougal (1993), and, as in the study of Strang *et al.* (1994*a*), those drug users who had injected temazepam most often prepared injections from the capsules, though a smaller number ground up temazepam tablets in order to inject the drug.

From 1996, GPs within the National Health Service have not been permitted to prescribe temazepam in capsule form, though other formulations of the drug continued to be available. At the same time as the Department of Health ban, the Home Office also implemented tighter regulations (including more secure storage at pharmacists) on all formulations of temazepam.

Cannabis

In Britain, as in many countries, cannabis is the most widely misused illegal drug. In the USA the 2000 National Household Survey on Drug Use estimated that 34 per cent of Americans aged 12 or older had used cannabis, and that 8 per cent had used it in the last year (SAMHSA 2001). A Canadian telephone survey of more than 11 thousand people (Williams, B. *et al.* 1992) showed a lifetime prevalence rate of 23 per cent, with 6.5 per cent having used in the last year. In New Zealand, Black and Casswell (1993) found a lifetime prevalence rate of 52 per cent of whom 24 per cent had used in the previous year.

Hall *et al.* (1994) suggest that daily or near daily cannabis use appears to put cannabis users at greatest risk of experiencing long-term health and psychological consequences of use, especially when this occurs over a period of years. They also suggest that chronic heavy cannabis users may develop a cannabis dependence syndrome with tolerance and withdrawal symptoms, and with users continuing to take the drug in spite of adverse consequences. Rounsaville *et al.* (1993) suggested that cannabis dependence was similar to that for other illicit drugs.

Although dependence upon cannabis can occur, it is rare for patients attending addiction treatment services to report cannabis dependence as their main problem. The use of cannabis is more relevant to clinical practice because it is so frequently used by patients receiving treatment for other drug problems. The observation that cannabis use by opiate addicts in treatment is common has been well documented. Hubbard *et al.* (1989) reported that cannabis was the most commonly used drug by patients both in the year before entry to treatment and while patients were in treatment. They also reported that rates of patients with daily cannabis use had increased from 15 per cent among patients in the 1970s to 35 per cent in the 1980s. In Australia, Darke and Hall (1995) reported that 84 per cent of heroin users had used cannabis in the previous 6 months.

In the USA Nirenberg *et al.* (1996) found that 78 per cent of their treatment sample were cannabis users, and Saxon *et al.* (1993) found that 45 per cent of a group of methadone maintenance patients were consistently positive for tetrahydrocannabinol (THC). Among opiate addicts in methadone treatment programmes in London and Edinburgh, Best *et al.* (1999*a*) found that 40 per cent were using cannabis every day, and more than three-quarters of the daily users were smoking more than four joints every day. Such levels of use are not trivial.

Few of the patients identified cannabis use as a problem or reported any desire to give up using cannabis, and it is likely that cannabis use remained an important feature of their drug-focused lifestyles. It is especially when drug-dependent patients seek to achieve a drug-free lifestyle that the significance of 'other' drugs such as cannabis may assume greater prominence.

However, opiate users in methadone programmes who were daily users of cannabis were found to be less likely to use either heroin or crack cocaine than those who had not smoked cannabis in the previous month; they were also less frequent drinkers than those who did not use cannabis. (Best *et al.* 1999*a*). This is consistent with studies of methadone maintenance patients in the USA where Saxon *et al.* (1993) also found that patients who consistently tested positive for cannabis were less likely to use illicit drugs. Reductions in the frequency of use of heroin, crack, and alcohol are positive treatment outcomes for methadone treatment (Simpson and Sells 1983; Hubbard *et al.* 1989; Ball and Ross 1991), and in this respect there is an apparently paradoxical finding that daily cannabis use among opiate addicts in treatment may be associated with a positive outcome in terms of reduced use of alcohol and other drugs.

Daily cannabis users have been found to be more likely to report higher levels of anxiety and depression, as well poor appetite, when compared to both occasional users of cannabis and non-users (Best *et al.* 1999*a*). Psychological problems including depression and anxiety are common among patients in substance use treatment programmes (Darke *et al.* 1994). Hall *et al.* (1994) also note that daily cannabis use is often associated with psychological problems in general populations, and Wiesbeck *et al.* (1996) also suggest that more frequent cannabis users are more likely to have psychiatric difficulties.

Volatile substances

Volatile substance abuse (VSA) is often, though less accurately, referred to as solvent abuse or glue sniffing. It differs from other types of drug problems in that it is primarily a problem of children and adolescents. Most volatile substance abusers tend to be aged between 12 and 17 years, though reliable estimates are difficult to obtain. It has been suggested that 3.5–10 per cent of adolescents may have at least experimented with volatile substances, and that 0.5–1 per cent of the secondary school population may be current users (Ashton 1990). As with many other drugs, recreational use of volatile substances is often a group activity (Richardson 1989). VSA sometimes occurs in localized clusters and in these circumstances the percentage of young people using these substances may be considerably higher.

The almost universal availability of volatile substances creates a special problem since it is impractical to prevent the abuse of these substances through restricting access to them. Volatile substances are appealing to adolescents for a number of reasons. They are legal, easily available, and relatively inexpensive. In addition, the average home contains dozens of substances which are capable of being abused, including aerosols, lighter fuel, petrochemicals, glues, thinners, and other solvents.

The method of use often involves 'sniffing' or 'bagging'. 'Sniffing' involves the inhalation of vapours directly from an open container or a heated pan. 'Bagging' refers to inhalation of vapours from a plastic or paper bag containing the desired substance. Habitual users generally begin with sniffing, and progress to bagging to increase the concentration of the inhalant and intensify or prolong the euphoric effect (Linden 1990; Henretig 1996).

There are differences in the types and degree of risk associated with different volatile substances. Two of the more risky forms of VSA appear to be the inhalation of cigarette lighter fuel and inhaling the contents of fire extinguishers (Gossop 1993). Both have been linked to fatalities. The level of risk to the user may also differ with the precise method of administration. Methods that involve the user putting a plastic bag over their head are risky and may lead to asphyxiation. In some instances, users may spray aerosol compounds directly into the mouth. This is also a dangerous method of use.

The high achieved with volatile substances occurs rapidly and disappears relatively quickly. This can allow the user to inhale these substances after school and still return home sober (Cohen 1977). Blood levels peak within a few minutes of exposure and the effects may include euphoria, excitation, and exhilaration similar to those with alcohol intoxication. Other acute systemic effects may include respiratory and gastrointestinal symptoms. Volatile substances can cause irritation to the mucous membrane, leading users to cough, wheeze, or salivate. VSA may also lead to more severe symptoms such as shortness of breath and difficulty in breathing, and heart palpitations. Users may also complain of nausea, vomiting, diarrhoea, or abdominal pain (Kurtzman et al. 2001).

Generally, the initial effects of volatile substances decrease as the substance is distributed to the CNS and absorbed by fat. Most volatile substances are diffusely toxic to the CNS, and the persistent use of volatile substances can lead to medical problems that require attention (Sharp and Rosenberg 1992). There is also concern about the toxic effects of volatile substance abuse upon other organ systems. Long-term and/or high-dose use of some organic solvents may cause polyneuropathy.

Volatile substances affect brain function in many ways, though most effects appear to be reversible. As with the sought-after intoxication effects, most adverse symptoms disappear relatively quickly and generally within a few hours. With more severe levels of intoxication, marked depression of the CNS may lead to slurred speech, tremor, visual changes, weakness, headache, delusions, disorientation, confusion, or visual hallucinations. The user may lose coordination. With excessive doses, depression of the CNS may lead to stupor, seizures, coma, cardiopulmonary arrest, or death (Shepherd 1989; Linden 1990). Death is rare but may occur as a result of asphyxia or disorders of cardiac function.

The risk of accidental injury is always a problem for young volatile substance users. Acute effects like drunkenness may be accompanied by confusional or hallucinatory states. A worrying feature of VSA is that the risk is not proportionate to the degree or the duration of involvement. First-time users may be at high risk. The number of young people who die as a consequence of volatile substance abuse is relatively small in comparison to the number of users but it is a matter for serious concern that there has been a steady increase in the number of deaths associated with these substances (Pottier *et al.* 1992). Tragically, many of these have involved children. Deaths have been recorded for 10 and 11 year olds, and the majority of deaths (60 per cent) are among people aged 17 or less.

Adolescents with histories of VSA are more likely than non-users to report a wide range of problems and disorders. These include poor family relations, disrupted living situations, school problems, involvement with substance-using peers and/or parents, and depressed mood and suicidal thoughts. Various forms of antisocial behaviour problems and delinquency are also linked to VSA (McGarvey *et al.* 1996; Howard and Jenson 1999).

Although many adolescents may experiment with volatile substances through curiosity or boredom, some may become habitual users. Young people often participate in these behaviours for reasons that are important features of normal adolescent development—to appear mature, to earn the approval of peers, or to demonstrate their autonomy from their parents (Jessor *et al.* 1991). However, since VSA poses risks to health and may be associated with delinquency and crime, it can jeopardize normal psychosocial or physical development. Among adolescents, VSA is generally only one problem within a pattern of behaviours that may constitute a 'risk behaviour syndrome' that reflects an adolescent's own concept of his or her lifestyle (Jessor *et al.* 1991). The treatment of volatile substance abuse may be more effective if it is designed to tackle the wider constellation of risk behaviours rather than concentrating on inhalant abuse alone.

Other drugs

Barbiturates and other non-benzodiazepine sedative–hypnotic drugs, such as methaqualone (Quaalude, Mandrax) have been misused at various times and in different countries. Many of the effects of these drugs are similar to those of alcohol. Problems associated with barbiturates and Mandrax were an important part of the national drug problem in the UK during the 1970s. These drugs can lead to full physical dependence with a severe withdrawal syndrome, which, if not properly treated, may include seizures (Gersema *et al.* 1987). The misuse of barbiturates carries a high risk of overdose and, when lying unconscious for prolonged periods, some users developed nerve damage with permanent sequelae. In a study of drug addicts between 1967 and 1981, Ghodse *et al.* (1985) reported that many of the overdose deaths during that period were associated with the use of barbiturates. When injected, barbiturates can also cause large abscesses. Barbiturate addicts were often among the most highly problematic groups of drug misusers. Jamieson *et al.* (1984) described them as typically being homeless, sleeping rough, regularly overdosing, and being resuscitated in Accident and Emergency departments. Barbiturate addicts were often stigmatized and avoided even within the drug subculture because of their unpredictability and reputation for violence.

Ghodse *et al.* (1985) suggested that the fact that prescribed and diverted drugs were causing the deaths of so many addicts demanded a response from the medical profession. It was in response to such concerns that the Campaign for the Use and Restriction of Barbiturates (CURB) was established in the UK during the late 1970s to reduce the availability of diverted barbiturates obtained from medical prescriptions. The campaign appeared to reduce the quantity of barbiturates being prescribed, though not the number of prescriptions (King *et al.* 1980). However, barbiturates did become much harder to obtain on the black market, and their use fell rapidly afterwards. Barbiturate addiction is not currently a major issue within the UK.

Recent years have seen great concern about the widespread 'recreational' use of MDMA (3,4-methylamphetamine, 'Ecstasy'). Current estimates have suggested that Ecstasy has been used by about one in ten of young people in the UK (Royal College of Psychiatrists and Royal College of Physicians 2000). Ecstasy is structurally related to amphetamine, though some of its effects are different. It acts as a stimulant, but also produces changes in mood, emotions, and states of consciousness. Many users find the experience very sensual. MDMA is not a new drug. It was first synthesized and patented in Germany in 1914, and was developed as an appetite suppressant, though it was never marketed.

Users often take doses in the range of 75–150 mg, and the effects start within about half an hour of taking the drug by mouth. The peak effects tend to occur over the next hour or so, and then fade over the next 2 hours.

There is still a comparative lack of information about the type and severity of adverse effects experienced by stimulant users. Williamson *et al.* (1997) found that stimulant users reported fewer adverse effects after taking Ecstasy than after using cocaine powder or amphetamines. Adverse effects associated with the use of Ecstasy include severe headaches, anorexia, insomnia, tachycardia, paranoia, depression, and panic attacks. Some of the more common side-effects of Ecstasy are tension in the jaw and grinding of the teeth. Anxiety, heart palpitations, and, in a few cases, paranoid delusions have been reported. As with 'bad trips' on LSD, 'talk down' methods have generally been sufficient to deal with these adverse effects. The drug also produces increases in blood pressure, and anyone with high blood pressure or heart problems would be well advised not to use it, as would people with a history of diabetes or fits.

One of the worrying but unresolved issues regarding Ecstasy is whether or not its use causes serious or irreversible neuropsychological impairment. The primary mode of action for MDMA is as an indirect serotonergic agonist, though the drug also affects 5-hydroxytryptamine (5-HT; serotonin)- and dopamine-containing neurons, as well as other neurotransmitter systems (McDowell and Kleber 1994). Studies with laboratory animals have found long-term serotonergic damage associated with the use of MDMA. Rats treated with MDMA developed serotonergic changes with a pronounced loss of 5-HT axon terminal markers (Ricaurte *et al.* 2000).

Serotonergic damage has also been found in human Ecstasy users. In a positron emission tomography (PET) scan study, McCann *et al.* (1998) found that a reduced density of 5-HT transporter sites was associated with the extent of past Ecstasy use, with serotonergic deficits occurring across a wide range of brain regions. There was also a gender effect, with women showing a greater 5-HIAA (hydroxy-indole acetic acid-5) reduction than men. During the days after taking Ecstasy the user may experience low moods with feelings of anhedonia, lethargy, and memory problems (Curran 2000). Memory and other cognitive impairments have been demonstrated on a variety of assessment tasks after controlling for potentially confounding variables (Verkes *et al.* 2001; Parrott 2002).

Ecstasy is often taken as a 'dance drug' to increase energy, physical stamina, and social confidence. Unfortunately, the pharmacological effects of the drug may be compounded by the exertion of hard and fast dancing. Among the complications that have been recorded are extremely high body temperatures, collapse, convulsions, and acute kidney failure. Dancers have been advised to wear loose clothing, to drink plenty of non-alcoholic liquids, and to stop dancing when feeling exhausted. Some club owners have provided 'chill-out' rooms with seating and air-conditioning to help cooling.

A good deal of public attention has focused on the physical health problems associated with use of MDMA, and especially on the possible acute toxicity effects. These rare but problematic toxic reactions to Ecstasy create challenges for hospital Accident and Emergency services. There have also been problems linked to excessive fluid intake by recreational users of MDMA. Whilst Ecstasy use is well known to produce dehydration, unlimited consumption of water during prolonged dancing in club/dance events that have high ambient temperatures can lead to acute cerebral oedema due to inappropriate levels of anti-diuretic hormone secretions (Matthai *et al.* 1996). There have been several highly publicized fatalities that have been linked to Ecstasy use (Dowling *et al.* 1987). Such extreme adverse effects are rare.

In practice, very few people present to addiction services to seek treatment for Ecstasy-related problems. Data on treatment samples collected during 1999, for example, indicate that only about 1 per cent of those in addiction treatment services reported Ecstasy to be their main problem drug (Department of Health 1999*a*). In addition, the majority of those who present to drug misuse treatment services with serious MDMA problems tend also to be long-term polydrug users.

The most widely used and the best-known hallucinogenic drug is LSD (lysergic acid diethylamide). This was discovered in 1943 by Dr Albert Hofmann at Sandoz Laboratories in Switzerland. LSD is extremely potent, and is measured in micrograms (μg, millionths of a gram). Doses as small as 20 μg produce effects similar to those of cannabis intoxication but, when it is taken for its full hallucinatory effects, doses of 50–250 μg are more usual.

Another naturally occurring hallucinogen is found in several different varieties of psilocybin ('magic') mushrooms. Most of these are insignificant tawny-brown toadstools that grow to a height of about 1 or 2 inches. These are common throughout Europe and America. An average hallucinogenic dose of psilocybin would appear to be in the region of 20–60 mg.

With the hallucinogens, and especially with LSD, visual perception is strikingly altered by the drug, leading to perceptions of patterns that are usually described as kaleidoscopic or geometric. With increasing intoxication, patterns become less symmetrical and more complex. When the eyes are opened, ordinary objects seem to glow as if they were illuminated from within. Colours seem to be deeper and more intense and, not infrequently, mundane objects seem to assume tremendous symbolic significance. At the peak of the drug experience, pseudohallucinations occur in which the person's visual perceptions are profoundly affected. True hallucinations are rare, though they do sometimes occur. Generally, they are linked to high doses of the drug, though some individuals may be more sensitive to LSD than others. Unlike the visual pseudohallucinations, in which the person is aware that their experiences are drug-induced, true hallucinations usually carry no such insight. The person mistakes their hallucinations for reality.

Thought processes are also altered by the drug. Thinking becomes non-logical, and often it has a strong magical quality to it. The person may believe that they can read the thoughts of other people or that they are able to transmit their own thoughts. The user may have pseudo-delusional thoughts—incorrect or irrational ideas—but with some insight into their strangeness. Although the person may believe that he or she is having profound or brilliant ideas, any attempt to express them usually reveals only banal or fragmented thoughts.

During the peak of the drug experience, LSD has strong effects on the personality of the user who may begin to lose a secure sense of their personal identity. Different people react to this in different ways. Some become euphoric or joyful, and regard the experience as a sort of mystical or religious revelation. Others are terrified by the apparent loss of their feelings of secure selfhood.

Acute adverse reactions may include anxiety or panic attacks ('bad trips'). In some cases, the user may experience strong feelings of persecutory anxiety with paranoid ideation. LSD is metabolized and excreted within 24 hours and, in the majority of cases, the anxiety wears off before medical attention is sought. Chronic adverse reactions may include 'flashbacks', which recreate some features of the altered state of consciousness of the drug experience. These may occur weeks, or even many months later. Flashbacks generally decrease in intensity and frequency with the passage of time, whether treated or not (Pechnick and Ungerleider 1997). In rare cases, a psychosis may develop and persist beyond the period of intoxication. There seems to be a very low probability that hallucinogens act as a direct cause of any such psychotic disorder, though for some users they may act as a trigger or catalyst. Among individuals who already have a psychotic disorder, the use of hallucinogens is clearly risky and can lead to acute disturbances of behaviour and mental state. Neither the acute nor the chronic adverse reactions can be reliably predicted.

Alcohol

The use of illegal drugs may be the primary and most conspicuous problem for drug addicts, but many also have problematic patterns of drinking. Among the drug users recruited to NTORS (National Treatment Outcome Research Study), more than one-third of those who were drinking at intake to treatment reported problematic or highly problematic patterns of alcohol consumption (Gossop *et al.* 2000*b*). Most of the heavy drinkers were drinking every day or almost every day, many reported problems of alcohol dependence, and more than a third of those who were dependent upon alcohol were regularly drinking 30 units or more per drinking day (30 units is equivalent to a bottle of spirits). In view of the excessive levels of alcohol consumed by some of the drug misusers, it is not surprising that many reported serious levels of concern about their dependence upon alcohol. Even among those who reported low levels of dependence upon alcohol, more than half were drinking very heavily (on average, 12 units or more) and relatively often (about every other day).

The problems of heavy drinking and dependent alcohol use among drug addicts are found in many countries. In Sweden, about three-quarters of a treatment sample of drug users were found to have been heavy drinkers at some time in their lives (Berglund *et al.* 1991). In the USA, studies have reported that 20–50 per cent of drug users in treatment are problematic drinkers (Belenko 1979; Hunt *et al.* 1986; Hubbard *et al.* 1989; Lehman and Simpson 1990).

Alcohol use and, in particular, excessive drinking can be an important and often underrated problem in the treatment of drug users. Drug users with concurrent polydrug use problems may require special consideration and treatment planning (Strain *et al.* 1991*a*). Excessive alcohol use by drug users may aggravate other drug-related and health problems, and may adversely affect outcomes after treatment. Alcohol use among drug users has been linked to increased levels of criminal activity (Roszell *et al.* 1986). Chronic alcohol abuse has been identified as an important cause of medical complications during methadone treatment and is frequently linked to the premature discharge of patients from treatment programmes (Kreek 1981; McLellan *et al.* 1983; Joe *et al.* 1991). Chatham *et al.* (1997) found differences in treatment response and treatment outcome among drug users who were alcohol-dependent and those who were non-dependent drinkers. Cocaine misusers who also have drinking problems have been found to be more likely to relapse to cocaine use after treatment, and drinking is often closely linked to relapse episodes (McKay *et al.* 1999).

The interrelationship of drinking and illicit drug use is not well understood. It has been shown that in some circumstances there may be an inverse relationship between the frequency of use of alcohol and drugs (Anglin *et al.* 1989*a*; Marsden *et al.* 1998a). Alcohol-dependent drug misusers have been found to be less frequent users of heroin and crack cocaine and more frequent users of stimulants such as cocaine powder and amphetamines, and of non-prescribed benzodiazepines (Gossop *et al.* 2002*c*). It has been suggested that some drug misusers may substitute alcohol for drugs (Simpson and Lloyd 1977; Hunt *et al.* 1986; De Leon 1987). It is unclear whether this is due to a deliberate choice to replace one substance with another, or whether it represents a gradual generalization of substance misuse patterns in which extra substances are incorporated within the drug-taking repertoire.

Drinking may also be linked to the use of different types of drugs. Lehman and Simpson (1990) found that heavy drinking was linked to the use of non-opioid drugs, and Chatham *et al.* (1997) found high rates of cocaine problems among alcohol-dependent drug misusers. Some of the most severely problematic drug addicts tend to be polydrug users, whereas those who confine their drug taking primarily to heroin tend to be younger and at an earlier stage of their drug-misusing careers (Gossop *et al.* 1998*b*). The finding that the most severely alcohol-dependent drug misusers are usually older may also suggest an age-related drift away from 'street' drugs such as heroin coupled with an increased use of alcohol.

The choice of alcoholic beverage by drug users is an interesting topic, though few studies have investigated this issue. In a study of drug addicts in the UK, Gossop *et al.* (2002*c*) found that one of the types of drink that was preferred by those addicts who were also dependent upon alcohol was extra strong beer. Those who were more strongly dependent upon alcohol were drinking, on average, about 19 units of alcohol per day just in the form of extra-strength beer.

Chapter 3

Consumption behaviours, problems, and dependence

Drug misuse is a complex and multifaceted phenomenon. A useful way of understanding its complexity is to conceptualize it as being represented along three dimensions. These are:

+ consumption behaviours;
+ problems;
+ dependence.

These dimensions can be regarded as being conceptually distinct and separate. In reality, of course, they tend to be related (sometimes closely) in a number of ways.

Consumption behaviour

The first of the dimensions refers to the behavioural parameters of drug taking. The most immediately obvious features of drug consumption behaviour involve frequency and quantity of drug use. Obvious or not, many misunderstandings arise in discussions of drug problems through a failure to distinguish between infrequent, frequent, and regular patterns of use, or between low-dose and high-dose use. Drug consumption behaviours are related to different types of risks and problems.

Route of administration is also an important feature of drug use. It is related to the effects experienced by the user, to dependence liability, to the risk of overdose, and to the risk of infections and other health problems. Surprisingly, route of administration has often been overlooked, and properties are sometimes attributed to the drug that are characteristics of the route of administration or of an interaction between the drug and the route of administration.

Routes of drug administration that are commonly used by drug misusers are:

+ oral (tablets, liquids);
+ intranasal/snorting/sniffing (e.g. cocaine powder, heroin powder);
+ smoking (cannabis, opium);
+ inhalation (chasing the dragon, volatile substances);
+ injection (intravenous, intramuscular, subcutaneous/skin popping).

Patterns of drug taking are sensitive to social, environmental, and interpersonal influences. As a consequence, there can be marked geographical differences in the types of drug being used, the amounts taken, or in routes of administration. The question of regional and local variations in patterns of drug misuse is both interesting and important. For example, cocaine users in South America often take very large amounts of the drug and experience severe levels of dependence. Many South American users take doses of more than 5 g/day compared to the 1–2 g reported by cocaine users in the USA and Europe (Ferri and Gossop 1999). Similarly, the doses of heroin used in a producer country such as Pakistan can often be in excess of 5 g per day (Gossop 1989b) compared to typical daily doses of about 1/2 to 3/4 g used by heroin addicts in the UK (Gossop *et al.* 1998a).

Patterns of drug taking can change with extreme rapidity. This has been demonstrated at the national level in the rapid growth of crack cocaine misuse in the USA during the 1980s (Kleber 1988), and the spread of heroin addiction after the appearance of the drug in Pakistan during the 1980s (Gossop 1989b). In the 1960s, all (or nearly all) heroin users in the UK injected it. A survey of heroin addicts at a London clinic during 1968 and 1969 found that all of them had started heroin use by injecting (Gardner and Connell 1971). Today, the situation has changed considerably, and virtually all heroin users in London start to use heroin by 'chasing the dragon' (Strang *et al.* 1992a). The changes in route of first use of heroin are shown in Fig. 3.1. This shows how

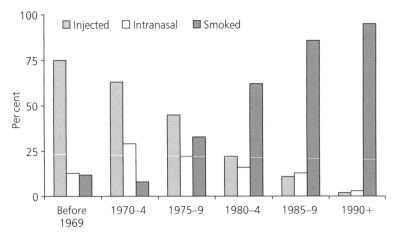

Fig. 3.1 The figure shows the steady increase in chasing the dragon as the preferred first route of heroin use in the UK between the mid-1970s and 1990. This replaced heroin injecting, which was the dominant route of use, including first use prior to 1975. The data are from the study of Strang *et al.* (1992a).

heroin chasing almost completely replaced injecting as an 'entry route' into heroin use in the years between 1970 and 1990.

Similar changes in routes of cocaine use occurred in many countries. The spread of smokable forms of cocaine in London during the 1980s was charted by Gossop *et al.* (1994*a*). Those who first took cocaine before 1986 had mostly started to take the drug by snorting (65 per cent) or injecting (30 per cent), with only 6 per cent having first used by smoking. Between 1987 and 1989, snorting remained the most common route of first cocaine use (65 per cent), though about a quarter of new users were now starting to smoke cocaine, with only 10 per cent injecting. After 1990, smoking became the most likely route of first use, with none of the drug users in the study sample first taking cocaine by injection. Similar changes have been reported in other countries. For example, a study in Brazil found that the percentage of cocaine users who smoked cocaine increased from 5 per cent in the years prior to 1986 to 65 per cent during 1995–7 (Ferri and Gossop 1999).

The two predominant routes of heroin administration among regular users in the UK are injection and chasing the dragon. Griffiths *et al.* (1994) found that injecting was preferred as the main route of heroin administration by 54 per cent and chasing by 44 per cent of heroin users. Although some users reported having taken heroin by snorting, this was not common and was not reported as a primary route by any users. Intranasal use of heroin has also been described among heroin users in New York (DesJarlais *et al.* 1992), and concern has more recently been expressed about changes in route of administration with increasing numbers of young people in the USA starting to use heroin by snorting rather than injecting (Office of National Drug Control Policy 1998).

Heroin can be smoked in different ways. The most marked difference is between methods in which the heroin is burnt in a cigarette (e.g. in a heroin joint), and methods in which the heroin is not actually burnt but is heated so that the vapours may be inhaled (as in chasing the dragon). Early reports of chasing the dragon in Hong Kong described how heroin was mixed with a base powder known as *daai fan*, which contained barbiturates. This mixture was placed on a piece of tinfoil and heated until it liquefied, after which the user would inhale the fumes that were given off from the liquefied mixture (Gossop *et al.* 1991*a*). Other reports from Hong Kong have described how heroin was also sometimes smoked in cigarettes (Mo and Way 1966). Heroin was placed on the powdered ash on the end of the cigarette to be heated (but not actually burnt).

Not all forms of heroin are equally suitable for smoking. Although it is sometimes believed that the suitability of heroin for smoking is primarily linked to purity, this is incorrect. A sample of 100 per cent heroin base and one of 100 per cent heroin hydrochloride (the most common salt of heroin) could both correctly be referred to as 'pure heroin'. However, the two forms of heroin would not be equally suitable for injection or for smoking. Drugs, such as heroin, can exist either as a base or as a salt. In both cases the active components of the drug are pharmacologically identical, as are their effects. However, the salt dissolves in water and has a high melting point; as a result the chemical is likely to decompose rather than become volatile on heating.

The base chemical on the other hand is fat-soluble. It does not dissolve in water and is not suitable for injection in the base form. It is more volatile and, on heating, the chemical forms a vapour rather than decomposing. Before it can be dissolved and injected, the heroin base requires a chemical transformation, commonly involving the addition of an acid such as lemon juice or acetic acid, to change it into a heroin salt. The salt form of heroin is not suited to smoking since it decomposes on heating.

The development of heroin smoking in the UK coincided with changes in the types of illicit heroin preparations being smuggled into the country (see Chapter 2). With the arrival of large quantities of cheap, good quality, and smokable heroin during the late 1970s and early 1980s, some of the negative social connotations of the drug were removed in a period characterized for many by mass unemployment and social alienation. As heroin smoking became more prevalent it attracted increasing attention. Chasing the dragon was first reported in the UK during the early 1980s, and reports of heroin chasing amongst drug users in treatment samples were seen from the mid-1980s (Parker *et al.* 1987; Gossop *et al.* 1988). In one of these early reports on the characteristics of these new heroin chasers, they were described as generally being younger than injectors, and having used heroin for a shorter period of time (Gossop *et al.* 1988). However many chasers had used heroin by this route for a considerable period of time—87 per cent for more than 2 years and 27 per cent for more than 5 years. Both chasers and injectors were found to be using similar amounts of heroin. Chasing the dragon became widespread as a route of heroin use amongst out-of-treatment samples of heroin users (Griffiths *et al.* 1994).

Chasing the dragon has been reported in other countries. It became established in the Netherlands during the 1980s, and by the late 1980s three-quarters of heroin users in the Netherlands were reported to be using heroin by smoking (Grund and Blanken 1993). The most common form of heroin smoking involved 'Chinesing' (chasing the dragon). Chasing continues to be overwhelmingly the main route of heroin use in the Netherlands (van den Brink *et al.* 2002). Chasing the dragon has also been reported in Spain (Lacoste Marin 1992).

Hunt and Chambers (1976) were among the first to explore the manner in which patterns of drug misuse spread across communities in the USA during the 1960s and 1970s. In their studies of drug use within England, Pearson (1991) and Pearson and Gilman (1992) investigated the manner in which drugs spread at the regional level (macro-diffusion) and at the local level (micro-diffusion). The spread of cocaine use among heroin users in Spain has been reported by Barrio *et al.* (1998). Preferences for certain drugs and for certain routes of administration may be associated with cultural or ethnic groups (Swift *et al.* 1999).

Although heroin users have clear preferences for specific routes of drug administration, preferred routes of administration may change. Although only two routes of heroin administration tend to be widely used in the UK, more than two groups of heroin users can be identified (Griffiths *et al.* 1994). These include heroin users who first took the drug by injection and who continued to inject (stable injectors), those who first used by chasing and continued to take heroin in this way (stable chasers), those who moved from chasing to injecting, and those who had previously been injectors and who moved to chasing. When compared to initial chasers who had made a transition to injecting, stable chasers were less involved with the heroin using subculture, they had more social contact with non-users, and they were much less likely to have friends who were heroin injectors. DesJarlais *et al.* (1992) described the transition from intranasal use to injection among heroin users in New York.

The progression from heroin chasing to injecting is not inevitable, and heroin chasing should not be seen merely as a first stage, or pre-injection phase of heroin addiction (Gossop *et al.* 1988). The majority of heroin chasers did not switch to regular injecting despite having used heroin in substantial doses for many years. Some chasers may also give up using heroin without ever moving on to injecting. However, there is a continuing risk of moving from chasing to injecting among those who continue to use heroin (Griffiths *et al.* 1994). Griffiths *et al.* (1994) found that nearly half of the heroin chasers (49 per cent) had previously injected, and 36 per cent had injected heroin at least once in the last year. Where a transition in route of drug use occurs, this is generally a significant personal event in the drug-taking career of the drug user. Most users remember when such changes occurred, whom they were with, and what was going on at the time.

Routes of drug administration may change as a result of the development of increased severity of dependence in the individual user, economic pressures to make more efficient use of available supplies of heroin, sociocultural factors, and changes in availability of drug preparations. A study of heroin users in London found that more than a third of them had made at least one transition in their preferred route of administration (Griffiths *et al.* 1994). More than half of those who were injecting heroin had previously used heroin by other routes. Most commonly, only one transition was reported—from chasing to injecting. This change of route is the one that is best known and has been a major target of HIV prevention interventions in recent years. Women were found to be less likely than men to make the transition from chasing to injecting. Interestingly, some heroin users made a reverse trans-ition from injection to chasing. About one in five of the heroin users had made this change from injecting to chasing. This change in route is much less well-known than the transition to injecting, and the reasons why it occurs are not well understood. Multiple transitions in route were found to be uncommon. When a main route of administration had been established, this was likely to remain the primary or even the exclusive route for a period of years.

Among drug users recruited from treatment services across England, Gossop *et al.* (2000*d*) found that rates of injecting varied between 5 and 58 per cent according to the specific

heroin, and, as in othe

approximately evenly div

were lowest for benzod

drug). Benzodiazepines

concern that has been e

benzodiazepines, it is s

indicated that the injec

valent than for other dr

transformed by drug m

(see Chapter 2), and th

by drug injectors of th

drugs.

There were also mar

the main routes by whi

benzodiazepines, coca

used (Gossop *et al.* 2000*d*). For example, the injecting of heroin and non-prescribed methadone was most prevalent in the areas around London and least prevalent in the north of England. There was no evidence of regional pockets where benzodiazepine injecting was especially high, though it was worrying that almost 10 per cent of the benzodiazepine users in the south-west of England reported recent use of the drug in this way. The injecting of cocaine powder was much higher in the north-west of England than in other areas, and lowest in the North Thames region. There were also regional differ-ences in the ways in which crack cocaine was used. Whereas smoking was the predominant route of use for crack in all regions, there were also areas where the injection of crack was relatively common. In both the south-east and the south-west of England as many as one in five crack users regularly injected the drug. In contrast, this practice was almost never used by crack users in the north-east of England. Since crack is essentially and purposely manufactured to be a smokable preparation of cocaine, it is interesting that some users are choosing to inject it. The injection of crack cocaine is a form of drug misuse that is not well understood. Few studies have reported it, examined the reasons for injecting crack cocaine, or looked at the risks associated with it.

The geographical variations in drug-taking practices raise questions about the wisdom of talking in general terms about 'national' drug problems. Pearson and Gilman (1994, p. 102) have noted that 'there is not truly a "national" problem . . . [but] a series of local and regional difficulties.' The maintenance of up-to-date information about changes in types of drug misuse and routes of drug administration requires that regular information on patterns of drug misuse is available through valid, relevant, and comprehensive monitoring systems.

In addition to having preferences for certain routes of administration for specific drugs, drug takers also tend to use specific routes for the administration of different drugs. In particular, once a drug user has started to take any drug by injection, this route of administration is likely to be used with other types of drugs. Gossop *et al.* (2000d) found a greatly increased likelihood that those users who injected heroin would also inject other drugs. Among the drug misusers who were current users of both heroin and crack cocaine, those who had injected heroin were almost 50 times more likely also to have injected crack during the previous 3-month period. Similarly, they were more than 30 times more likely to have also injected illicit methadone, nearly 20 times more likely to have injected benzodiazepines, and 10 times more likely to have injected amphetamines.

These differences in route of drug administration have implications both for preventive and treatment interventions. In areas where the prevalence of drug injecting is relatively low, it may be appropriate to design and deliver interventions specifically targeted to prevent transitions to injecting routes of drug administration (Strang *et al.*, 1994b; Hunt *et al.* 1999). However, it is not known whether such interventions are effective or what is the most effective way to provide them. Similarly, where injecting is more prevalent, services should ensure that both clinical staff and users are aware of how overdoses occur and what sorts of response are appropriate to overdoses (Hall 1999). One possible option is that antagonist drugs such as naloxone could be made available to opiate misusers as a public health measure (Strang *et al.* 1999b).

Problems

The problems of drug misuse must be assessed in terms of risk as well as actual harm. Injecting drugs carries a number of risks, and it is the route of administration that causes greatest concern. One obviously risky type of behaviour is the sharing of injecting equipment with other drug users. Because heroin chasing avoids the obvious dangers of injecting, many users, especially new and naive users, see it as a safer way of taking drugs. However, regular heroin chasers and cocaine smokers may develop respiratory problems as a result of the inhalation of high-temperature vapours. Heroin chasers are much less likely to take an overdose. In one study, only 2 per cent of heroin chasers had overdosed compared to 31 per cent of heroin injectors (Gossop *et al.* 1996). Heroin injectors are also at greater risk and are more likely to carry blood-borne infections such as HIV and hepatitis C (Gossop *et al.* 1994c).

The risks to the physical and psychological health of the user and the dangers of overdoses are closely linked to route of drug administration with injectors being at much higher risk. These issues are dealt with at length in Chapter 4. Indeed, the problems associated with drug misuse are a recurrent theme of this book and are dealt with in many other chapters. This section therefore outlines just some of the problems that are linked to drug taking.

Where significant behavioural, social, or health problems are found among drug addicts, it is common to assume that the problems have occurred as a result of the drug taking. This is simplistic and it may be incorrect. Although there are a number of relationships that link drug misuse and some types of problems, these relationships seldom apply to all cases, and there are many instances in which the direction of effect appears to differ. In an earlier discussion of this issue, Edwards *et al.* (1997) suggested that the assumptions underlying attempts to make such attributions of direction of effect are generally so dubious that, wherever possible, this search for 'causes' should be avoided. Others have been more optimistic about identifying the associations and direction of effect that may exist between substance use and problems (Drummond 1992).

What is clear is that some problems arise or are exacerbated because of the illegality of drugs. On a weight-for-weight basis, heroin is vastly more expensive than gold (Reuter 1997), and the regular use of illicit drugs places an excessive economic burden upon the user that, in most cases, cannot be met by normal means. The main options for supporting a drug habit tend to be crime, drug dealing, and prostitution.

The links between drug addiction and prostitution have been known for many years. Goldstein's (1979) review suggested that 30–70 per cent of female drug users were also prostitutes, and that 40–85 per cent of prostitutes were also drug users. Some drug-dependent men also support their habit through prostitution. Other studies have reported similar findings both in the USA and Scotland (Thomas *et al.* 1989; DesJarlais *et al.* 1987; McKeganey *et al.* 1990). Some studies have found lower rates of prostitution among drug users. In a study of female prostitutes in Sydney, Philpot *et al.* (1989) reported that about 12 per cent had used drugs intravenously. A study of a non-clinical sample of heroin users in London found that 17 per cent of the women and 6 per cent of the men had been involved in some sort of prostitution and that it was the more severely dependent heroin users who were most likely to be involved in prostitution (Gossop *et al.* 1993*a*). Since unsafe drug injection and unprotected sex are two of the primary routes of HIV transmission, drug injectors and prostitutes are both potentially at great risk of contracting and transmitting HIV and other serious infections as a result of their behaviour. Prostitutes who also inject drugs may, therefore, be at especially high risk in this respect.

There are several possible links between drug use and prostitution. The use of drugs and the development of drug dependence may precede prostitution. Under such circumstances prostitution may be used by some women as a means of financing their use of heroin or other drugs, and the primary link between addiction and prostitution may be the economic necessity of obtaining the finances to buy heroin (Goldstein 1979; Weisberg 1985). Equally, prostitution may precede drug use and drug problems. Where this occurs, drugs or alcohol may be used in an instrumental manner to cope with the often stressful, anxiety-provoking, and unpleasant demands of working as a prostitute. It is also possible that prostitution and the use of drugs may develop independently. For instance, some prostitutes work in settings or areas where there is high availability and acceptance of illicit drug use. Under such circumstances, the association between drug misuse and prostitution may be, at best, indirect.

A study of drug taking and sexual behaviour among women working as prostitutes in south London found that more than three-quarters of them were current users of heroin (Gossop *et al.* 1994*b*). Most of the women (more than two-thirds) used heroin either every day or on most days. Even among those who used less than every day, about one-quarter had at some time in their lives been daily users. Many of the women in this study were using comparatively high doses of heroin. One of the reasons most commonly given for working as a prostitute was the need to buy drugs and, specifically, to buy heroin. Almost two-thirds of them said that they only worked as prostitutes in order to fund their use of drugs (predominantly heroin), and that they would not continue working as prostitutes if they were not still using drugs. The more severely dependent upon heroin they were, the more likely they were to report these links between heroin use and prostitution.

However, the association between heroin use and prostitution was not straightforward. Many of the women started to use heroin at the same time that they started to work as a prostitute (at about age 19) and about half of the women in our sample said that they first started to work as a prostitute in order to pay for drugs. However, there was also a group of women who began to work as prostitutes prior to using heroin. Clear differences were found between those women who worked as prostitutes in order to pay for heroin and women whose prostitution and heroin use were not linked in this way. The latter group tended to be less severely dependent upon heroin, and they did not describe their involvement with prostitution as being driven by the need to maintain a supply of heroin. These women were also more likely to report that they would continue to work as prostitutes whether or not they stopped using heroin. It was primarily those women who began to use heroin prior to prostitution and who were more severely dependent on heroin who described themselves as being trapped in prostitution by the need to maintain a supply of heroin. On average, these women had used heroin for about 2 years before they started prostitution. These women in particular were more likely to report that they used drugs to help them cope with their work as prostitutes and that they would not have continued to work as prostitutes if they had been able to stop using heroin.

Many studies have found high levels of criminal activity among drug-misusing populations (Inciardi 1979; Jarvis and Parker 1989; Ball et al. 1983). In the UK, recent police estimates suggested that about half of all recorded crime may be drug-related with costs to the criminal justice system alone of at least £1 billion per annum (Central Drugs Coordinating Unit 1998). However, crime among drug misusers may also be related to factors other than drug taking. Many drug misusers tend to have been involved in crime before they started taking drugs (Nurco et al. 1993), and crime and drug use often share common links with psychological and social lifestyle factors associated with social deviance (Hammersley et al. 1990). High levels of crime and drug use often coexist in economically disadvantaged and socially deprived neighbourhoods (Nurco et al. 1984; Pearson and Gillman 1994).

Acquisitive crimes involving theft are also among the most frequent ways of obtaining drugs, or of obtaining money for drugs (Hammersley et al. 1989; Stewart et al. 2000a). Income-generating crimes are often linked to the dependent use of heroin and cocaine. However, it is important to note that crime and addiction do not inevitably go together. Half of the patients recruited to NTORS (National Treatment Outcome Research Study) had not committed any acquisitive crimes during the 3 months prior to admission, and, of those who were involved in crime, the majority were relatively low-rate offenders. The vast majority of acquisitive crimes were committed by a small minority of the drug users, with 10 per cent of them committing 76 per cent of the crimes (Stewart *et al.* 2000*a*). Those who were most heavily involved in crime were the drug users who were most severely dependent on heroin and cocaine.

The onset of addictive drug use has been found to be associated with increased levels of criminal behaviour, which continues during periods of addiction (Ball *et al.* 1983). Speckart and Anglin (1985) found that heroin addicts were charged with a higher number of property crimes than non-addict criminals, and Ball *et al.* (1983) found that crimes involving theft were the most common offence among heroin addicts. Many heroin addicts report financing their habits largely through acquisitive crime (Jarvis and Parker 1989). The patients in the NTORS programmes reported committing a very large number of acquisitive crimes (more than 17 000) during the 90-day period prior to treatment intake (Gossop *et al.* 1998*b*). Shoplifting was the most common type of offence, both in terms of total number of crimes and in terms of percentages of drug users committing that offence.

Ball *et al.* (1983) found drug selling to be second to property crime in frequency of offences. Among the NTORS patients, such offences were among the most frequent crimes. The cohort of just over 1000 addicts reported more than 39 000 drug-selling offences during the 90 days prior to treatment. However, as with acquisitive crimes, the majority of the drug users were not involved in selling drugs. Fewer than one-third reported selling drugs and, for the majority of those who were selling drugs, selling was an infrequent and occasional activity. Even among such long-term, dependent, and problematic drug users, drug selling can be an atypical behaviour. Reuter *et al.* (1990) also found that most drug sellers sold drugs infrequently and that most drug sellers at the lower end of the chain of supply made very little money.

Heroin is mostly sold by those who themselves use the drug (Johnson *et al.* 1985), and most illicit drug sellers also use the types of drugs that they sell (Clayton and Voss 1981). Half of the drug sellers in the study of Reuter *et al.* (1990) reported purchasing drugs for their own use, and dealers tended to use the same drug that they sold with particularly high correlations for selling and use of heroin and crack cocaine. Multiple drug sellers tended to be multiple drug users.

A minority of the drug users within NTORS were highly active as drug sellers. The involvement of these drug users with drug selling was of a different order to that of the other drug sellers. Seventy-one (7 per cent) of the patients reported almost 35 thousand offences during the 90 days prior to admission. By any standards, this is a very large number of offences. Frequency of drug selling was related to frequency of heroin use, and the high frequency of heroin use among this group could be seen, at least partly, as a consequence of their ready access to the drug through dealing. This is consistent with the observation of Reuter *et al.* (1990) that, the larger the quantity of drugs consumed by the user, the greater the gain from being a seller. Gains are associated both with being able to buy drugs more cheaply in bulk, and the ability to cream off a percentage of the drug by passing on cost to lower-level buyers.

The term 'drug selling' refers to a range of different activities that are conducted by a range of different types of people (Caulkins *et al.* 1999). It is possible that the involvement of the most highly active drug sellers reflects their more professional approach to dealing. Reuter *et al.* (1990) have calculated that the income from drug selling is often much greater than earnings from other crimes or from legitimate sources and that, for this reason, successful drug sellers may see property crime as a relatively unattractive option. Speckart and Anglin (1985) have also suggested that there exists a hierarchy of illegal activities with dealing as the preferred means of support followed by nonviolent crimes such as theft.

Dependence

Progression from occasional to dependent use of drugs is not inevitable. Nonetheless, many people who have started to use drugs find the effects rewarding and continue to do so, sometimes with increasing frequency and regularity, until they are taking drugs every day and several times a day. When this happens, the amount that they take usually also increases, and often they begin to run into many types of social, psychological, and physical problems associated with their drug taking (increased financial costs, legal and criminal risks, and dangers of infection and ill-health).

Initially, people may use drugs for many reasons but the decision to use or not to use drugs represents a voluntary choice. With the development of dependence, the relationship between the user and his or her drug is altered. The person become increasingly preoccupied by the drug and feels some degree of compulsion to use it. The initial reasons for drinking or taking drugs may or may not still be present but, with the development of dependence, new factors are added that complicate the picture and increase the likelihood, intensity, and persistence of drug taking. The use of drugs seems to develop a life of its own so that, even when the user wants to cut down the amount or to give up using altogether, they experience great difficulty in giving up the habit.

They may have withdrawal reactions and become unwell when they stop taking the drug, and they become preoccupied with thoughts about it. Despite their wishes to stop using, they frequently fail in their efforts to do so and go back to taking drugs again. The phenomena of craving, compulsion, and impaired ability to control drug use have been known for many years. During the nineteenth century, there was a period during which different addictive behaviours were seen in the form of 'manias'—morphinomania, dipsomania, and narcomania.

Dependence is an important clinical reality. The behaviours underlying 'addiction' or 'dependence' are the most frequent reasons for drug users seeking treatment, and dependence is a phenomenon that all therapists should fully understand.

The term 'dependence' was introduced as an alternative to 'addiction' by the World Health Organization in 1964. This reformulation carried with it an attempt to differentiate the physical and psychological components of dependence. In some circumstances physical dependence is seen in a relatively 'pure' form. One such example is the surgical patient who receives opiates for pain relief. The patient may require increased doses of opiates to manage his or her pain and may also show withdrawal symptoms when the drug is stopped. If the patient shows no desire to continue taking the drug after treatment, the existence of the physical signs of dependence would not justify the patient being described as 'addicted'. Usually the physical and psychological components are more closely linked.

Various attempts have been made to define more precisely what is meant by dependence. Edwards *et al.* (1981) suggested that dependence should be regarded as a syndrome in which the use of a particular drug, or even of a wide range of drugs, assumes a much higher priority than other behaviour that once had a higher value. Dependence occurs as part of a wider pattern of behaviour in which not all the components of the dependence syndrome need be present, nor always at the same intensity. Among the various cognitive, behavioural, and physiological effects that are said to make up the dependence syndrome are the following:

- a feeling of compulsion to take drugs;
- a desire to stop taking drugs;
- a relatively stereotyped pattern of drug taking;
- signs of neuroadaption (tolerance and withdrawal symptoms);
- the salience of drug-taking behaviour relative to other priorities and the tendency to return to drug taking soon after a period of abstinence.

For many years the concepts of tolerance and withdrawal provided the twin pillars that supported the concept of addiction. This was largely due to their being among the most readily observable and objective features of addiction. It can be readily demonstrated that the repeated administration of certain drugs leads to progressive decreases in some of their effects. This occurs with the euphoric and analgesic effects of opiates such as heroin and methadone. Early studies of addiction identified the development of tolerance with the tendency of addicts to increase the dose they were taking or to increase the frequency with which they took the drug.

The suggestion that addicts go on using ever-increasing doses of the drug with the development of tolerance is only partly supported by the evidence. Because of their regular and repeated use of drugs, addicts do become physically tolerant to them, and they increase their consumption to levels far greater than those that would be safe for a non-tolerant user. On the other hand, although it is seldom explicitly described in the literature, it is also found that almost all addicts reach a dose plateau. Most UK heroin addicts stabilize their daily dose of street heroin at levels between 0.5 and 0.75 g (Gossop *et al.* 1998*b*). Very few go on to take doses greater than 1.5 g. The extent to which users escalate their dose can be strongly influenced by environmental factors such as drug availability or cost. In producer countries where drugs are more easily available, users often take much higher doses.

With the growth of tolerance, symptoms of withdrawal often are found when the drug is discontinued. In the case of the classic drugs of addiction such as heroin and alcohol, a fairly predictable set of symptoms occur that make up the 'withdrawal syndrome' of that drug (see Chapter 7).

Although tolerance and withdrawal were once seen as the defining characteristics of physical dependence, tolerance also occurs to drugs that are not physically addictive in the traditional sense, such as amphetamines and cannabis. Similarly, there are withdrawal-like responses to the discontinuation of these drugs after regular use (Gossop *et al.* 1982*a*). Whether or not one calls these responses 'withdrawal symptoms' could be regarded as a semantic rather than a scientific question. Both tolerance and withdrawal have been observed in relation to habitual behaviours that do not involve the use of drugs at all. Compulsive gamblers, for instance, tend to 'escalate the dose' and may also show symptoms of withdrawal such as irritability, restlessness, anxiety, sleeplessness, depressed mood, and poor concentration (Wray and Dickerson 1981). Similar responses are also found among compulsive eaters under dietary control.

The phenomena of tolerance and withdrawal have been more precisely delineated as neuroadaptation (Edwards *et al.* 1981). The physiological processes of neuroadaptation are just a part of the cluster of factors that may be associated with the dependence syndrome.

Although tolerance and withdrawal may no longer be regarded as essential defining features of dependence, their clinical significance should not be underestimated. The development of tolerance affects the requirements for any subsequent prescription of drugs, either as part of an addiction treatment programme (e.g. methadone maintenance) or for the treatment of other medical conditions (e.g. for relief of pain). Drug withdrawal symptoms can also be a clinically important issue. For many physically dependent drug users, the prospect of withdrawal can provoke serious anxiety (Phillips *et al.* 1986). Fear of withdrawal may serve to perpetuate drug use to avoid onset of withdrawal symptoms, and it can be a barrier to entering treatment. If not properly treated, the discomfort of withdrawal may interfere with broader treatment plans and may lead the patient to drop out of treatment.

Neither of the two international diagnostic nosologies has achieved a fully satisfactory classification of the addiction disorders. Such approaches have focused upon specific substances without sufficiently recognizing the variability and complexity of consumption behaviours, problems, and dependence. The earlier nosologies also tended to give undue emphasis to the concepts of tolerance and withdrawal as essential characteristics of drug dependence. DSM-III (*Diagnostic and statistical manual of mental disorders*, 3rd edn), for example, stated that 'the diagnosis [of dependence] requires the presence of physiological dependence' (Kuehnle and Spitzer 1981). The attempt to confine the social and psychological complexities of the dependence disorders within such narrow physiological boundaries proved unsuccessful.

More recent nosologies have attempted a broader approach to diagnosis. The criteria for dependence as defined by both the American Psychiatric Association in DSM-IV (1994) and by the World Health Organisation in ICD-10 are very similar (see Table 3.1). For a diagnosis of dependence, both systems require that three or more specified symptoms/behaviours should have occurred within a 12 month period.

The two psychiatric classification systems make little reference to the notion of severity of dependence. Their view of dependence is as a categorical disorder.

Table 3.1 Dependence criteria as proposed by DSM-IV and ICD-10

Symptom	DSM-IV	ICD-10
Strong desire or compulsion to use	Yes	Yes
Difficulties in controlling use	Yes	Yes
Withdrawal	Yes	Yes
Tolerance	Yes	Yes
Increased dose or extended periods of use	Yes	Not specified
Neglect of other activities	Yes	Yes
Persistence despite problems	Yes	Yes

This conceptualizes dependence as a state (is this person dependent/addicted?), and represents a contrasting approach to assessment to that which regards dependence as being distributed along a dimension (how severely dependent/addicted is this person?). The dimensional view is more in keeping with current understanding of dependence disorders as learned behaviours.

There are both practical and theoretical limitations to the categorical formulation of dependence. If dependence is a learned behaviour that develops over time and that feeds upon repeated exposure to the reinforcements of drug taking, it may be expected to exist in varying degrees of strength, and should be assessed as such. Where something can be assessed by means of a dimensional measurement system, this provides more useful information. Dependence may, therefore, be more appropriately assessed using a dimensional formulation to determine not just whether there are signs of dependence but, more usefully, the degree of its development and its severity.

The psychiatric nosologies rely upon multiple criteria for the identification of a dependence disorder. However, a strong case can be made for the centrality of the desire or compulsion to use drugs. The essence of dependence is the psychological desire for drugs (Edwards *et al.* 1981). Gossop (1989*a*) noted that, of these elements, 'the sense of compulsion would seem to be an essential ingredient. It contradicts our understanding of what we mean by an "addiction" that someone could be said to be addicted to something but not experience a strong need for it.' In this respect, dependence must ultimately be regarded as a psychological phenomenon.

The International Classification of Diseases (ICD-10 1992, p. 76) also recognizes that:

> It is an essential characteristic of the dependence syndrome that either psychoactive substance taking or a desire to take a particular substance should be present; the subjective awareness of compulsion to use drugs is most commonly seen during attempts to stop or control substance use.

Multiple substance use, and particularly multiple dependence, complicates both the assessment and understanding of the phenomenon (Gossop 2001). For example, where dependence on several substances occurs, does this constitute a single problem or a collection of problems? Are these problems directly related, indirectly related, or unrelated? Is the overall degree of dependence established by the more severe of two dependencies? Does the user have a more severe dependence problem than if they took only one drug? Is severity of dependence upon each drug additive or interactive?

ICD-10 (1992, p. 6) states that clinicians should record 'as many diagnoses as are necessary to cover the clinical picture. When recording more than one diagnosis, it is usually best to give one precedence over the others by specifying it as the main diagnosis.' This assumes that the precedence given to the 'main diagnosis' can be used to guide further treatment interventions. However, it does not adequately deal with the questions raised above.

Relatively few studies have investigated multiple substance use with specific attention to severity of dependence upon more than one substance. Rawson *et al.* (1981) suggested that dually (drug and alcohol) dependent patients may have worse treatment outcomes than those who are not heavy drinkers, and co-dependence upon alcohol among opiate users in methadone treatment programmes has been found to affect treatment response and treatment outcome (Chatham *et al.* 1997). Some recovering drug addicts turn to alcohol as a substitute (Simpson and Lloyd 1977; Hunt *et al.* 1986; De Leon 1987).

In a study of multiple substance dependencies, Gossop *et al.* (2002c) found no association (a zero correlation) between severity of dependence upon alcohol and drugs. This lack of association between the two forms of dependence is interesting in view of the fact that the sample comprised drug misusers with a wide range of severe and often long-standing drug-related and other problems (Gossop *et al.* 1998b; Stewart *et al.* 2000a; Marsden *et al.* 2000). In such a sample, it might be expected that the possibilities of a general predisposition towards a 'chemical dependency' might be more evident. Our results provide no support for this with regard to a generalized dependence upon alcohol and upon drugs.

Research into the addictive behaviours has drawn an increasingly clear distinction between drug-related problems and dependence. The view that alcohol problems and dependence constituted two separate dimensions was stated by Edwards and Gross (1976) and developed by Edwards *et al.* (1981). The view that consumption behaviours, problems, and dependence should be seen as separate dimensions extends this formulation and serves as a useful device to emphasize the conceptual independence of these three aspects of drug misuse. In practice, however, they cannot easily be formulated as unidimensional constructs, and they are often related.

Many people run into social, legal, psychological, and health problems as a result of their drug taking without being dependent. Examples might include the first-time user of Ecstasy who is unfortunate enough to have a toxic reaction to the drug, or the inexperienced heroin injector who is unfortunate enough to take an overdose. First-time injectors are especially likely to share injecting equipment, and many drug takers become infected with hepatitis or HIV within the first few weeks of starting to inject drugs (and at a time when they are unlikely to be seriously dependent upon drugs).

Some drug users may also become dependent upon drugs but without experiencing significant harm. A frequently cited example is Dr William Halstead, a renowned nineteenth century American surgeon and a founder of the prestigious Johns Hopkins Medical School, who was able to continue his successful medical career despite being a dependent user of morphine for most of his life. Many of the opiate addicts in Britain during the first half of the twentieth century were doctors or nurses who were able to continue working despite their addiction. Even among the heroin addicts who approached the clinics after their inception in 1968, some of the heroin addicts were described as 'stable' (Stimson 1973) and tended to be in work, with little or no involvement in crime and leading a relatively 'normal' life. On the two dimensions of problems and dependence, they would score high on dependence but low on problems.

More often, there are positive associations between severity of dependence and problems. The stereotypical 'junkie' tends to be severely dependent as well as having many drug problems. The chronic heroin addict with an extensive criminal record and who is infected with HIV or hepatitis B and C provides one such example. In his description of the more chaotic heroin users in his study, Stimson (1973, pp. 178–9) noted that 'The Junkies emerge as the opposite to the Stables in nearly every respect. Nearly all . . . support themselves by stealing . . . their drug use involves . . . the sharing of equipment with which to inject themselves . . . they report the highest incidence of physical complications . . . they eat poorly.'

The regular and dependent use of drugs such as heroin and cocaine has been found to be strongly related to certain types of crime, psychiatric comorbidity, impaired social functioning, accidents, physical health, and deaths. Drummond (1992) found that substance-related problems and dependence were still correlated even after controlling for such consumption behaviours as quantity of consumption, but that there was no relationship between problems and consumption after controlling for dependence. Drummond suggested that the frequently observed relationship between problems and dependence exists independently of the quantity of consumption, and that dependence may act as an intervening variable in the consumption–problems relationship.

Severity of dependence has been found to be related to a range of different problems, including injecting risk and sexual risk behaviours for blood-borne infections (Gossop et al. 1993a,b). The congruence of consumption behaviours, dependence, and problems is well illustrated in the use of dangerous injection practices by addicts such as attempts to inject into the femoral vein, or the use of other inappropriate and dangerous injection sites (Cunningham and Persky 1989). Attempts to inject into the femoral vein may lead to serious infections and infected femoral artery aneuryms with a significant risk of the need for amputation of the leg (Reddy et al. 1986).

Chapter 4

Psychological health, physical health, and mortality

Drug users who present for treatment often have physical and psychological health problems in addition to their drug problems. Many dependent drug users have generally poor health associated with their lifestyles, and many physical health problems are directly associated with drug use. Intravenous drug users can develop respiratory complications from granuloma formation after injecting insoluble adulterants (Glassroth *et al.* 1986), and the inhalation of high-temperature vapours such as those of heroin, crack, or free-base cocaine can also cause respiratory disease or damage (Hughes and Calverley 1988), especially when the drug contains contaminants (Tashkin *et al.* 1987). Regular cannabis smoking can lead to respiratory symptoms such as wheezing, shortness of breath, and tightness in the chest. Such symptoms are similar to those induced by cigarette smoking but can occur (independently of cigarette smoking) even after a relatively short duration of cannabis use (Taylor *et al.* 2000).

Use of cocaine is associated with cerebral vasoconstriction and this may lead to cerebrovascular dysfunction (Kaufman *et al.* 1998). Seizures are among the more common of the serious neurophysiological reactions to cocaine, and seizures are especially dangerous if these occur repeatedly (Dyll 1990). In a study of patients presenting to a hospital in San Francisco with cocaine-related complications, Lowenstein *et al.* (1987) found seizures, headache, and transient loss of consciousness were among the main neurological complications, with anxiety, depression, and paranoia among the psychiatric complications. Psychological and physical health problems are often found together among drug misusers. The close association between physical health and psychiatric symptoms has been reported by Darke *et al.* (1994) and Marsden *et al.* (2000).

In many cases, the decision to seek treatment may be influenced more by the accumulation of health problems than by drug problems (Ward *et al.* 1998). However, for both comorbid physical and psychological health problems, there are often difficulties in determining the nature and direction of the relationship between the disorders (e.g. which disorder has preceded the other and which is the more severe). Physical health problems, for example, are often aggravated by the poor nutrition and health care of dependent drug takers (Best *et al.* 1998). It should also be borne in mind that comorbid physical and psychological health problems may develop independently of drug misuse.

Psychological problems and psychiatric comorbidity

Anxiety and depression are relatively common disorders. A useful distinction should be made between two different types of anxiety state (Barlow and Lehman 1996; Clark 2000). Panic attacks consist of intense feelings of apprehension. Typically, they are of sudden onset, and are associated with distressing physical sensations (e.g. breathlessness, palpitations, dizziness, and feelings of unreality). A different type of anxiety state is characterized by generalized, unrealistic, or excessive worries, usually involving thoughts of not being able to cope, anticipating negative evaluation from others, and diffuse somatic concerns. Many people with anxiety states experience both types of anxiety (Clark 2000).

In the general population, Weissman and Merikangas (1986) found a 1-year prevalence rate of 0.5–3 per cent for panic disorder and 3–6 per cent for generalized anxiety disorder. Patients with panic disorder are among the most frequent users of out-patient mental health services (Boyd 1986). Lader and Marks (1971) suggested that approximately 8 per cent of all psychiatric out-patients suffer from anxiety states. Lifetime prevalence estimates for depression may be as high as 25 per cent for women and 12 per cent for men (Feinberg 1999). Depression can be a normal mood response, a symptom of other mental and physical disorders, and a specific syndrome, and includes adjustment disorders, grief reactions, and dysthymia, as well as severe incapacitating reactions.

Anxiety and depressed mood are more prevalent among drug users in treatment than in the general population, and many people who present to drug use treatment services have these sorts of problems (Rounsaville *et al.* 1982; Regier *et al.* 1990; Kessler *et al.* 1994; Farrell *et al.* 1998; Marsden *et al.* 2000). Around half of opioid- or cocaine-dependent drug users in treatment have a lifetime depressive episode, while a third have depressed mood at intake to addiction treatment (Kleinman *et al.* 1990*b*). In a national study of treatment admissions in the USA, Hubbard *et al.* (1989) found that, depending on the treatment modality, between a quarter and a half of their sample reported depressive and suicidal thinking. Rounsaville *et al.* (1982) found that more than half (54 per cent) of a clinical sample of 533 opiate addicts had a lifetime history of a depressive disorder, and about a quarter (24 per cent) of them were experiencing an episode of major depression at the time of the study.

Khantzian and Treece (1985) also suggested that about two-thirds of the opiate addicts in their study met lifetime criteria for a mood disorder. However, although depressed mood may increase the risk of opiate use among some individuals, both the acute and the chronic use of opiates can also produce and/or exacerbate depressive states (Mirin *et al.* 1976). Weiss *et al.* (1992) concluded that, while depressive symptoms may play a role in opiate abuse, major depression was seldom a primary determinant of the initiation of heroin drug use.

About one in five of the NTORS (National Treatment Outcome Research Study) patients had previously received treatment for a psychiatric health problem other than substance use (Marsden *et al.* 2000). Staff in both psychiatry and addiction treatment settings may need enhanced training to improve their ability to detect, assess, and respond to those with comorbid or dual diagnosis disorders (Scott *et al.* 1998). There is a strong case for suggesting that much more could be done to establish and strengthen the links between substance use and mental health services. Drug misusers with psychiatric problems also have relatively high rates of contact with various sorts of health-care services (Alterman *et al.* 1993).

Undoubtedly there are many missed opportunities for improved coordination between addiction, general medical, and mental health services. A further, organizational problem is that the mental health needs of drug users are often not properly met by treatment services that specialize in treating either mental disorders or substance use disorders (Hall and Farrell 1997). Where drug users present with both psychiatric and substance use problems, failure to address their mental health problems leads to poorer outcomes (McLellan *et al.* 1983). However, a word of caution is required. The use of the term dual diagnosis implies more similarities within this population than may actually exist (Weiss *et al.* 1992). As with drug addicts in general, people with drug dependence and coexisting psychiatric disorders are also a diverse group.

Drug use disorders are often found in conjunction with various types of psychological and psychiatric disorders, and the presence of both substance use and psychiatric problems within the same individuals is increasingly recognized as among the more difficult issues to be tackled by psychiatry (Schuckit and Hesselbrock 1994; Johnson 1997; Hall and Farrell 1997). Improvement in psychological well-being and functioning is an important treatment goal for people with drug dependence (Task Force to Review Services for Drug Misusers 1996), but the nature and course of psychiatric symptoms and disorders among dependent drug users (drug addicts) remain underresearched.

Psychiatric disorders and drug misuse can coexist with varying degrees of association or independence. Some disorders may be due to physiological changes that occur during chronic intoxication, or during acute or protracted withdrawal states. Psychiatric disorders may be secondary to psychosocial factors that are associated with addictive behaviour. Problematic drug use and psychiatric disorders may also coexist by chance since both disorders are relatively common. Nonetheless, even in these circumstances, psychiatric problems are likely to influence the course and outcome of drug misuse disorders, and may require a specially tailored treatment approach.

Drug misuse can also induce and perpetuate psychiatric disorders. Cocaine, amphetamines, and cannabis, for instance, may induce anxiety states or panic attacks during acute intoxication (Deas-Nesmith et al. 1998). Cocaine can produce a pharma_____enon of kindling involv_____trical stimulation of the_____. This may lead to increa_____recip-itate panic attacks_____order (Aronson and Cra_____

The presence o_____ers is generally associate_____1986, 1987), as is the sev_____et al. 1999). Interesting_____toms, Carroll et al. (1995_____omes than the drug use_____gs of other studies that_____pres-sion fare less well_____than their non-mood_____991). However, the prov_____ric or psychological disc_____aville and Kleber 1985). Patient–treatment matching, based on assessment of comorbid psychiatric disorders, has also been found to improve treatment outcome (McLellan et al. 1983, 1997a).

At one time drug misuse disorders were widely believed to represent attempts to self-medicate underlying psychological and psychiatric disorders. One implication of the self-medication hypothesis was that effective treatment of the underlying disorder would lead to a resolution of the substance use disorder. The literature suggests that the effective treatment of comorbid disorders does not necessarily translate into improvements in drug use outcomes. Carroll et al. (1995) found that reductions in depressive symptoms could occur without reductions in cocaine use, and, conversely, reductions in cocaine use occurred without reductions in depression.

The association between psychiatric symptoms and substance use may be indirect or conditional. Marsden et al. (2000) found that, for opiate-dependent drug users with relatively low levels of polydrug use, pre-intake levels of drug use were not correlated directly with the presence or severity of psychiatric symptoms. Psychiatric symptoms were more often found among opiate users who were also frequent users of stimulants, benzodiazepines, and/or alcohol. Yet again, these findings point to the importance of assessing polydrug use patterns. In addition, drug users with more severe physical health symptoms, those with more severe substance use dependence, those who had previous psychiatric treatment, and those who reported higher levels of conflict in their personal relationships were all more likely to have severe psychiatric problems. Treatment service personnel should undertake a thorough assessment of the psychological health problems of polydrug users who may need special consideration and treatment planning (Strain *et al.* 1991*a*).

Where drug misusers with a psychiatric disorder present in an acutely disturbed state, it is good clinical practice to use a period of abstinence for observation and assessment before a diagnosis of a comorbid, non-substance-induced psychiatric disorder is made. The persistence or remission of psychological and psychiatric symptoms during periods of abstinence may help to clarify matters. The continuation of psychological problems during periods of abstinence increases the probability that the problems are not due to drug misuse. Where psychological problems are reduced or disappear during periods of abstinence, this points to a drug-related disorder.

In many cases, anxiety and depressive symptoms may be closely associated with drug use and will remit with abstinence. Strain *et al.* (1991*b*) found reductions in the majority of depressive symptoms reported by heroin-dependent patients within the first week of methadone maintenance treatment and subsequent to abstinence from heroin. The finding that depressive symptoms improved despite continued opioid (methadone) administration suggests that the depression was, in some cases, a consequence of the heroin use, possibly mediated by psychosocial and/or pharmacological factors.

The course of depressive symptoms among opiate-dependent patients was investigated over a 6-month period by Rounsaville *et al.* (1982). More than half (60 per cent) reported depressive symptoms at intake, but only 11 per cent after 6 months. Of those patients with major depression at intake, most improved without receiving any specific treatment for their depression, again suggesting the importance of initially focusing treatment on the addiction rather than on the depression. Nonetheless, although treatment of drug dependence may be regarded as the first priority, careful assessment of persistent or emergent depressive symptoms is also required. More than a quarter of the NTORS patients reported suicidal thoughts before treatment (Gossop *et al.* 1998*b*). Drug-dependent patients who report current suicidal ideation or a history of suicide attempts may require special and immediate treatment response. Again, clinical services should be alert to this issue and should conduct a careful assessment where there are indications of suicidal risk.

Severe mental illnesses such as schizophrenia are less often found than anxiety and depressive disorders among *drug-dependent* patients, though substance abuse problems are relatively common among patients with primary psychotic disorders. Community mental health services and other psychiatric services encounter many patients, including those with very severe mental illnesses, who also use illegal drugs (see Chapter 13). The lack of association between psychosis and *addiction* may be largely due to the difficulties of living what is, in its own way, an extremely demanding addict lifestyle with its requirements to maintain a regular and expensive daily supply of illegal drugs, and to avoid arrest by the police.

One of the psychotic states that may be found among drug misusers is a direct consequence of drug use. Stimulant psychosis may occur after high-dose and/or prolonged use of any of the stimulants, but is more often associated with amphetamines than cocaine because of the shorter duration of effect of cocaine and the greater difficulties of sustaining chronic, high levels of cocaine (King and Ellinwood 1997). Stimulant psychosis typically starts with suspiciousness; this may be followed by beliefs about being watched or followed (Ellinwood 1967). Suspiciousness and paranoid delusions develop in a clear sensorium (i.e. the patient is alert and oriented). This is followed by overreaction to stimuli in the peripheral field of vision, and finally by a confusional state and hallucinations, sometimes including tactile hallucinations (formication). Full hallucinations, however, tend to be reported by only a minority of stimulant abusers (Siegel 1978).

Stimulant psychosis has some similarities with an acute schizophrenic disorder but it differs in other ways. Schizophrenia tends to have a relatively slow onset and to be accompanied by a stable, somewhat bland mood (Goodwin and Guze 1988). The onset of a stimulant psychosis is rapid and is often accompanied by an agitated or manic mood state. Also, the schizophrenic seldom shows abnormal physical findings whereas a patient with stimulant psychosis may have severe weight loss, needle marks, and excoriations (from scratching at 'cocaine bugs'). One of the main differences is that the treatment of stimulant psychosis is relatively straightforward. If the person is out of contact with reality, it may be necessary to hospitalize him or her. In general, the patient should be placed in a situation with a quiet, non-threatening atmosphere, and should be treated in a manner that would be appropriate for the management of any patient with paranoid ideation (e.g. not performing any procedures without first offering a thorough explanation, not touching the patient without their permission, and avoiding sudden movements in the patient's presence).

When stimulant use is discontinued, a stimulant psychosis would be expected to clear within days, with the hallucinations disappearing first and the delusions later (Schuckit 1989). It has been suggested that a few drug misusers with a stimulant psychosis may continue to have some residual symptoms for up to a year or more, though in his monograph on amphetamine psychosis Connell (1958) suggested that the continuation of psychotic symptoms after the drug has ceased to be excreted (usually within a maximum of 7 days) should be viewed with 'grave suspicion', and that such cases should be regarded not as stimulant psychoses but as of possible schizophrenic aetiology.

Blood-borne infections

Injecting drugs can lead to many health problems. One of the first reports of infections transmitted between heroin injectors was of an outbreak of malaria during the 1920s (Biggam 1929). Injecting can cause skin and soft tissue infections (Levine 1991), endocarditis, and bone and joint infections (Contoreggi *et al.* 1998). Repeated injection in the same sites can cause progressive sclerosis of the veins. The adulterants in street drugs may also cause problems. In a recent outbreak of deaths due to 'unexplained illness' among injecting drug users, the responsible agent was subsequently identified as the bacterium *Clostridium* (Ahmed *et al.* 2000). Injecting problems may be aggravated by the injection of insoluble particles (Scott *et al.* 1997), and problems have also been reported due to the addition of acids to increase the solubility of drugs (Hunter *et al.* 1995; Strang *et al.* 1997c). Injection is also associated with a greatly increased risk of overdose (Gossop *et al.* 1996; Fugelstad *et al.* 1997; Powis *et al.* 1999).

In addition to the risks associated with injection, the shared use of injecting equipment gives rise to serious concern because of its role in the transmission of HIV and other blood-borne infections. Injecting drug use was rapidly identified as one of the principal factors implicated in the spread of HIV infection. During the early phase of the epidemic, 6.6 per cent of all cases reported in the European countries were among drug users. By 1986, this had increased to 20.6 per cent. In 1988, it had gone up further to 34.5 per cent, and by 1991 it had reached 38.2 per cent (World Health Organization 1993).

The appearance of HIV/AIDS had a dramatic impact on the behaviour of drug users. The urgent need to respond to the threat of HIV/AIDS also radically changed the addiction treatment agenda, produced many changes in national responses to drug problems, and forced a rethinking of the nature of the problem and of the appropriateness and effectiveness of existing services.

In many countries, the HIV issue led to a reappraisal of national aims and practices and, in certain respects, to a reversal of trends. Treatment services were forced to re-examine the need for harm reduction responses aimed at goals other than drug-free functioning. The reluctance to provide longer-term, maintenance type prescribing which was a feature of British clinical practice during the 1970s and early 1980s (Mitcheson 1994) was strongly challenged and reversed. There was an increased awareness of the acceptability of reducing the harm that drug users may suffer as a result of their drug taking. Concern about AIDS also increased political willingness to provide money to support drug treatment and support services. It is unfortunate that it took such a tragic development to produce these changes.

During the period immediately after HIV was identified, the Advisory Council on the Misuse of Drugs (ACMD 1988) stated that 'HIV is a greater threat to public and individual health than drug misuse'; that 'the first goal of work with drug misusers must therefore be to prevent them from acquiring or transmitting the virus'; and that 'prescribing may serve two . . . purposes directly related to our goal of containing the spread of HIV', namely, 'attracting more drug users to services and keeping them in contact' and 'facilitating change away from HIV risk practices'.

For several years after its identification, concern about HIV tended to over-shadow other drug problems, including other serious blood-borne infections about which there is now an increased awareness, such as the viral hepatitis infections, and especially hepatitis C (HCV). These infections are not directly caused by drugs or by drug dependence. They are the result of drug consumption behaviours, specifically the use of injecting equipment that has been previously contaminated by infected blood.

Increasing concern has been voiced about hepatitis C infection and its extremely high prevalence among drug injectors (Crofts *et al.* 1997; Alter *et al.* 1999; Best *et al.* 1999*b*). A review of HCV and HBV (hepatitis B virus) sero-prevalence in drug users in Europe found HCV prevalence rates of 59–83 per cent and HBV rates of 22–69 per cent (Vingoe *et al.* 1997). Australian studies have reported prevalence rates of 60 and 67 per cent for HCV and 23 per cent for HBV (Loxley *et al.* 1997; Crofts *et al.* 1997). Other surveys reported HCV antibody prevalence rates ranging from 65 to 95 per cent (Hagan 1998). A study of methadone maintenance patients in London found rates of seropos-itivity of 86 per cent for HCV and 55 per cent for HBV (Best *et al.* 1999*b*). HCV positive patients are usually older, have been injecting for longer, and have had more contact with treatment services (Noble *et al.* 2000). One of the strongest predictors of hepatitis seropositive status is the number of years of injecting drugs. The association between years of injecting drug use and hepa-titis infection rates is shown in Fig. 4.1.

Although drug users are generally aware of the risks of HCV and HBV, their beliefs about their own viral status are frequently inaccurate.

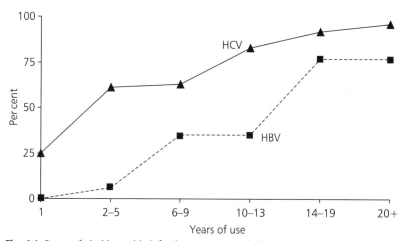

Fig. 4.1 Rates of viral hepatitis infection are extremely high among drug injectors. This figure shows the steady increase in seropositivity rates for hepatitis B (HBV) and hepatitis C (HCV) plotted against the number of years for which the user had been injecting drugs. Almost all drug injectors who had been using for more than 14 years had been infected with the hepatitis C virus. The data are from the study of Noble *et al.* (2000).

Best *et al.* (1999*b*) found that addicts tended, mistakenly, to believe that they were not infected with HBV or HCV when they were, in fact, seropositive for one or other of these infections. This misapprehension may lead to behaviours that have serious public health consequences. Clinicians should encourage testing in all injecting patients and use this as a catalyst for interventions.

Injecting and the shared use of injecting equipment are both highly problematic behaviours, and the reduction of public health threats associated with injecting risk behaviours has been identified as an appropriate treatment goal (McLellan *et al.* 1997*b*). Research into the injecting practices of drug users has led to an improved awareness of the injection-related activities that put them at risk of infection.

'Needle sharing', for instance, involves several different behaviours and practices. Hall *et al.* (1993*b*) distinguished between the 'borrowing' and 'lending' of needles and syringes. Injectors often regard 'sharing' as referring only to using a syringe borrowed from another person, but not as lending a used syringe to others (Koester 1994). In addition to the shared use of needles and syringes, there are other risky but indirect forms of sharing linked to the preparation and the act of injection that also involve contact with blood and infective agents. Preparation frequently involves the use of a spoon, or 'cooker', and a water container to flush syringes before use, and/or from which water is drawn to dissolve substances for injection (Booth *et al.* 1991). The shared use of these items carries a risk of infection from infective viral material (Chitwood *et al.* 1990; Heimer *et al.* 1996).

Injectors are more likely to share spoons and water containers than syringes, and they show less discrimination in the sharing of such paraphernalia than with needles and syringes. Almost all (86 per cent) of the drug users studied by Gossop *et al.* (1997*b*) reported having used a syringe to add water to the spoon in which they were preparing their heroin. Since drug users may use their own syringe to inject but share a mixing spoon, this represents a potential risk of viral transmission. The hepatitis C virus has been found to be surprisingly robust and is able to survive for considerable periods of time in the environment (Heimer *et al.* 1996) and the infection may be communicable through the sharing of spoons and other injecting equipment other than the needles and syringes. The HIV virus has also been found in some circumstances to survive for considerable periods in used syringes. It is certainly possible that the widespread sharing of injecting paraphernalia could account for some of the transmission of hepatitis C amongst drug injectors. Drug users and drug workers should be aware of the risks of sharing all items of injecting equipment that have been in contact with blood or other infective material.

Drug injectors tend to be reluctant to share syringes when these are from people who are not well known to the user but the sharing of spoons and water appears to be treated in a less discerning manner (Gossop *et al.* 1997*b*). It is likely that sharing syringes is treated with greatest caution partly because of the obviously (and literally) intrusive quality of using needles and syringes and because of the success of preventive messages that have been published about 'needle sharing'. In contrast, the sharing of spoons and water does not have such an intimate or intrusive quality and the risks associated with sharing such types of injecting paraphernalia have been largely omitted from prevention messages.

Less is known about HIV awareness among early, non-dependent and episodic users, than among dependent, treatment samples. Knowledge of HIV/AIDS has been found to be lower among early injectors (less than 2 years) than among more experienced users (Kleinman *et al.* 1990*a*). Drug injectors who are in contact with drug intervention services often show good awareness of injecting risk issues (Stimson 1991). It is likely that the opportunities for exposure to harm reduction messages among early heroin users are less than for more severely dependent, clinical samples of heroin users who have been more directly targeted for such harm reduction interventions.

Most drug injectors have been exposed to multiple risks of infection with blood-borne diseases (Gossop *et al.* 1997*b*). About three-quarters of the injectors had been exposed to more than one risk factor and more than half had been exposed to three or more risk factors. Not surprisingly, drug-related risks were frequently reported (with 69 per cent of the sample having injected drugs at least once). However, as in other studies (Donoghoe *et al.* 1989; Klee *et al.* 1991), sexual risks factors were also common, and the majority of heroin users in this sample (83 per cent) reported having been exposed to infection risk factors that were not directly related to the injection of drugs.

Some drug users are also exposed to increased risk of infection through the additive effects of drug risk and sexual risk factors through having a sexual partner who injects drugs. Particular risks are often associated with the unprotected sex that was frequently reported between two injecting drug users. Because each of these people was likely to have been exposed to many different sorts of infection risk, the overall probability of one of them carrying HIV or HBV infection was greatly increased. Women may be at higher risk in this way. In a sample of London heroin users, 60 per cent of the women were living with a drug user as compared to 34 per cent of the men (Gossop *et al.* 1994*c*). In the USA women infected with HIV by a drug-using partner are the second largest group of women with AIDS (Cohen 1991), and HIV rates are especially high among female drug injectors who have had multiple sexual partners (Schoenbaum *et al.* 1989).

Preventing infections

The health risk behaviours of drug users have been the focus for various preventive activities. Dissemination of information about the transmission of HIV and other blood-borne infections is one of the least controversial prevention responses. This has been widely used and in some circumstances such measures may be effective (Selwyn *et al.* 1987).

Needle and syringe exchange schemes have been more controversial, though these have now been established in many countries throughout the world (Stimson *et al.* 1990). Some critics have regarded the idea of providing needles and syringes to drug injectors as an unacceptable means of trying to prevent drug problems, and some countries (notably the USA) have shown great reluctance to implement such measures. Some countries have actively intervened to restrict the availability of injecting equipment.

In the USA many states have used 'drug paraphernalia' laws to limit the availability and possession of syringes by drug users, or required prescriptions to permit the sale or possession of syringes (Pascal 1988). Sweden used laws against 'facilitating drug abuse' to prevent the sale of syringes to addicts. In New South Wales, Australia, it was a criminal offence until 1986 to carry equipment for the purpose of injecting drugs (Wolk *et al.* 1988). Even where national laws permit it, there have also been professional actions to restrict the availability of injecting equipment. In the UK, during the period 1982–86 (at a time when unidentified HIV infection was spreading), the Royal Pharmaceutical Society of Great Britain recommended that pharmacists should not supply injecting equipment to known or suspected drug injectors (Sheridan *et al.* 2000).

The rationale for syringe distribution is that, since many drug injectors at some time could be expected to share injecting equipment and since HIV and other blood-borne infections can be transmitted through blood products, the shared use of injecting equipment puts the user and others at serious risk of infection. In a study of more than 400 London heroin users, Gossop *et al.* (1994*c*) found that nearly a quarter of those who were injecting heroin (23 per cent) had shared needles and/or syringes in the previous year. There are many reasons why people share syringes, but one of the most obvious is the lack of availability of sterile equipment. Stimson *et al.* (1988) suggested that problems of restricted availability were reported as a reason for sharing syringes by almost half of the injectors in their survey.

Syringes have been supplied to users in a number of ways. There are, essentially, two types of services. Some services provide needles and syringes (either free of charge or for sale) but make no requirement for the return of used equipment. In other services, needles and syringes are provided on an exchange basis (either on a one-for-one, or some other agreed basis). All services make suitable and safe arrangements for the safe disposal of returned used needles and syringes. Used equipment is not generally handled by staff, and clients are asked to place their equipment in a sharps bin.

The best known system involves the provision of needles and syringes to injectors on an exchange basis. This addresses public health concerns about used and possibly infected needles being left in public places, or otherwise disposed of in ways that may put others at risk. Exchange schemes were opened in the UK very swiftly after the identification of HIV among drug injectors. Some syringe exchange schemes were operating in the UK as early as 1986. It was as a consequence of the success of the initial pilot needle exchange projects that there was a rapid expansion of needle exchange schemes in the UK during the following years. By the end of 1989, it was estimated that there were about 120 such schemes (Stimson *et al.* 1990) and, by the mid-1990s, there were over 300 dedicated syringe exchange schemes in England (Stimson 1996). With this sort of exchange system, it has been found that syringes can be distributed with return rates of around 62 per cent in the UK (Stimson *et al.* 1988), 41 per cent in New South Wales (Wolk *et al.* 1988), and 70–95 per cent in Amsterdam (Stimson *et al.* 1990).

Needle exchanges in the UK are most often located in drug treatment agencies and in community pharmacies. Although pharmacists are not obliged to provide needle exchange as part of their National Health Service contract, over 12 000 community pharmacies are currently providing sterile injecting equipment, either as needle exchange, or for sale 'over the counter' (Sheridan *et al.* 2000). One worrying finding about the use of pharmacy-based schemes is that Sheridan *et al.* (2000) found that only around one-third of the injecting equipment given to users was returned to pharmacy-based exchange schemes. This is potentially a major weakness of such schemes, since it is not known what methods of disposal are actually used.

Some exchange schemes also offer pre-prepared packs that contain a variety of needles and syringes. Sometimes these contain other items such as swabs and condoms. Some schemes permit clients to choose from a range of items, and this option is preferred by most clients. Drug injectors also make use of other items of equipment in their injecting practices, such as filters, sterile water, and citric or ascorbic acid which is used to help dissolve the poorly soluble heroin base (Sheridan *et al.* 2000). Since it is illegal in the UK to supply injecting paraphernalia other than needles and syringes, those services that provide such items could, in law, be liable to prosecution. In practice, however, many services do provide these items.

In some countries needles and syringes can be obtained from pharmacies. In Austria they have been available in this way since 1985 (Fuchs *et al.* 1988), and in France since 1987 (Stimson *et al.* 1990). There have been a few instances in which needles and syringes have been supplied from vending machines. Such initiatives have been described in Bremen and Copenhagen (Gossop *et al.* 1993). This method is anonymous and is available 24 hours a day. Among the disadvantages of such schemes are that there is little or no control over who obtains the syringes and, for the user, these methods do not provide direct access to information or counselling services.

A number of commentators on the needle exchange schemes have suggested that they have played an important and effective role in helping to keep HIV seroprevalence at a relatively low level in the UK (Durante *et al.* 1995; Stimson 1995). HIV prevalence rates amongst drug injectors in London declined from about 13 per cent in 1990, to 10 per cent in 1991, and to 7 per cent in 1993 (Stimson 1995), and the low and stable HIV prevalence rates across most cities in the UK have been attributed, in part, to the early introduction of harm reduction interventions and syringe exchange schemes. However, any complacency about the successful prevention of HIV should be offset by the continuing problem of needle sharing and the extremely high prevalence of hepatitis C infection rates among injecting drug users (Garfein *et al.* 1996; Gossop *et al.* 1997*b*; Best *et al.* 1999*b*).

When the needle exchange services first opened, it was thought that those drug injectors who used them would do so repeatedly. This tended not to happen, and one feature of the schemes has been their high turnover of clients (Stimson *et al.* 1990). Stimson suggested that there could be positive as well as negative reasons for this high turnover. Among the possible positive outcomes were admission to formal treatment programmes or cessation of injecting. The possible negative ones included continued injection without a regular supply of clean equipment, imprisonment, or death.

Since drug injectors often contract hepatitis infections very early in their injecting careers, hepatitis vaccination programmes can be useful and should be targeted towards early-stage drug users. Vaccination may be especially appropriate for those drug takers who have not yet injected drugs but who are using drugs that are likely to be taken by injection such as heroin, amphetamines, and powder cocaine. Regardless of local injection prevalence rates, hepatitis vaccination can play an important role. In areas where rates of heroin injecting are known to be high, it is likely that the injection of other drugs will also be common, and services should be alert to the needs of injecting users who may take non-opiate drugs and of those who may not be in contact with treatment services. In such areas, needle and syringe exchange schemes may provide a valuable harm reduction service to drug misusers who would otherwise have no contact with treatment services.

Conventional addiction treatment services also play an important role in tackling blood-borne infections. Most drug treatment programmes have incorporated interventions targeted at the injecting risk and sex risk behaviours of their patients. Methadone maintenance treatment has been found to lead to reduced levels of HIV risk behaviours and to lower HIV seroconversion rates (Gibson *et al.* 1999; Marsch 1998; Ward *et al.* 1998; Sorensen and Copeland 2000). Needle sharing has been found to be lower among patients in methadone maintenance programmes than among those not in treatment, even after controlling for injection frequency and user characteristics (Longshore *et al.* 1993), and patients who remained continuously in methadone maintenance have been found to be less likely to seroconvert than those who did not (Williams *et al.* 1992; Metzger *et al.* 1993; Friedman *et al.* 1995). Moss *et al.* (1994) also found that HIV seroconversion rates were lower among methadone maintenance patients than among patients in detoxification programmes. Higher methadone doses and longer duration of treatment are two specific treatment factors that have been found to be related to lower rates of HIV infection (Hartel and Schoenbaum 1998).

In a review of 33 studies conducted with more than 17 000 drug users, Sorensen and Copeland (2000) noted that 'what the field knows about the protective effect of drug abuse treatment against HIV infection is largely based upon studies in MMT [methadone maintenance treatment]'. Less is known about changes in health risk behaviours after treatment in residential programmes. Reductions were found by Hubbard *et al.* (1989) in drug injecting after treatment in both residential and out-patient treatment programmes. McCusker *et al.* (1997) also found reduced rates of HIV risk behaviour after patients were randomly allocated to treatment in one of two residential treatment programmes (a therapeutic community and a relapse prevention programme). Both programmes produced reductions in injecting risk and sex risk behaviours.

The NTORS outcomes for injecting and sharing of injecting equipment showed that injecting, sharing injecting equipment, and having unprotected sex, were all substantially reduced 1 year after treatment entry (Gossop *et al.* 2002*a*). Of those drug users who were sharing needles or syringes at intake, less than 15 per cent had done so during the posttreatment follow-up period. Reductions were found among the drug users admitted to methadone treatment programmes and among those admitted to the residential treatment programmes.

The risks associated with sharing may be amplified or attenuated by the beliefs and behaviours of drug misusers. Moss and Chaisson (1988) found that injectors were able to incorporate cleaning and sterilizing practices into their drug-using repertoire, and Gossop *et al.* (1993*b*) found that more than half of those who shared injecting equipment reported always cleaning it before use. There are, however, doubts about the effectiveness of the cleaning methods used by injectors (Hartgers 1990). Also, whereas some injectors only share drugs with individuals who are well known to them (Gossop *et al.* 1993*b*), injectors are frequently unaware of their own viral status with regard to hepatitis B and hepatitis C infection and are even less certain of that of their sharing partners. Many drug users have been found to believe they were seronegative when they had already been infected with such viruses (Best *et al.* 1999*b*). In such circumstances, sharing only with known persons gives no protection.

Overdose and mortality

Deaths among drug users have many causes, including accidents, suicide, violence, AIDS, acute toxic reactions, and various drug-related and other illnesses (Rivara *et al.* 1997; Rossow and Lauritzen 1999; Hulse *et al.* 1999). The use of 'dance drugs' such as MDMA/Ecstasy (3,4-methylenedioxymethamphetamine) is linked to a small number of deaths each year. Such deaths typically occur among people who are not dependent upon drugs and not in contact with treatment services. The most common acute complication associated with MDMA deaths is hyperthermic collapse (overheating) due to dancing for long periods in a hot environment without adequate fluid replacement

(ACMD 2000). Deaths have also occurred as a result of excessive fluid intake, possibly due to a mistaken interpretation of harm limitation messages. Excessive drinking can produce vomiting, drowsiness, agitation, and convulsions, in effect leading to death by water intoxication. When deaths occur soon after MDMA ingestion, these may be due to cardiac arrhythmias.

In addition to a number of less serious medical problems, cocaine can also cause cardiac arrest (heart attack), cerebral haemorrhage (stroke), and seizures. In most cases, the possibility of death as a consequence of cocaine use is not predictable. Death has occurred in first-time users as well as in chronic users, and in low-dose as well as high-dose users (Washton 1989). In a study of cocaine-related strokes, Klonoff *et al.* (1989) found intracranial haemorrhage to be more common than cerebral infarction: the mean age of these cases was 33 years. The use of cocaine by those with undiagnosed medical conditions, including heart conditions, can lead to an elevated risk of fatal reactions.

Despite the greater attention that is generally given to HIV/AIDS as a potential cause of death among drug misusers, drug overdose continues to be one of the most frequent causes of death in this group (Ghodse *et al.* 1978; Hall and Darke 1998; Powis *et al.* 1999; Strang *et al.* 1999*a*). In a Scottish study, for instance, Frischer *et al.* (1993) found that more than 90 per cent of deaths among drug misusers were due to drug overdose or suicide, and only 2 per cent to HIV/AIDS.

In several countries there have been consistent increases in overdose deaths among young adults in recent years. Neeleman and Farrell (1997) noted a 9-fold increase in opiate-related deaths in England and Wales between 1974 and 1992, and in Australia Hall (1999) described a 55-fold increase in drug overdose deaths between 1964 and 1997. Heroin has frequently been associated with fatal overdoses, though the concurrent use of other drugs, and particularly benzodiazepines has also regularly been found to be related to overdose deaths (Strang *et al.* 1999*a*; Darke and Ross 1999; Risser *et al.* 2000).

A 20-year follow-up of addicts in the USA (Vaillant 1973) reported a yearly death rate of 1 per cent and, in a study of UK drug misusers, Oppenheimer *et al.* (1994) reported a mortality rate of 1.8 per cent per year. Ghodse *et al.* (1998) noted that mortality rates differ considerably throughout the world. A comparatively high death rate has been reported in Australia by Darke *et al.* (1996*b*) who suggested that 2–3 per cent of heroin users die each year.

The mortality rate of the drug users in the NTORS cohort was 1.2 per cent. This is substantially greater (by about 6 times) than that of their peers in the general population (Gossop *et al.* 2002*b*). These findings are consistent with those of other studies (Joe and Simpson 1990; Oppenheimer *et al.* 1994; Darke *et al.* 1996*b*; Ghodse *et al.* 1998). Simpson and Sells (1983) found the death rates of drug users (predominantly heroin users) to be 3–14 times higher than those of their peers of the same age. The majority of deaths (68 per cent) were associated with drug overdoses. Opiates were the drugs most commonly detected during post mortem examinations. Mainly these showed the presence of heroin (in two-thirds of the overdose cases), though methadone was also found in almost half of the overdose deaths.

Among the reasons given by opiate misusers for overdoses are taking a higher dose than usual, taking stronger heroin than usual, and using heroin after detoxification and loss of tolerance (Gossop *et al.* 1996). The mechanism by which opiate overdose leads to death is generally attributed to respiratory depression mediated by inhibition of medullary centres (White and Irvine 1999). However, there is some uncertainty about the exact causes of overdose and similar blood morphine levels have been reported among fatal heroin overdose victims and among current heroin users (Darke and Zador 1996; Darke *et al.* 1997).

Although fatal and non-fatal overdoses are commonly attributed to the use of opiates, these are seldom due simply to the use of opiates. As with many other problems, the risk of overdose is strongly linked to, and increased by polydrug use. Overdoses that are attributed to heroin are more likely to involve the combined use of opiates and alcohol or other sedatives (Darke and Zador 1996; Gossop *et al.* 1996; Best *et al.* 1999*c*), and the same factors have been found to be associated with both fatal and non-fatal overdoses (Gossop *et al.* 2002*b*; Stewart *et al.* 2002). As with other drug problems, alcohol often operates as a 'hidden drug' and exacerbates the severity of the problem.

In a study of American drug users, Joe and Simpson (1990) found heavy drinking to be associated with increased risk of mortality, as did Ruttenber and Luke (1984). The Australian studies of Darke *et al.* (1996*b*, 1999) found that fatal overdoses were associated with polydrug use, use of benzodiazepines, and higher levels of alcohol consumption. In their study of drug-related deaths in Scotland, Hammersley *et al.* (1995) found that mixtures of heroin, temazepam, diazepam, and alcohol were common. Risser and Schneider (1994) reported that, whereas 30 per cent of the overdose deaths in Austria involved a single substance overdose, 56 per cent involved more than one drug. Polydrug use and drug and alcohol combinations have also been found to be common among drug users taking non-fatal overdoses (Gossop *et al.* 1996; Powis *et al.* 1999).

Because of the high rates of hepatitis C infection among problem drug users, heavy drinking is also an independent risk factor for mortality because of its adverse effects upon the physical health of the user. For individuals chronically infected with HCV, heavy drinking is especially risky, but even low levels of alcohol consumption have been found to be associated with increased risk of viraemia and hepatic fibrosis (Pessione *et al.* 1998).

In the deaths among the NTORS cohort, benzodiazepines and alcohol were frequently detected during post mortem examinations. In the majority of cases, more than one drug was detected. Indeed, a single substance was found after death in only about one in five of the cases. In more than half of the overdose deaths, three or more different drugs were detected. The most common drug combinations associated with death involved opiates and alcohol, opiates and benzodiazepines, or a mixture of all three of these drugs. Polydrug use in general, but this sort of mixture of substances in particular, was found to lead to a significant increase in the risk of mortality. The most risky combination of all undoubtedly involves a mixture of all three of these substances (opiates, benzodiazepines, and alcohol) and this was detected in one-fifth of the overdoses.

Treatment can reduce the risk of overdose. Insofar as treatment has been shown to lead to increased abstinence from drugs and to reduced frequency of illicit drug use (Simpson and Sells 1983; Hubbard *et al.* 1989; Gossop *et al.* 1998*a*), it is reasonable to expect that treatment will also lead to reductions in drug overdoses taken accidentally. Reductions in drug use after treatment have been found to be associated with a reduced risk of overdose, and cessation or reduction in frequency of injection was strongly related to reduced risk of overdose with drug injectors being 10 times more likely to overdose (Stewart *et al.* 2002). Overdose has also been found to be less frequent among drug misusers in treatment than among out-of-treatment samples (Capelhorn *et al.* 1994; Darke *et al.* 1996*b*).

Most overdoses (fatal and non-fatal) occur in the presence of other people, generally other drug users. Powis *et al.* (1999) found that more than half of their sample had been present when another person had taken an overdose, and more than three-quarters had themselves taken a non-fatal overdose in the presence of another person. Strang *et al.* (1999*b*) found that a third of their sample had been present when another user had taken a fatal overdose. Under such circumstances, the ability of other drug users to identify and respond to an overdose may have a potentially life-saving effect. When an overdose occurs, the drug users who are present often make some sort of attempt to help. Unfortunately, the types of responses by other drug users may be ineffective or even counterproductive (Darke *et al.* 1996*b*; Best *et al.* 1999).

When asked about overdoses, many drug users expressed a willingness to intervene and to use such active resuscitation measures as placing the overdose victim in the lateral recovery position to reduce the risks of inhalation of vomit and asphyxia and even to apply mouth-to-mouth resuscitation (kiss of life) (Strang *et al.* 2000*a*). Resuscitation measures of this sort require prior information or training. It seems appropriate that treatment services should provide information or educational sessions to provide drug users with the knowledge and skills to implement appropriate resuscitation measures in the event of someone taking an overdose in their presence.

Strang *et al.* (1999*b*) found that only about one-third of the drug users in their study had heard of the opiate antagonist drug naloxone. However, when the effects of the drug were explained, most thought that increased availability of naloxone was a good thing, and 89 per cent of those who had witnessed an overdose stated that they would have administered it. Strang *et al.* (1999*b*) estimated that as many as two-thirds of the witnessed fatal drug overdoses could potentially have been prevented by making naloxone available to drug users.

In a survey of the drug-related problems seen in London casualty departments during a 1-month period, Ghodse and Rawson (1978) noted 1706 separate incidents. Overdoses (accidental, suicidally intentioned, and addiction-related) were among the most common problems. In more than a quarter of these cases the patients were dependent on drugs, and most of them were admitted for treatment of a drug overdose, generally as the result of multiple drug use (Ghodse 1977). The attitudes of ambulance personnel and of the casualty staff towards patients who took accidental drug overdoses were more favourable than towards patients who did so in a deliberate suicidal attempt. Attitudes were least favourable towards those who took an addiction-related overdose (Ghodse 1978).

In reality, it is often extremely difficult to draw a clear distinction between accidental and deliberate, or between intentional and non-intentional overdoses, especially when these occur among drug misusers. Drug misusers may take (sometimes extremely) high doses of drugs in their search for intense states of intoxication, and their behaviour is sometimes willfully reckless. Nonetheless, some overdoses among drug abusers reflect deliberate suicide attempts. Among the NTORS deaths, it was clear in at least two cases that a fatal overdose of drugs was taken with suicidal intent. A significant minority of the drug misusers who seek treatment for addiction problems have been found to have thoughts of killing themselves (Gossop *et al.* 1998*b*). Another study of opiate addicts who had taken a non-fatal overdose found that 10 per cent reported that the overdose had been taken deliberately (Gossop *et al.* 1996). A study of suicide attempts and life-threatening overdoses in Norway found that 37 per cent of a sample of drug addicts had attempted suicide (Rossow and Lauritzen 1999). Similarly, 31 per cent of the deaths among a Swedish sample of drug users were found to be due to suicide (Wahren *et al.* 1997). Rossow and Lauritzen (1999) also found that drug users who had previously attempted to commit suicide reported more severe psychiatric problems. Farrell *et al.* (1996) suggested that official data collection systems may tend to underestimate the prevalence of suicidal fatalities among addicts because of the requirement of clear evidence of intent.

Chapter 5

The relationship between the
drug user and treatment

The role of treatment

The role played by treatment in helping addicts to give up drugs is complex, and the evidence about the effectiveness of specific treatments is often difficult to interpret. To understand the effectiveness of treatment it is necessary first to ask the right questions. The apparently straightforward question, 'what is the most effective way to treat opiate addiction?', is misleading and cannot be answered directly. The problems of drug misuse cannot be fitted within a single unitary category. Instead, they are a diverse range of different problems and clusters of problems. Similarly, addiction treatments consist of many different procedures and interventions. It makes no more sense to ask what is the most effective treatment for drug abuse than it does to ask what is the most effective treatment for mental illness. In order to respond to such questions it is necessary to restate them in order to create more precise definitions of the problem with a clearer specification of who is being treated and what they are seeking from treatment.

The treatment of physiological withdrawal symptoms and the treatment of psychological dependence, for example, are profoundly different processes and require fundamentally different types of interventions. Nonetheless, the treatment of drug addiction is always a collaborative enterprise. Drug problems cannot be treated without the co-operation and commitment of the patient. Treatments cannot be applied mechanically. Indeed, the traditional notion of a 'treatment' delivered by expert clinicians to a 'patient' (i.e. a passive recipient) is misleading in this context. Rather than being an event that happens to the addict, the treatment of drug abuse problems is a process in which the patient takes an active role. This is true even for the pharmacological treatment of drug withdrawal, which is perhaps the most straightforward form of treatment and the one that most closely approximates the medical model. But, even here, the characteristics of the patient, the nature of their problems, and their beliefs and intentions remain important factors that affect the probability that the treatment will be effective.

Treatment can be influenced by the patient's sociodemographic characteristics, their personal resources, health and cognitive status, and the chronicity and severity of their problems and impairment. Other relevant factors include the individual's expectations and preferences regarding treatment. Most patients are able to exercise some choice about which treatment programme they go to, and these sorts of factors and the interactions between them affect further factors such as programme participation and treatment engagement that are also likely to influence subsequent outcomes.

The interventions that occur during treatment are merely a part of a much wider range of factors that can influence outcome. In many cases, treatment may be neither the most important nor the most powerful influence upon outcome. Environmental supports and stressors can influence outcomes. Social factors, such as peer and family relationships, unemployment, and living arrangements, can have an important effect on the individual's chances of success. The gains produced by an effective treatment programme can be undermined or neutralized by adverse social and environmental factors.

Edwards (1987) has warned about the limitations of treatment and suggested that excessive enthusiasm about treatment effectiveness can be misguided: such enthusiasm may be 'constrained to the point of tunnel vision if it assumes that treatment influences are so paramount that all that has to be asked is "Does treatment work?" with every other influence . . . discounted.' Treatment usually makes only a small and time-limited contribution to the lives of the people who receive treatment. For this reason alone, its influence may be limited and short-lived. Treatment takes place within a much broader context and can be more accurately conceived as being 'a timely nudge or whisper in a long life course' (Edwards 1987).

To state this is not to demean or play down the role of treatment. Treatment provides an important and sometimes vital opportunity to intervene and interrupt the psychological, social, and biological processes that are acting to trap the person within a destructive pattern of addictive behaviour. Even where treatment factors do not act as direct determinants of change, treatment still generally provides an important facilitative setting in which behavioural improvements can take place (Simpson and Sells 1983). What is urgently needed is a better understanding of the processes underlying effective treatment. To achieve a fuller understanding of the factors that influence the patients' psychosocial functioning in the community, we need to see their problems within the wider social context of their family and work settings and their broader life circumstances (Moos *et al.* 1990).

Moos (1997) has sought to identify the connections between treatment factors and patient characteristics, and suggested how the patient's adaptation in the community is mediated by the social climate of treatment programmes and by the patient's responses during treatment. The diversity of treatment programmes includes both objective and psychological factors. In addition to the treatment interventions, features of treatment include the physical design, policies, and services of the treatment service, the institutional context, and the overall characteristics of the patient and staff groups.

We still know surprisingly little about what actually happens during treatment, or how treatments are applied in day-to-day clinical practice. In most respects, we have only a broad and generalized understanding of the components and processes of treatment. Hubbard *et al.* (1989) noted that 'The complexity of treatment is difficult to conceptualize and even harder to define and quantify.' We have yet to identify and define the relevant variables, much less to accurately assess them. This gap in our knowledge of the components, processes, and dynamics of treatment has often been referred to as the 'black box', in which the people, events, and interactions that are incorporated within such labels as 'therapy,' 'counselling,' 'referral', and 'rehabilitation' remain largely unspecified. As a consequence, many of the variations in treatment delivery that affect treatment effectiveness are also unspecified (Lipton and Appel 1984).

Moos (1997) also noted that: 'Although most behavioral scientists endorse the idea that both personal and environmental factors determine behavior, evaluation researchers have typically conceptualized the treatment program as a "black box" intervening between patient or staff inputs and outcomes. Thus, these programs often are assessed only in terms of broad categories.' Research into the ways in which treatment process factors actually operate has been neglected. We need to know more about the effective components of treatment. Many treatment factors could be related to outcome, although few of these have been identified. Indeed, there is still a need for basic systematic descriptions, classifications, and measurements of treatment factors.

What the drug user brings to treatment

Drug users are a diverse and heterogeneous group of people. When seeking treatment, they bring with them a range of factors that may help or hinder the processes of recovery. Some of these factors may be social. A major influence upon young people is that of their friends and close companions. A person who mixes with other drug takers is at greatly increased risk of taking drugs simply because of this. Some factors may be environmental. Drug cultures thrive within deprived inner city areas amid poor housing, crime, alienation, and unemployment.

Some of the factors that the user brings to treatment are psychological. Examples could include a predisposition to drug taking because of anxiety or depressed mood, or possibly as a result of a low threshold for boredom and a tendency towards seeking extreme and exciting experiences. Cognitive factors, including the beliefs, attitudes, expectations, and intentions of the user, are also relevant to treatment. The user's expectations of treatment may range from immediate relief from physical symptoms, to short-term resolution of current crises, to long-term changes in their lifestyle (McLellan *et al.* 1997*b*).

Drug users present to treatment with complex mixtures of substance use and other problems. The range and severity of these problems present challenges for those services that have responsibility for their management and treatment, and the nature, severity, and complexity of the problems are likely to affect the ways in which treatment is provided. The most common presenting problem in the UK tends to be long-term heroin dependence. This typically occurs in conjunction with polydrug and/or alcohol problems (Gossop *et al.* 1998*b*). Stimulants, especially crack cocaine, are also frequently used, as are benzodiazepines (Strang *et al.* 1994*a*). The severity of the drug problems, including type of drug(s) used, duration of use, and route of administration, can all have an impact upon the options for change.

Patients often present to treatment with various psychological and physical health problems. They also typically have a range of social behaviour problems. Among the most conspicuous of these is involvement in crime. High rates of criminal behaviour are common among drug-dependent patients. The most common types of crime often involve some form of theft linked to the need to obtain drugs. One of the most frequent offences, for example, is shoplifting (Stewart *et al.* 2000*a*). The high rates of criminal behaviour are reflected in similarly high rates of contact with the criminal justice system. This criminality and the associated demands upon the criminal justice system represent a considerable burden for society.

Many attempts have been made, with relatively little success, to predict post-treatment outcomes in terms of patient variables at the start of treatment. Some of the variables associated with poor posttreatment outcome include more frequent pretreatment use of drugs, greater severity of dependence, psychiatric problems, a diagnosis of antisocial personality, and lack of family and social supports (McLellan *et al.* 1980, 1983; Schuckit 1985; Rounsaville *et al.* 1986; Alterman and Cacciola 1991; Havassy *et al.* 1995).

Men and women may differ in their patterns of drug and alcohol use, health status, personal relationships, and addiction treatment histories (e.g. Marsh and Simpson 1986; Chatham *et al.* 1999). Women have been found to use lower quantities of drugs (Powis *et al.* 1996), to be less likely to be multiple drug users (Darke and Hall 1995), and to be less likely to use drugs by injection (Gossop *et al.* 1994*b*; Powis *et al.* 1996). When they do inject, women may engage in more risky injecting practices (Camacho *et al.* 1996; Gossop *et al.* 2002*a*). Women are also more likely to have a drug-using partner, to be responsible for looking after children (Hser *et al.* 1987; Weiss *et al.* 1997), and to have more physical and psychological health problems than men (Swift *et al.* 1996; Marsden *et al.* 2000).

Drug-using partners can have a strong and unhelpful influence upon women's drug use and their lives. Women injectors are more likely than male injectors to be given their first injection by a sexual partner (Powis *et al.* 1996). Partners also have an influence upon women's treatment outcomes. Women with supportive partners are more likely to enter (Eldred and Washington 1976) and remain in treatment (Ravndal and Vaglum 1994). Unfortunately, many women drug users are in unsupportive and abusive relationships (Powis *et al.* 1996; Swift *et al.* 1996).

Despite differences in their pretreatment problems, it is interesting that treatment outcomes are very similar for men and women. The lack of association between pretreatment gender differences in problems and treatment outcome has been described by Fiorentine *et al.* (1997) as 'the gender paradox'. Among large samples of methadone patients, Chatham *et al.* (1999) and Mulvaney *et al.* (1999) found no gender difference in treatment response across a wide range of variables including drug and alcohol use and medical, employment, and legal problems. Among the patients in NTORS (the National Treatment Outcome Research Study) treatment programmes, both men and women showed improvements across a range of outcome measures (Stewart *et al.* 2003). Frequency of use of heroin, benzodiazepine, and cocaine was greatly reduced at 1 year follow-up, with no significant differences between men and women in the rate of change. Psychological and physical health problems also improved with no differences between men and women in rates of change.

Not all drug addicts fit the stereotype of the street 'junkie'. Washton *et al.* (1984) described a treatment programme for drug-dependent business executives. Health-care professionals, such as medical students, doctors, dentists, nurses, and pharmacists, are also at risk of developing drug problems (Ghodse and Howse 1994; Trinkoff and Storr 1994; Gossop *et al.* 2001*b*). The prevalence of such problems is not known, but increasing attention is being paid to the identification and treatment of impaired health-care professionals in many countries. A report by the British Medical Association estimated that one doctor in 15 could develop drug- or alcohol-dependence problems (BMA 1998).

In a study of 1000 physicians, Talbott *et al.* (1987) found that alcohol was the most commonly used problem drug, followed by meperidine and diazepam. The physicians most likely to develop substance misuse problems were working in anaesthetics and general practice. Younger physicians were more likely to be multiple drug misusers. Although more is known about alcohol misuse among health-care professionals, those working in medical and related professions have long been known to be also at risk of developing drug problems. Prior to the 1960s, a substantial number of the addicts notified to the Home Office (about one-third in 1956) were in health-care professions (Stimson *et al.* 1984).

There are several possible reasons why doctors and other health-care professionals may develop drug problems. By the nature of their work, doctors, nurses, and others who work in medical settings have knowledge of and easy access to many types of drugs. Misuse of drugs by health-care professionals may begin with a 'legitimate' reason such as insomnia, depression, back pain, or chronic headache. Health-care professionals often diagnose and treat themselves, sometimes inappropriately (Chambers and Belcher 1992). Also, the years of medical training are characterized by intense competition, excessive workload, social isolation, and fear of failure, and there are few occupations that face such intense and continuous stresses as the daily practice of medicine.

Self-change

Treatment is not always necessary for recovery. Not all drug users (not even all users of heroin or crack) go on to become addicted and, even among those who do, some will stop using drugs without formal treatment. There is a growing interest in the changes in drug-taking patterns, including cessation, that occur without any formal treatment. The processes of self-change are interesting in their own right. They may also be more common than is usually believed. Without doubt, the majority of cigarette smokers who give up smoking do so without treatment (Schachter 1982). Many people with alcohol problems also give up without treatment (Tuchfeld 1981). Studies of the natural history of drug use or the 'careers' of drug users have contributed to our understanding of how drug addiction develops, how it is maintained, and how it is terminated.

Biernacki (1986) investigated a group of heroin addicts who had deliberately chosen not to become involved in treatment as a way of giving up. The majority believed either that there was no need for formal treatment because they could take care of themselves, or they thought that treatment would not help. For Biernacki's subjects, breaking away from addiction was often accomplished by moving away (geographically) from the location in which the drug-taking patterns had been established. In other cases, the moving away was achieved by the person putting a 'social distance' between themselves and their previous drug-using friends and environments.

A study of self-detoxification by heroin addicts found that almost all had previously made at least one self-detoxification attempt (Gossop *et al.* 1991*b*). Most had made repeated self-detoxification attempts without treatment assistance, and many reported having managed to complete at least one such detoxification attempt and become drug-free. However, the longer-term success rate was rather poor with only 14 per cent of the attempts leading to even a few weeks continued abstinence from opiates. Various different self-detoxification approaches were employed. Abrupt cessation of opiates ('cold turkey') was one of the most commonly reported methods. Benzodiazepines were also commonly used to help alleviate withdrawal symptoms, and addicts described benzodiazepines as being quite effective in this role. Some also reported using non-pharmacological strategies such as distraction and avoidance to help them cope with withdrawal symptoms.

Whether behaviour change is attempted with or without treatment support, the user's beliefs and confidence about their own abilities to achieve change play an important role in influencing their health behaviours. This issue has been discussed in detail by Bandura (1997) with regard to addiction and a range of other health problem behaviours. Self-efficacy beliefs may influence the individual's capacity for self-regulation, their motivation to change, and their motivation to seek treatment. More importantly, the impact of therapeutic interventions on health behaviours is partly mediated by self-efficacy (Bandura 1997). Where individuals are not convinced of their personal efficacy, this may undermine their efforts and coping responses when they are faced by difficult situations. Measures of self-efficacy have been found to provide one of the predictors of posttreatment abstinence from heroin among a sample of opiate addicts receiving in-patient treatment (Gossop *et al.* 1990). The more support they received from friends and family and the more they engaged in supportive activities, the stronger their belief in their ability to exercise control.

However, for many dependent drug misusers, neither external pressure from others nor internal motivation to change is sufficient to produce effective change (McLellan *et al.* 1997*b*). Their addiction may be sustained for many years, and they may require long-term treatment and support. Patients in the UK were found to have been using heroin for 9 years, on average, at the time of admission to treatment (Gossop *et al.* 1998*b*). Long-term follow-up studies of addicts have found that some addicts persist with their drug use for decades. Hser *et al.* (1993), for example, assessed the outcome of 581 male heroin users over a 24-year period. At the final follow-up, about a quarter (23 per cent) of the original cohort were still using opiates. It is not uncommon for drug careers to last for extended periods of time (sometimes for decades) and, while dependent drug use continues, the costs to the individual, to those around them, and to society, are massive.

Treatment contact

The problems and needs of individual patients have been found to be broadly reflected in the types of treatment programmes that they approach. The ways in which different drug users make contact with treatment services may be due to a mixture of self-selection and more formal service referral processes. These processes vary according to the ways in which national (and regional) service systems operate. Patients in UK residential treatment modalities such as rehabilitation and in-patient units have been found to have more serious problems at intake than patients in out-patient methadone programmes (Gossop *et al.* 1998*b*). The rehabilitation patients had the longest heroin careers, were more likely to be regular stimulant users, and were more likely to share injecting equipment. They were more likely to have had pretreatment drinking problems in addition to their drug problems, to have been actively involved in crime, and to have been arrested more times than the other patients. Drug users in methadone reduction programmes tended to be younger, had used heroin for the shortest time, were more likely to confine their drug use to heroin, and were less likely to have broad patterns of poly-drug or alcohol use and to share injecting equipment.

Drug users who approach treatment services often report having made either a previous unsuccessful attempt to deal with their problems without treatment or having had some previous treatment episode. It is not unusual for earlier brief flirtations with treatment to be followed by later, more committed treatment episodes. In many programmes half or more of those starting a particular treatment are likely to be repeat admissions to that programme, without counting time spent in other programmes (Institute of Medicine 1990*a*). Repeat admissions are often found in methadone treatment programmes where as many as two-thirds of the patients may be second or later admissions (Hubbard *et al.* 1989).

The treatment histories of dependent drug users usually include multiple episodes and often long periods of treatment. The form of treatment most commonly reported by the NTORS patients involved the prescription of some sort of substitution drug. Although treatment in residential services was less often reported, it is still of interest that more than a quarter had previously been treated in either an in-patient or a rehabilitation unit. The contribution of services such as Narcotics Anonymous (NA) and Alcoholics Anonymous (AA) are also of considerable importance within the UK (Wells 1994). Almost one in five of the NTORS patients had attended NA in the 2 years prior to intake (Gossop *et al.* 1998*b*).

Problem drug users come into contact with many treatment services and agencies other than the specialist addiction services. The NTORS cohort, for example, were regular consumers of medical and psychiatric as well as addiction treatment services. A substantial minority had received previous psychiatric treatment for a problem other than drugs prior to the current addiction treatment episode (Gossop *et al.* 1998*b*). Almost half had been treated in an Accident and Emergency Department during the previous 2 years. This represents an extremely high rate of contact with emergency services. Similarly, a quarter of the patients had received treatment requiring admission to a general hospital bed. If these findings were representative of the utilization of such services by other addicts, they point to a substantial use of these treatment resources by problem drug users.

Moos (1997) has emphasized the complex interrelationships between the problems of the drug taker and the processes of treatment, and suggested that greater emphasis should be placed on the drug user's adjustment to the treatment environment and how this affects outcomes. In particular, Moos suggested that more attention should be paid to the ways in which treatment environments vary in their impact on patients with different levels of impairment, and with different chronicity and severity of problems.

Readiness for change

A number of stages of change models have been proposed. Such models can be useful in drawing attention to issues such as resistance to change, ambivalence, and commitment to change. De Leon (1996) described 10 stages of change. Six of these are pretreatment stages, and four stages relate to treatment.

De Leon's pretreatment stages are the following.

1 *Denial.* Continued drug taking with no recognition or acceptance of problems.

2 *Ambivalence.* Some recognition of problems but with inconsistent awareness of their consequences for self and others.

3 *Extrinsic motivation.* Some recognition and acceptance of problems, but with these mostly attributed to external factors.

4 *Intrinsic motivation.* Acceptance and recognition of drug use and associated problems.

5 *Readiness for change.* Willingness to look at options for change but without seeking treatment.

6 *Readiness for treatment.* Acceptance of the need for treatment to achieve change.

The treatment-related stages proposed by De Leon are the following.

7 *De-addiction.* Cessation of drug use/pharmacological and behavioural detoxification.

8 *Abstinence.* Stabilization of drug-free state.

9 *Continuance.* Sobriety plus resolve to acquire or maintain drug-free behaviours, attitudes, and values.

10 *Integration and identity change.* The sum of treatment influences, recovery, and life experiences resulting in self-perceived changes in social and personal identity.

One of the best known of the models of change is the transtheoretical model proposed by Prochaska and DiClemente (1982). Most of the early work upon which the transtheoretical (stages of change) model was built, draws upon studies of cigarette smokers, but the model has often been assumed to apply to all addictive behaviours. As originally outlined, the stages of change were described as precontemplation, contemplation, action, and maintenance. Slight variations in these stages have since been described, and Prochaska *et al.* (1992) defined the stages as:

◆ *precontemplation:* no intention to take action within the next 6 months;

◆ *contemplation:* intending to take action within the next 6 months;

◆ *preparation:* intending to take action within the next 30 days and having made some behavioural moves in this direction;

◆ *action:* having changed behaviour for less than 6 months;

◆ *maintenance:* having changed behaviour for more than 6 months.

Precontemplation is characterized by lack of awareness of the nature and extent of the problem, or an unwillingness to change the problem behaviour. Individuals in precontemplation are not aware (or not sufficiently aware) of their problems, though others (family, friends, doctors) may be acutely aware of them. When precontemplators seek treatment, they usually do so under pressure from others.

In contemplation the person is aware of their problem and starting to think about the need for change. Some people may remain stuck in the contemplation stage for long periods. During the preparation stage, there is greater clarity about the problem, about what is required for change, and some plans may be made for change in the near future. The action stage involves the implementation of a plan for change and some behavioural changes. If these changes are sustained, the person moves to the maintenance stage in which the changes are integrated into their lifestyle.

The transtheoretical model has enjoyed much recent popularity among researchers and practitioners. Its popularity is largely due to its simplicity and intuitive appeal. It provides a compelling metaphor and has been widely used in professional training programmes. Even critics of the model have acknowledged its intuitive appeal and heuristic value. On the other hand, the evidence to support the notion of distinct stages of change is weak and inconsistent, and the model is descriptive rather than explanatory (Joseph *et al.* 1999).

Sutton (1996) suggested that the model does not even provide an accurate description of how people actually change. Although the model states that the stages of change are 'sequential', there is little to support the assumption that changes in addictive behaviour involve an ordered movement through a sequence of stages. In the study of Prochaska *et al.* (1991), few cigarette smokers (16 per cent) showed a stable progression from one stage to the next in the sequence (e.g. precontemplation to contemplation) without suffering any reverses, and none appeared to move through three or more adjacent stages. More than a third of them remained in the same stage throughout the entire study. More worryingly for the model, some who were categorized as being in a specific stage could equally have been seen as being in two different stages at once (Sutton 1996). If this interpretation is accepted, the concept of stage loses its meaning, and it may be more useful to think of 'states of change' rather than stages since states of change does not imply ordering or sequence. Bandura (1997) has also criticized the transtheoretical model as mistakenly describing pseudostages as if they were genuine transitions.

Nonetheless, the model has been useful in reinforcing the view of recovery as a process that may require several attempts at change over a (possibly prolonged) period of time before a behavioural goal is achieved. It has also provided a reminder that treatment should serve not just those who are already committed to change (action stage), but that it should also include those who are either unsure (contemplation) or who are not currently thinking about change (precontemplation). The model draws attention to the needs for different types of treatment and suggests how different types of interventions may be required at different stages of change. It also helps to suggest how therapists might adapt their approach to enhance motivation for change (see also Chapter 8). For example, patients in the precontemplation stage should be helped to recognize and develop an awareness of their problems rather than being guided directly towards behavioural change. For patients in the contemplation stage, consciousness-raising interventions (such as self-monitoring procedures or educational methods) may be appropriate, and patients at this stage may still be resistant to the interventions of a directive action-oriented therapist. During the action stage, patients are likely to require practical help with behaviour change procedures, such as skills training, practice, and rehearsal.

Coercion

One issue that has again begun to attract attention is whether or not drug users can benefit from treatments delivered under coercion. Coercion can occur in various forms (Kothari *et al.* 2002). One of the least formal (and most common) types of coercion involves pressure from families, spouses, or friends. Coercion may also involve formal pressures from social agencies (Rotgers 1992), and may involve referrals to treatment by employers or professional regulatory bodies. The most formal type of coercion may come from within the criminal justice system. This may involve deferment or reduction of sentence if a drug user convicted of an offence agrees to participate in a treatment programme.

The compulsory treatment of drug misusers dates back many years—at least as far as the 'narcotics farms' in Lexington, Kentucky, and Fort Worth, Texas during the 1930s. The narcotics farm is interesting as one of the earliest examples of a national response to the treatment of drug addicts. These services were originally established as prison hospitals for drug addicts, though an increasing number of their patients were eventually voluntary. There is relatively little evidence that they were effective, and rates of relapse to drug use after discharge were very high (Maddux 1988).

Pressure from the criminal justice system is often among the reasons for seeking treatment. Studies in the USA have found that, among drug users who entered out-patient and residential programmes between 1979 and 1981, more than a third (40 per cent) were directly referred by the criminal justice system (Hubbard *et al.* 1989; Anglin *et al.* 1989*b*). However, direct referral is a relatively insensitive measure of the influence of the criminal justice system. Between one-half and two-thirds of these patients were facing some form of legal pressure such as parole or probation.

As a result of the Crime and Disorder Act 1998, the UK is currently looking at forms of coerced treatment using Drug Treatment and Testing Orders. These were based upon the US 'drugs courts'. They involve a community sentence imposed by magistrates or crown courts and administered by probation services. The drug user is required to attend a treatment programme for between 6 months and 3 years and to provide urine specimens for testing. An early government report (Turnbull *et al.* 2000) reported positive findings and expressed enthusiasm for this system.

It is unclear, at this time, what are the clinical implications of coercion. It has been suggested that legal pressures can be used productively. Studies of treatment given as a consequence of mandatory referrals from criminal justice authorities have found that mandated drug misusers may remain in treatment for longer periods than non-mandated drug users. This has been found both for length of stay in residential and in community treatment programmes (De Leon 1988; Collins and Allison 1983).

However, the results of research studies are inconsistent. Marlowe *et al.* (2001) found improved outcomes after coerced treatment. Many studies have found little evidence of differences in drug use outcomes between coerced and non-coerced groups (Anglin 1988; Collins and Allison 1983; De Leon 1988; Simpson and Friend 1986). Some studies have found that coercion may lead to worse outcomes (Friedman *et al.* 1982). The heroin users in NTORS who were facing pressure from the criminal justice system at intake to treatment were found to have worse heroin use outcomes at follow-up (Gossop *et al.*, 2002*d*). Studies from other countries have also found poor outcomes among drug users processed through drug courts (Vermeulen and Walburg 1997; Belenko *et al.* 1994).

The negative consequences of drug dependence (both the physical health problems and other factors associated with the addict lifestyle), and social pressure from a family member, some other closely related person, or an employer, are among the most commonly reported reasons for attempting to give up drugs. Pressure on the user often comes from more than one of these sources (Polcin and Weisner 1999).

In a study of people who had given up problem drinking without treatment, Tuchfeld (1981) suggested that the change process was rarely if ever 'spontaneous' in the sense of developing without external influence. Some addicts stop using heroin because of a perceived need to change their lifestyles or because of external pressures and responsibilities (Biernacki 1986; Joe *et al.* 1990). Health concerns are one of the most frequent reasons given by ex-cigarette smokers for stopping (Pederson and Lefcoe 1976). This point is made more colourfully by Orford (2001) who noted that change often occurs at times of crisis and cited the aphorism that drinkers give up their drink only because of livers, lovers, livelihood, or the law.

What treatment gives to the user

To take account of the diversity among drug users, treatment interventions must be responsive to their differing problems and needs. The treatment or treatment setting that may be appropriate for a 35-year-old heroin injector with a long history of dependence may be inappropriate or even contraindicated for a 14-year-old schoolboy sniffing glue. Similarly, the 50 year old who has become addicted to relatively low doses of benzodiazepines prescribed by her family doctor is likely to require a quite different type of treatment intervention to that for the 25 year old who is a compulsive binge user of cocaine.

Matching

The US Institute of Medicine (1990b, p. 143) recommended that the simplistic question of whether a treatment works should be redefined as:

> Which kinds of individuals, with what kinds of . . . problems, are likely to respond to what kinds of treatments by achieving what kinds of goals when delivered by which kinds of practitioners?

Although the search for matching criteria has been going on for many years, doubts have been expressed about how well this can be achieved in practice (at least, given our current state of knowledge). Simpson and Sells (1983) noted that the evidence from the DARP (Drug Abuse Reporting Programme) research was opposed to the possibility of finding optimal matches of patients with treatments. They further suggested that this lack of evidence for optimal matching of patients and treatments, as well as the lack of outcome differences between treatment agencies, was likely to be contrary to the clinical judgement of many others.

Discussion of how substance misusers are likely to respond to different types of treatment often touches upon Project MATCH. This study was exclusively concerned with the treatment of drinking problems and not with drug addiction. Nonetheless, its findings are interesting and relevant. It represents the largest and most expensive clinical trial of substance misuse treatments yet conducted (costing US$27 million or $15,643 per patient). The study involved 1726 patients recruited from nine treatment facilities throughout the USA. It attempted to find out whether certain types of patients respond better to specific psychological treatments for alcoholism.

Three treatment conditions were evaluated in this randomized clinical trial.

♦ Twelve-step facilitation (TSF) consisting of 12 weekly sessions in which the therapist introduced patients to the first 5 of the 12 steps of Alcoholics Anonymous (AA), and encouraged them to become involved in AA. Although this was based upon the 12-step principles, it differed in the important respect that it was a professionally delivered, individual therapy (unlike the peer support system of normal AA meetings), and was not intended to duplicate or substitute for traditional AA.

♦ Cognitive behavioural therapy (CBT) with relapse prevention methods. Patients received 12 individual treatment sessions in which they were taught skills to cope with high-risk situations and emotional states associated with relapse.

◆ Motivational enhancement therapy (MET) consisting of four individual sessions in which therapists used motivational interviewing techniques to encourage patients to consider their problems and to develop and implement a plan to stop drinking.

In all three treatment conditions, procedures were specified in detailed treatment manuals, and the individual therapy sessions were delivered by trained and supervised professionals. A range of patient characteristics was investigated including severity of alcohol involvement, cognitive impairment, conceptual level, gender, readiness for change, severity of psychiatric problems, social support for drinking, alcohol dependence, anger, antisocial personality, prior involvement with AA, religiosity, self-efficacy, and social functioning.

Patients received extremely intensive assessment using interviews and tests, to collect information about demographic characteristics, drinking behaviour, personality, predisposing factors for alcohol problems, and personal and medical effects of drinking. The pretreatment assessment took about 8 hours (Project MATCH Research Group 1997). Further intensive assessments were conducted during the five follow-up sessions that took place every 90 days following treatment.

The assumption of Project MATCH was that the randomization of patients to the treatment conditions would lead to some of them being 'correctly matched' and others being 'mismatched'. It further assumed that correct matches ought to have a better outcome than mismatches (Drummond 1999).

The study found improved drinking outcomes among patients in all treatment conditions, but little evidence of matching effects. However, Marlatt (1999) suggested that it is misleading to conclude that the study showed that treatment matching does not work, or that any one type of treatment works as well as any other. A major problem was that the study randomly assigned patients to the treatment conditions. Marlatt (1999) commented that 'As a way of assigning patients to treatment, nothing could be more opposite than random assignment (assigning patients on a random basis similar to a coin toss) and treatment matching (assigning patients based on a professional therapist's knowledge and skills).'

The method of treatment assignment used in Project MATCH may not be an efficient way of allocating patients to treatment, and it is very different from circumstances in the real world where patients make active choices between the treatments that they approach. Bale et al. (1980) randomly assigned opiate-dependent patients to therapeutic community programmes or to methadone maintenance for 1 month. After this time, they were able either to remain in that programme or to change to the programme of their choice. Of those who were assigned to the therapeutic communities, only

18 per cent chose to remain in that modality, and only 29 per cent of those in methadone maintenance remained in that programme.

Negrete (1999) noted that Project MATCH failed to study some of the matching issues that are most relevant to clinicians. Its treatments were individually based, out-patient, and relatively short-term. Treatment selection questions, such as who was suitable for group therapy (the standard option in most services), who would benefit more from treatment in a residential setting, or which patients would do better if given more than 12 weeks treatment, were not tested.

The project also differed from the ways in which treatment is generally provided in normal clinical practice, where therapists often use a variety of interventions. The constraints of the controlled trial design do not permit the therapist to tailor the treatment interventions to the specific individual needs and treatment responses of the patient. In almost all types of addiction treatment, a number of complex interactions take place between the patient and the treatment intervention.

Such criticisms were summarized by Glaser (1999) who observed that, whatever the merits and validity of the project's experimental design, a study of matching in which none of the patients was actually matched to a particular treatment lacked persuasiveness.

A different approach to matching involves 'stepped care'. Less intensive interventions are offered prior to more intensive treatments. Where patients fail to respond to less intensive interventions, they are subsequently offered more comprehensive or more intensive interventions. This has been seen as a potentially resource-efficient way of delivering treatment, and it is also able to take account of the dynamic interaction between the needs and problems of the patients and their responses to treatment (Drummond 1999). A treatment system that provides a continuum of care offers one way of engaging a variety of people at different points in their addiction careers, and can thus address their differing needs and resources, the type of severity of their problems, and the context in which their problem occurs.

The Patient Placement Criteria of the American Society of Addiction Medicine (ASAM 2001) provided guidelines for matching patients to different treatment options. Six domains on which patients should be assessed and subsequently matched to an appropriate level of treatment were:

◆ acute intoxication and withdrawal;

◆ biomedical condition;

◆ emotional and behavioural problems;

◆ acceptance of or resistance to treatment;

- relapse potential;
- recovery environment.

The placement criteria seek initially to provide the least intensive level of care with this being increased if the response is poor. This is consistent with the principles of a stepped care framework in which the recommended treatment should be the one that is least intensive but likely to resolve the problem, with more intensive treatments being reserved for those with more severe problems (Sobell and Sobell 1999). If the patient responds poorly to the initial treatment, further assessment takes place with the decision about what to do next being based on the individual's case characteristics, what has been learned from the failure to respond to treatment, and what clinical judgement and research suggest as the most appropriate next phase of treatment, and, if indicated, the next level of care.

The ASAM criteria and the placement recommendations offer a useful working tool to conceptualize and manage the problem of matching patients to treatments. One risk of such criteria is that, given the present state of knowledge (or ignorance) about treatment matching for individual clinical cases, they rely upon a 'best guess' rather than empirical evidence. They also carry a risk of misuse in that some practitioners may apply them mechanistically and to the detriment of individual patients whose specific circumstances and problems may require exceptional measures.

As with the random allocation procedures of some research trials, a major concern about these sorts of matching procedures is that they differ in important respects from the 'consumer choice' paradigm in which drug users assess the treatment options and then seek treatment from an agency of their choice. Attempts to impose a type of treatment or treatment method upon the patient undoubtedly have an appeal for the bureaucratic minds of treatment planners and purchasers, but this may not be an especially efficient or productive way to achieve patient/treatment matching. One of the more common treatment delivery problems is the widespread practice of offering a standard treatment package to all patients. It is possible that this problem could be compounded within the 'levels' of a stepped care system.

Treatment engagement and the therapeutic alliance

If no single treatment can be universally effective for drug dependence and a range of different interventions is required, this challenges many of the existing service delivery systems that tend to offer a fixed package of treatment components. Despite widespread recognition of the importance of providing treatments that are appropriate to the diverse needs and problems of patients, many programmes offer only a single type of treatment. This Procrustean system expects all patients to fit into the services provided rather than making the adaptations and adjustments needed to identify and respond to the specific needs of the individual. In such situations, those patients who are a good fit for a given approach are more likely to remain in treatment, and those who are less well suited are more likely to drop out (Carroll 1997).

The patient's views about treatment are important because they influence the individual's willingness to approach and use treatment services. Where treatment is tailored to the specific needs of the patient, this is likely to lead to increased patient satisfaction and treatment engagement, and it can also affect treatment compliance. Among the treatment factors that affect treatment satisfaction are accessibility, adequacy, contact, and impact of services received (Marsden *et al.* 2000*b*). Relatively few studies have investigated the impact of treatment satisfaction on outcome, and these have produced mixed results. In a study of methadone maintenance, Joe and Friend (1989) found only modest associations between satisfaction, time in treatment, and outcome. In a study of patients in day-care and residential settings, Chan *et al.* (1997) found that treatment satisfaction was correlated with treatment retention and with several measures of outcome at 6-month follow-up.

The various and related issues of adherence to the treatment regime, compliance with programme rules and requirements, and retention in treatment have often been discussed as patient responses. They are more appropriately seen as interactions between treatment and patient factors.

These issues have also sometimes been identified as if they were peculiar to the treatment of addiction problems. This is incorrect. Treatment noncompliance or non-adherence is common in most areas of medical and mental health treatment. Treatment non-adherence may take various forms, including failure to keep appointments, premature dropping out of treatment, insistence on discharge against medical advice, and failure to comply with prescribed treatment regimens, and it is regularly listed by doctors as one of the most distressing features of their clinical practice (Haynes 1979).

In an out-patient drug dependence clinic, Love and Gossop (1985) found that almost half (44 per cent) of the referrals failed to attend their first appointment. Studies of general medical and general psychiatric patients have also found that 20–50 per cent of patients may fail to turn up for their scheduled appointments, although the rate of appointment keeping tends to be higher when patients initiate the appointments themselves (Sackett and Snow 1979). After starting treatment 20–60 per cent of patients who receive prescribed medication will stop taking their medication before they are instructed to do so, and 19–74 per cent will not follow instructions about how to take their medication (Stimson 1974). It has been estimated that, of the 750 million new prescriptions written each year in England and the United States, there are over 520 million cases of partial or total non-adherence (Buckalew and Sallis 1986).

Drug addiction shares many features with other chronic illnesses. It has been found to be difficult to convince patients with anaemia to take iron supplements, atherosclerotic patients to take cholestyramine, epileptics to take anticonvulsants, hypertensives to take diuretics, or psychiatric patients to take psychopharmacological drugs (Masek 1982). Estimates of treatment non-adherence typically vary from 30 to 60 per cent, though these may vary enormously with ranges as extreme as 4 and 92 per cent being reported (Masek 1982).

In a study of diabetic patients, Cerkoney and Hart (1980) found that only about 7 per cent adhered to all of the stated treatment requirements considered necessary for good control of their condition. Among hypertensive patients, up to 50 per cent of patients failed to follow referral advice, over 50 per cent dropped out of care within 1 year, and only two-thirds of those who remained in treatment took sufficient medication to control their blood pressure adequately (Eraker et al. 1984; Vetter et al. 1985). In renal dialysis treatment, only 50 per cent of patients complied fully with the treatment regimen (Finn and Alcorn 1986).

McLellan et al. (2000) compared drug dependence with hypertension, diabetes, and asthma. These three chronic medical conditions are disorders for which treatments are effective but dependent on adherence to the medical regimen. Less than 60 per cent of adult patients with diabetes mellitus fully adhere to their medication schedule (Graber et al. 1992), and less than 40 per cent of patients with hypertension or asthma adhere fully to their medication regimens (Clark 1991; Dekker et al. 1993). The problem is even worse for the behavioural and diet changes that are so important for the maintenance of gains in these chronic illnesses. Less than a third of patients with adult-onset asthma, hypertension, or diabetes adhere to prescribed diet and/or behavioural changes that are designed to increase functional status and to reduce risk factors for recurrence of the disorders (McLellan et al. 2000). As a general rule of thumb, Podell and Gary (1976) suggested that one-third of patients take their medication as prescribed, one-third sometimes do so, and the remaining third almost never follow the treatment regimen.

For most chronic medical illnesses, adherence (and ultimately outcome) is often poorest among patients with low socio-economic status, a lack of family and social supports, or psychiatric problems (Clark 1991; Dekker et al. 1993). The highest rates of treatment non-adherence tend to be found among patients with chronic disorders, when no immediate discomfort or risk is evident, when broader lifestyle changes are required, and when the treatment is aimed at prevention rather than symptom alleviation or cure (McLellan *et al.* 2000).

Noncompliance occurs even when the patient knows it can have serious consequences. Among patients being treated for glaucoma, some were told that 'they must use eye drops three times a day or *they would go blind*'. Vincent (1971) found that more than half of them still did not follow these instructions closely enough to produce the desired outcome. Even when patients were at the point of becoming legally blind in one eye, adherence improved only from 42 to 58 per cent.

The therapeutic alliance is also increasingly recognized as an important element within the treatment process (Martin *et al.* 2000). Although the original concept of the therapeutic alliance originated in early psychoanalytic theories, it has re-emerged in a revised form and with a sounder empirical base. The therapeutic alliance is generally seen as comprising:

- ◆ the collaborative relationship between the patient and the therapist;
- ◆ the emotional bond between patient and therapist;
- ◆ agreement between patient and therapist about treatment goals and tasks.

The alliance has been found to be related to treatment outcome (Horvath and Symonds 1991; Margison *et al.* 2000). In a meta-analysis of 79 studies, Martin *et al.* (2000) found a consistent, positive, and moderately sized relationship between therapeutic alliance and treatment outcome. However, in a study of cocaine-dependent patients, Barber *et al.* (2000) failed to show any association between alliance and drug use outcomes though alliance was related to retention in treatment.

The revival of interest in the therapeutic alliance has been partly influenced by the inability of researchers to find clear and consistent differences in the effectiveness of different types of treatment interventions. This failure to demonstrate consistent differences between treatment types is not limited only to the treatment of the addictions. It is also an issue within the broader context of the evaluation of psychotherapies for other mental health problems (Lambert and Bergin 1994; Stiles *et al.* 1986). As a consequence, there has been an increased interest in processes that are common to different therapies. The therapeutic alliance is one such common factor. It has been suggested that the quality of the alliance may be more important than the type of treatment in predicting positive treatment outcomes. The alliance has even been described as a 'quintessential integrative variable' of therapy (Wolfe and Goldfried 1988).

The therapeutic alliance may itself be an active ingredient of treatment (Henry *et al.* 1994) and, where an effective alliance is established between patient and therapist, this may be effective in inducing change regardless of other psychological interventions. It has also been suggested that the effect of the therapeutic alliance on outcome may be indirect or that the alliance may interact with specific interventions (Gaston 1990). Differences between types of addiction treatment may be less important than whether the treatment is competently delivered by skilled therapists operating within an efficient service delivery organization (Orford 1999). The variations in outcomes achieved by different therapists within a treatment modality may be greater than those between different treatment modalities (Luborsky *et al.* 1985).

Chapter 6

Assessment and setting treatment goals

This chapter considers two things that almost all therapists think they can do well. In fact, assessment is frequently done rather poorly and goal setting is often neglected.

Few would disagree with the proposition that assessment should be thorough and comprehensive. This is a truism. No one would argue the case for a casual and superficial assessment. What is more important than thoroughness, however, is relevance. The mere accumulation of information is no substitute for an effective and focused assessment. Overestimating the virtues of thoroughness can lead to assessments that take too long to complete and that collect too much irrelevant information.

What are the governing principles of an effective assessment of addiction problems? For what reason is the information being collected? Assessment should provide a detailed and coherent account of the presenting problem(s). This requires a careful analysis of the drugs used, the ways in which they are used, and the social and psychological circumstances in which they are used. This information provides the basic grounding for a treatment plan.

One of the most frequent errors of assessment is to become bogged down in an increasingly detailed, retrospective analysis of the presenting problem. Few instruments are easier or more satisfying to use than the retrospectoscope. Clinical staff should avoid the temptation of using assessment to try to explain how the patient got from some point in their past to their present state. Assessment proves its worth by providing clear guidance about future action. How will the assessment information help the therapist and the patient in the move towards recovery? How does the information help to set in motion the processes of recovery? How does it support recovery? What are the obstacles to recovery? Assessment should be firmly and clearly directed towards the possibility of change.

Most people who seek treatment for addiction problems present with long-standing patterns of drug misuse, generally involving several different types of drugs, and typically accompanied by other related, indirectly related, and unrelated problems. In addition to their drug problems, many will be drinking heavily and eating poorly; frequently they will have many social problems including poor housing arrangements and criminal convictions; they will also often have medical and psychiatric problems, some of which may be serious. There is no shortage of clinically relevant material that can be uncovered by even the novice assessor. The mere fact that there is so much material can lead the assessment into endless diversions. Any or even all of the problems that may emerge during assessment may be important and require attention. But the main purpose of the assessment of addiction is to chart the pathways for recovery and to identify barriers to change.

Conducting a focused assessment

Assessment can be made more difficult by the fact that people who seek treatment often present with generalized complaints linked to an undifferentiated array of difficulties. It is fairly typical, for example, for many drug addicts to present to treatment with the vague intentions of 'getting off drugs', 'getting myself sorted out', or 'getting my head together'. Not infrequently, this is accompanied by generalized complaints of feeling that life is not worth living, getting no pleasure from any activity other than drug taking (and often not even from that), self-loathing, and hopelessness. This is often expressed in terms of a pervasive sense of weariness or melancholy, a cumulative and demoralizing realization that the increasing trouble that comes with regular drug use and dependence is not worth it.

It is one of the roles of the therapist to help to clarify and differentiate the presenting problems so that these can be made explicit and reduced to manageable proportions. In this way, the assessment can help to introduce some optimism by helping the patient begin to see that change and recovery may be possible.

The therapist is required to create some sort of order out of what may sometimes be a chaotic or highly unstructured presentation and to identify relevant issues and collect information that can be used to direct and support further treatment. For all types of drug problems that require treatment, the intervention should be tailored to the needs and circumstances of the individual. This apparently simple and uncontentious statement turns out to have complex and far-reaching implications for policy and services if it is seriously applied in clinical practice. There is not, nor can there be expected to be any single best treatment for these problems. Both aetiology and outcome are influenced by a broad range of different factors. A thorough assessment should identify, for each individual case, the nature of the problem, and appropriate and achievable goals for treatment. Also, the treatment process should identify as early as possible, those particular factors (often outside the treatment setting) that will assist or hamper the achievement of the treatment goal(s).

Among the most basic issues that need to be explored are the following. What types of drugs are being used, by which routes of administration, and with what sorts of associated problems? What are the relevant contextual variables, both for drug use, and for seeking treatment? Why has the person sought treatment? Why at this particular time? In what ways do they feel better or different when they take drugs? Many people have quite definite beliefs about how drugs improve their ability to function. How do they expect to feel when they have stopped using drugs? Do they want to give up all drugs? Or do they just want to stop taking one drug that is seen as causing particular problems? Many heroin addicts, for instance, do not see the use of either alcohol or cannabis as in any way related to their difficulties and intend to continue using these substances after giving up heroin. Do they believe that they can learn how to regulate their problem drug use in future and that they can return to being a 'recreational' user?

Other important questions that need to be asked concern the obstacles to maintaining change once the person has stopped using drugs. The factors that assist or impede the initial stages of change (getting off) may be quite different to those that assist or impede the maintenance of change (staying off).

Drug users may give various reasons for seeking treatment (Anglin *et al.* 1989*b*; Hubbard *et al.* 1989). In many cases, the person will present with distressing and sometimes urgent problems. These may involve physical or psychological problems (a serious infection, chronic depression), social pressure (an imminent court case, pressure from a partner), or some other factor that

Table 6.1 An example of a 'drugs grid'

Drugs	Ever used	Age first used	Number of days used in last month	Typical amount used per day	Route of administration
Heroin					
Other opiates/opioids					
Crack cocaine					
Cocaine powder					
Amphetamines					
Benzodiazepines					
Cannabis					
Other drugs (specify)					

draws attention to the costs of continued drug use. In many cases, although the person may be aware of the need to change, they are also ambivalent both about drugs and about treatment (Orford 2001).

From about the 1950s and early 1960s clinicians and researchers started to view many of the phenomena of abnormal psychology as being due to, or strongly influenced by maladaptive conditioning or learning rather than as symptoms of some more general underlying psychopathology or personality disorder. Clinical and research interests became increasingly focused upon specific problem behaviours. One of the important contributions of psychological approaches to the treatment of addiction problems has been to direct attention towards the addictive behaviours themselves as the main target for treatment.

An assessment of addiction and other drug misuse problems can be largely achieved by conducting a cognitive–behavioural assessment. The principles of such an assessment are relatively simple. Addictive behaviours and problems are powerfully influenced by immediate situations and events, and by the individual's perceptions and interpretations of them. This perspective provides a main point of focus for the assessment. The emphasis remains firmly upon specific problems rather than upon generalized entities.

A cognitive–behavioural assessment has two general aims (Kirk 2000):

- to identify and formulate the target problems and reach an agreement with the patient on the nature of the problems;
- to obtain sufficiently detailed information about the factors that are maintaining the problem to be able to design and present a treatment plan.

In seeking to determine how the problem is currently being maintained and what are the barriers to change, a behavioural assessment is used to identify the contexts in which the problem behaviour occurs, the factors that influence the intensity of the problems, and to assess the consequences of the behaviours.

One conceptual device that has been used to identify what is maintaining the problem, and what can be changed, is in terms of what have been termed the A-B-Cs (O'Leary and Wilson 1975):

- *antecedents*;
- *behaviours and beliefs*;
- *consequences*.

The task of the therapist during assessment is to identify and understand the antecedents (environmental, emotional, and cognitive) of episodes of addictive behaviour, and the consequences that maintain the behaviour. The task of treatment then involves testing individualized treatment strategies, capitalizing on those that work, and abandoning those that fail. Assessment should determine to what extent each of these factors increases or decreases the probability that the target behaviour will occur. For any drug misuse problem, it should be possible to make changes in any or all of the antecedents, behaviours, or consequences.

The assessment of drug-using behaviour is itself not straightforward (Wells *et al.* 1988). Most problem drug users will report multiple drug use, and there is no accepted way of combining different drugs into a single summary measure. Measures are, therefore, required for each of the different drugs. A thorough and informed assessment requires good information about types and quantities of drugs used, patterns of use, the social and psychological circumstances, and consequences of drug use prior to treatment, throughout treatment, and after treatment.

It has been recommended that the minimum requirement for assessment of drug use should involve measurement of types of drugs currently (or recently) being used, measures of quantity and frequency of use, routes of drug administration, and duration of use. A commonly used device is some sort of 'drugs grid' (see Table 6.1). This can be expanded to meet specific programme needs. Extra drugs (including alcohol and tobacco, if necessary) can be added to the rows. Extra substance use measures (such as age of first use, main problem drug identified by the patient) can be added to the columns. The use of a grid of this sort provides a concise summary of a good deal of information within a single page. It also provides a reminder to the assessor of the information required.

Frequency of consumption, for example, is often assessed for specified drugs during specified time periods (e.g. during the past 3 months), with the classification of drug use by pattern and history usually involving measures of the heaviest or most problematic level of use within a given period (Simpson and Sells 1983). Weighted indices can be developed by combining the 'seriousness' (or dangerousness) of drugs with their frequency of use (Clayton and Voss 1981). The use of constructed composite measures of this sort is of uncertain clinical value. Drug use and problem severity have often been assessed using standardized instruments that include measures of the type, quantity, and frequency of drug use, with wider measures of functioning in other areas (McLellan *et al.* 1980).

A distinction should be made between assessment and screening. Screening involves the use of a procedure to identify those individuals who have a specific health disorder requiring treatment. In general medicine this normally involves the identification of a risk factor, a marker of the condition, or some early-stage symptom(s). Screening tests should be simple, precise, and validated.

They should also be acceptable to the population being tested and should link with further procedures for diagnostic assessment. In methadone treatment programmes, for example, screening may involve determining whether an individual meets a set of criteria for that particular treatment (McPherson and Hersch 2000). This usually involves detecting the presence of the signs and symptoms of opioid dependence, and may involve either self-report, or biological investigations, or both (Wolff *et al.* 1999).

As part of the assessment, the patients should be asked about specific situations they have encountered that are associated with their use of drugs. In what sorts of situation do they usually take drugs? What sorts of situations help them to stay off or to reduce their intake of drugs? They should be asked about physiological states, cognitions, and interpersonal factors, as well as about overt behaviour, and about how each of these groups of variables relates to the problem.

Properly directed assessments can have an educational role by helping to focus the patients' attention on internal and external variables that they may not previously have seen as being relevant to their problems. The identification and clarification of such functional relationships plays a crucial role in helping the addict to learn to take some control of his or her own drug-taking behaviour.

Treatments for addictive behaviours have many points of contact with the principles of self-help, and are best conducted within a collaborative therapeutic relationship. This should be explained to the patient during the early stages of treatment, since he or she may be expected to take an active role by helping to collect information, giving feedback on the effectiveness of techniques, and making suggestions about new strategies.

As part of the assessment process, patients may be asked to monitor, or even keep a 'diary' of their behaviour. The process of self-monitoring has important theoretical implications and practical consequences. Social-learning theory suggests that self-monitoring may lead to self-evaluations of performance standards, and that perceived discrepancies between performance and self-prescribed goals or standards are likely to lead to a negative self-appraisal that may motivate corrective changes in behaviour (Wilson 1980). Self-monitoring of personally important behaviours such as using illegal drugs or drinking heavily may be associated with self-evaluative processes that constitute an important cognitively based source of motivation in social-learning theory (Bandura 1977).

It will be unfamiliar to some patients to see their addiction problems as being related to identifiable, internal and external situations and events, rather than as due to unknown and uncontrollable forces. To the extent that drug-taking behaviours and variations in drug taking are predictable, they may also be controllable. Patients may not readily identify the functional relationships that exist between their addiction and such events. Indeed, it is a key feature of addiction that it feels like something that is uncontrollable or, at least, something over which the individual has serious difficulty in exercising control.

Assessment of dependence

The vast majority of those who seek help from addiction treatment services have drug problems that are chronic and severe. They tend to seek treatment as the result of pressures and selection processes that may not be fully evident at the point of presentation. Typically, they have already made failed attempts (either on their own or with the support of others) to moderate or to give up drugs (Gossop *et al.* 1991*b*). Many people whose drug use is less problematic, less severely dependent, and/or less deeply embedded in their lives, and those who have better resources to support behaviour change are able to stop using drugs without help and often do so (Sobell and Sobell 1998).

In practice, the assessment of dependence need not be complicated. In most clinical circumstances, the assessment of dependence typically involves the taking of a drug use history, an examination for physical signs of drug injection (e.g. venopuncture marks and scarring), and noting signs of drug intoxication or withdrawal. When conducted by experienced clinicians, this form of assessment probably provides the best and most practical method for assessing dependence and most other drug problems.

Where the assignment of a formal psychiatric diagnosis is required, this is done by reference to the criteria of one or other of the diagnostic systems (DSM-IV or ICD-10). DSM-IV (1994) distinguishes between two groups of disorders: *substance use disorders* (substance dependence and substance abuse) and *substance-induced disorders* (intoxication, withdrawal, and drug-induced psychosis).

DSM–IV also specifies six further options that may be used to categorize the status of treatment and recovery. These are:

- early full remission (no signs of dependence or misuse for at least 1 month but less than 1 year);
- early partial remission (one or more criteria of dependence or abuse not seen for at least 1 month but less than a year);
- sustained full remission (no criteria seen for 1 year or more);
- sustained partial remission (full criteria for dependence not met for 1 year or more but one or more criteria are seen);
- receiving agonist therapy (e.g. methadone maintenance);
- in a protected environment (e.g. hospital or residential rehabilitation facility).

The four remission specifiers can only be applied after none of the criteria for dependence or abuse has been seen for at least 1 month.

In day-to-day clinical practice, what is often required is an assessment of dependence that has practical utility in guiding decisions about courses of action with regard to the prescribing of drugs within treatment programmes. For this reason, assessment tends to be focused upon the extent of physical dependence and, more specifically, upon levels of tolerance or the likelihood of clinically significant withdrawal symptoms after discontinuation of a drug. For such purposes, severity of physical dependence (tolerance and withdrawal) is generally assessed by reference to drug consumption behaviours, and the indicators that are used in this assessment are primarily dose, and frequency and duration of use.

The best indicators of the extent of physical dependence to a particular drug are current (or very recent) drug-taking behaviours, and information about this is usually obtained mainly by history taking. Where issues concerning the validity of self-reported drug use are of special concern, information may be sought from other sources or by other means (e.g. analysis of urine samples). An accurate assessment of tolerance is of particular importance when a patient is first prescribed a drug (e.g. at the start of a methadone maintenance programme). In some circumstances, and especially where the patient's history is uncertain, it may be necessary to require that the initial doses are taken under observation in a clinical setting. The miscalculation of tolerance levels can have serious consequences if relatively high doses of a drug are prescribed to a non-tolerant drug misuser. In rare circumstances this has led to tragic consequences. In 1992, two police doctors in the UK were convicted of manslaughter for recklessly causing the death of a 23-year-old heroin addict through prescribing what were subsequently determined to be excessive doses of opioids and other drugs (Brahams 1992). Fortunately, such cases are extremely rare, and should always be avoidable if appropriate assessment and observation procedures are followed.

Where objective measures are required, urine samples can be tested for the presence of drugs. Urinalysis can establish recent use of these drugs, but provides little information about the extent of use or dependence. A more radical and less often used method of testing for the presence of physical dependence involves the administration of an antagonist challenge.

The first use of naloxone was reported by Blachly (1973). Where an antagonist is administered either by intramuscular or subcutaneous injection to individuals who are physically dependent on opiates, this provokes an immediate withdrawal syndrome that lasts for several hours. Patients are usually assessed before and then 20 to 30 minutes after administration of naloxone. Despite its apparent objectivity, this method may not be entirely reliable, especially for low levels of dependence. Some individuals who have received therapeutic doses of morphine for 2–3 days and who would not otherwise show a withdrawal syndrome if opiates were discontinued have been found to do so when given naloxone (Jaffe 1985). There are also opiate misusers who are psychologically dependent and compulsive users of opiates who do not show signs of neuroadaptation (Resnick 1983). It has been suggested that the naloxone challenge gives undue weight to the physiological aspects of dependence (Ward *et al.* 1998).

Without doubt, one of the main disadvantages of the naloxone challenge is the discomfort for the patient. It is not obvious that the discomfort involved in such procedures is necessary when a careful history and physical examination would be sufficient. The use of a challenge may also create an unhelpful and confrontational relationship between the patient and therapist.

The procedures by which initial doses of methadone are prescribed have changed little since the inception of methadone maintenance. It is generally agreed that, based on a careful assessment of the patient, the first dose should be in the range 10–40 mg (Dole and Nyswander 1967; Ward *et al.* 1998). The initial dose should seek to prevent withdrawal without producing intoxication.

Split or serial dosing may be useful where there is doubt about the extent of tolerance. For patients with low levels of physical dependence and where lower first doses are indicated, it may be useful to prescribe serial or split dosing with observation of patient responses for 3–4 hours. This may also be indicated where unusually high doses seem to be required. Methadone usually reaches peak plasma concentrations within 2–6 hours after oral administration (Kreek 1997*a*). Methadone has a long elimination half-life of 24–36 hours, and methadone doses may have cumulative effects. For this reason, dose increases should be prescribed with care. Patients with severe liver dysfunction should also be dosed with care.

As in other areas of science, the development of useful concepts is intimately linked to measurement, and various attempts have been made to measure dependence. Dependence has been assessed both in terms of categories (is this person dependent or not?), and as a dimensional assessment of severity (to what extent is this person dependent?). The categorical assessment method is the one that has been used by the two main psychiatric diagnostic systems. In the earlier DSM-III-R (1987), criteria were included for rating the severity of substance dependence. Severity of dependence is not assessed in DSM-IV.

Where dependence is regarded as a learned state, it is also seen as a condition that develops through repeated reinforcements and that can exist in varying degrees of intensity. This view supports the notion that dependence can be seen as being distributed along a dimension rather than as a categorical state. However, since dependence has both psychological and physical components, it can be useful to retain this conceptual distinction since these have different implications for treatment.

Research and theory tend to be more interested in the assessment of psychological dependence, which provides a measure of habit strength and which has drive properties. The assessment of psychological dependence can also be used to help select appropriate treatment goals and in the planning of relapse prevention interventions. It may also have longer-term implications for the outcome of the patient in terms of the risk of relapse even during the period long after the components of physical dependence have completely disappeared.

The Severity of Dependence Scale (SDS) provides a short, easily administered scale that can be used to measure the degree of psychological dependence experienced by users of different types of illicit drugs (Gossop *et al.* 1995). The SDS contains five items, all of which are explicitly concerned with psychological components of dependence: these are specifically concerned with the users' feelings of compulsion to use and impaired control over their own drug taking, their preoccupation with drugs, and their anxieties about drug taking. The SDS includes instructions that require a response relating to a specified period of time. This can be varied depending upon the purposes of the assessment, but could be 'during the past month', 'during the past year', or even, if a very time-specific assessment were required, 'during the past 24 hours'. The SDS is easy to understand and can be completed for a specified drug within a matter of minutes. One advantage of the SDS is that the same scale items can be readily adapted to measure dependence upon different types of substances.

The SDS is primarily a measure of *impaired behavioural control* and *compulsion to use*. These are essential ingredients of what we mean by an addictive behaviour. It contradicts our understanding of what we mean by an 'addiction' that someone could be addicted but not experience a strong need for it or have difficulties in controlling their consumption (Edwards *et al.* 1981; Gossop 1989a; West and Gossop 1994). In this respect, the SDS measures the central components of dependence.

Any assessment of an addiction problem must address the question of the severity of dependence. This should be differentiated from other types of problematic drug taking. Edwards *et al.* (1981) suggested that these could include *unsanctioned use*—the use of a drug that is not approved by a society or by a powerful group within that society. Alternatively, the hazardous use of drugs represents another form of problematic use. This involves the use of a drug that could be expected to have harmful consequences for the user (either in terms of psychological dysfunction or to physical damage). It is possible to use illicit drugs, and even to use them by injection without experiencing any actual harm, but it is known to be hazardous. Other forms of problematic use include *dysfunctional use*—use of a drug that leads to impaired psychological or social functioning (e.g. loss of job or marital problems)—and *harmful use*—use of a drug by a person to whom it is known to have caused physical or psychological problems.

Each of these categories of drug problems may cause difficulties for the drug taker and each may require different sorts of intervention. The use of illegal drugs (unsanctioned use), particularly when it occurs among very young people, may cause enormous concern; it may lead to serious social sanctions, including being expelled from school, loss of job, or imprisonment; and it may cause great anxiety among the family and friends of the user. However, it need not in itself be associated with clinical problems. Equally, drug taking may lead to many different types of problem. Acute intoxication often leads to hazardous behaviours and not infrequently to actual harm. This sort of behaviour may or may not be a cause for intervention by the addiction therapist.

Assessment methods

For most clinical purposes, the main source of information during assessment is the clinical interview. This is heavily reliant upon the self-reported problems and behaviours of the patient, typically obtained during semi-structured interviews that may or may not also include some use of structured instruments. The apparently straightforward matter of determining the drug or alcohol usage of the patient can be complicated by the belief of some clinicians that drug misusers are unreliable informants.

Although there are undoubtedly some occasions on which drug misusers may distort or conceal information (Morral *et al.* 2000), many research studies have found that both drug addicts and alcoholics can be reliable informants with regard to a wide range of different types of information (Ball 1967; Sobell and Sobell 1978; Del Boca and Noll 2000). Although drug misusers may underreport their substance use in certain circumstances, Weiss *et al.* (1998) found self-reported use to be consistent with urine screen results 95 per cent of the time and, when the two sources of information did not agree, 89 per cent of the time it was because subjects reported more substance use than was detected by the urine screens. Others have found that self-reported drug misuse can have high validity that correlates well with objective measures such as urine analysis (Sherman and Bigelow 1992; Zanis *et al.* 1994), and hair analysis (Wolff and Strang 1999). Weiss *et al.* (2000) also found a high level of agreement between self-reported drug use and collateral informant reports.

In general, it seems that researchers are more likely to regard addicts and alcoholics as reliable informants and clinicians are more likely to distrust them. This may be due in part to the different demand characteristics of the research and clinical situations. Babor *et al.* (2000) suggested that, in clinical research studies, biochemical tests and collateral informant reports usually did not add sufficiently to the measurement accuracy of self-reports to warrant their routine use.

Self-report remains an essential tool (Carey and Correia 1998). In many circumstances it is the most practical way to obtain information, and in some circumstances it is the only possible way of obtaining information (as with internal states). Despite the suspicion that has been voiced about the use of self-report data from drug users, there is a substantial literature that points to the reliability and validity of such information in most circumstances. A more productive approach to the discussion of the accuracy of self-reports from drug users might consider the respondent and situational variables that influence the accuracy of self-reported information (Babor *et al.* 1990).

These include the following.

♦ *Intoxication.* Where the user is intoxicated at the time of assessment, this is likely to be associated with lower reliability and validity of self-reported information (Brown *et al.* 1992). Intoxication may produce sufficient cognitive impairment to have a serious effect on the person's ability to provide accurate self-reports.

♦ *Motivated deception.* Drug users, like other people, may provide information that is selectively presented or manipulated to serve their own interests. Concerns about confidentiality can reduce the accuracy of self-report, especially when this may lead to negative consequences (legal or housing). Overreporting may be due to a desire to obtain a higher dose prescription or access to treatment, and underreporting to maintain treatment privileges. Del Boca and Noll (2000) suggest that self report can provide useful estimates of drug consumption, especially when conditions are designed to increase accuracy. Research interviews that provide assurances of confidentiality have been found to elicit good quality information about drug use and other problem behaviours.

In some circumstances, it can be helpful to use objective measures to determine the presence or absence of one or more drugs. Drugs can be detected in body fluids or tissues. The choice of screening method will be influenced by the pharmacokinetics of the drugs that are being investigated, and will also depend on the questions being asked (Wolff *et al.* 1999). Among the biochemical methods that can be used are analysis of blood, breath, saliva, urine, sweat, and hair samples for direct metabolites of abused substances, or indirect evidence of biological changes related to prolonged use of drugs.

In clinical practice, urine screening is the most commonly used method of assessing illicit drug use, though analysis of blood samples may give a more accurate measurement of recent drug use. Urinalysis provides information over a broader time frame but with less quantitative accuracy. Urine testing provides a good biological screening tool for assessment periods relating to the previous 24–72 hours. Urine can be easily collected and usually contains metabolites as well as the parent drug. However, urine testing is of little use for quantitative analyses of drug use.

The analysis of blood samples may be a more effective method for quantitative analyses. The disadvantage of obtaining blood is that this can be a potentially problematic procedure among drug misusers. Special care must be used in the collection, transport, storage, and analysis of such samples because of the risks of blood-borne infections. Some chronic drug injectors have extensive damage to their superficial veins, and obtaining blood may require higher levels of expertise than with non-injectors. There may also be risks in demonstrating new potential injection sites to users who have problems with venous access, or in showing new techniques of drug use to non-injecting drug misusers.

Testing hair samples for misused substances is a relatively new biological tool. It offers the potential for assessment of drug use over an extended period of time, but is not suitable for assessment of current drug use. There are several difficulties concerning the analysis of hair. The factors affecting the incorporation of drugs into hair and the rate at which this occurs are not properly understood (Henderson 1993). Hair analysis does not necessarily widen the range of detectable drugs, and it can be problematic because drug compounds are found in very low concentrations (Cassani and Spiehler 1993). There are also practical difficulties. The collection of scalp hair for drug screening is not a straightforward process. Maintaining hair alignment and securing and identifying the cut ends are critical if quantification of time with drug concentration is required (Marsh 1997). The use of shampoos and conditioners may alter drug levels in hair (Welch *et al.* 1993).

On their own, the biological tests are incomplete as measures of drug taking. Metabolites may remain in a person's system for varying periods of time after drug use, and they may be insensitive or poor indicators of patterns of drug taking, though, where repeated positive results are obtained, this can help to suggest drug use patterns. Where drug use is infrequent, such tests may produce false negative results if there is a substantial delay between last use and testing. Biological tests are frequently unable to detect the use of extra drugs of the same type as those being prescribed (as with diverted methadone). There are, at present, no laboratory tests that provide adequate identification of drug dependence, though a naloxone challenge can be used to determine neuroadaptation among opiate users (Loimer *et al.* 1992).

Biochemical tests can be of value when used to support broader assessment procedures, and where the consequences of error are potentially serious. The interpretation of laboratory findings should take place in conjunction with other contextual data. Self-report and laboratory tests can also be used interactively. Hamid *et al.* (1999) found that rates of agreement between self-reported drug use and urinalysis increased when urine was taken for testing prior to interview.

Although structured instruments are not widely used in routine clinical assessment, they provide a useful means of collecting information and can help to avoid omitting questions about important behaviours and problems. Structured instruments can be particularly useful where there is a need for a systematic assessment of problems and of changes over time (Institute of Medicine 1990*a*). Several such instruments are available.

The Addiction Severity Index (ASI) can be used to make a multidimensional assessment of substance use disorders (McLellan *et al.* 1980, 1985, 1992). The ASI is a standardized, structured, 45-minute clinical research interview that assesses problem severity for drug and alcohol use, medical, legal, employment, family/social, and psychiatric problems. In each of these areas, the ASI assesses the number, frequency, intensity, and duration of problems in the 30-day period preceding admission to treatment. ASI measures can also be taken for lifetime problems.

Another structured instrument that has been used is the Opiate Treatment Index (OTI; Darke *et al.* 1992). The OTI contains measures from six domains: drug use; HIV risk-taking behaviour; social functioning; criminality; health status; and psychological adjustment. Drug use is recorded by the patient on the last 3 days use for each of 11 classes of drugs: heroin, other opiates (including illicit methadone), amphetamines, cocaine, tranquillizers, alcohol, cannabis, barbiturates, hallucinogens, inhalants, and tobacco.

One problem with these instruments is that they require a relatively lengthy completion time (approximately 45 minutes) and, partly for this reason, they have not been widely used in clinical settings.

The Maudsley Addiction Profile (MAP) was developed as a brief, interviewer-administered questionnaire that could be used to assess recent problems of drug misusers and problem drinkers. The MAP was specifically developed to be easily and rapidly administered, and to minimize practical and administrative problems for clinical staff. For most subjects, the interview can be completed in about 12 minutes. The items were designed for simple

In general, the identification and setting of goals should occur as early as possible within the treatment process. However, there are many cases in which drug misusers present with complex and multidimensional problems. This may make it very difficult to reach firm decisions about implementing a comprehensive treatment plan after a single assessment interview.

Despite the undoubted importance of both the therapist and the patient agreeing upon the goal(s) of treatment, this does not mean that the therapist cannot aspire to goals more ambitious than those set by the patient. However, it does imply that, where the therapist wishes to set a goal beyond that which is immediately acceptable to the patient, this is likely to create certain tensions and will require careful management.

Setting goals at an early stage of treatment increases the possibilities of change by helping the patient to focus upon the possibilities and attainment of improvement rather than being dragged down by the burden of what may be chronic and severe problems. Whenever possible, goals should be stated in positive terms, so that the patient (and therapist) is clear about what it is that treatment is seeking to achieve and what the patient is moving *towards*, rather than what he or she is trying to give up.

Specific and short-term goals are more effective in motivating behaviour change than generalized or long-term goals. Bandura and Simon (1977) suggested that 'Explicitly defined goals regulate performance by designating the type and amount of effort required to attain them, whereas general intentions provide little basis for regulating one's efforts or for evaluating how one is doing.'

Clearly defined goals also impose a structure on the treatment programme and keep the treatment focused. This reduces the risk that treatment will be diverted into a series of *ad hoc* crisis interventions. The marked and often unacceptable variation in programme delivery leads to a situation in which key elements of treatment may be neglected or even omitted. Where treatment takes place over a prolonged period, there is a risk that the focus of treatment may drift away from the originally agreed problem to other problems that arise over time. Of course, there may be occasions on which it is appropriate that goals should be re-negotiated. But, again, the re-negotiation should be done explicitly, together with the patient, in order to avoid the risk that the patient and therapist start to pursue different agendas.

Different people approach treatment services and enter treatment programmes with different expectations of what the therapeutic process will entail. To the extent that there may be incongruities between what the patients expect and what they receive, this is likely to interfere with progress or reduce treatment adherence (Meichenbaum and Turk 1987).

scoring and interpretation. The MAP was not intended as a replacement for other clinical assessment procedures. It was designed to be easily incorporated within routine clinical practice, and to be used in association with other assessment protocols. Marsden *et al.* (1998*a*) recommend that the instrument be used as part of a *modular* approach in which a primary set of measures is recorded, with others included as required.

The MAP is a reliable and valid instrument that can be easily administered at intake, during, and after treatment. It contains 60 self-report items measuring behaviours and problems in four domains. These are: substance use behaviours; health risk behaviours and health problems; and various aspects of personal and social functioning. Like the ASI, the MAP assesses problems during the 30-days before treatment.

Initial ratings of problem severity as measured by both the ASI and the MAP have been found to be highly correlated with treatment outcome and can be used to determine the need for specialized psychiatric, vocational, or medical interventions (McLellan *et al.* 1997*a*; Marsden *et al.* 1998*a*). These (and other similar) instruments can also be used to monitor the effects of treatment and changes in the patient's functioning.

The wider role of assessment

Assessment should not be seen as an impersonal and routine procedure to be completed as quickly as possible before moving on to the more interesting and important business of treatment. Assessment has several different functions. Its central and key purpose is to obtain information that can be used to guide the processes of treatment. Assessment also has other functions. It can be used for determining suitability for treatment, for evaluating patient needs, for diagnosis, and for devising a treatment plan. If carried out properly it becomes an important first stage of the therapeutic process. The drug taker is actively involved in his or her own addictive behaviour and must be actively involved in his or her own recovery. It is the responsibility of the therapist to use assessment as an opportunity to encourage that involvement in recovery.

Assessment has a *pragmatic* function. As a first point of contact, the assessment session(s) should be concerned with practical issues. The assessment should seek to identify the nature and extent of the presenting problems, the reasons why the person is making contact, and why at this particular time. It is possible that this may be due to some sort of objective or psychological crisis. Some of those seeking treatment may have emergency needs that require immediate attention. The individual seeking treatment may, for example, have an acute medical illness, be feeling acutely depressed, or have suicidal thoughts.

Assessment also has *psychological* and *therapeutic* functions. It is possible that the patient's reason for seeking treatment is that their drug misuse is a cause for concern to others. Ambivalence is often a characteristic of substance use from the earliest stages through to later addictive phases (Orford 2001). Where the user may be ambivalent or resistant to change, assessment provides an opportunity for the application of motivational enhancement procedures to generate greater willingness for change. Where the user is more fully committed to change, assessment should clarify and agree the goals, and move on to identify the barriers to change as well as actual or potential supportive factors.

The assessment should be used to establish empathy and rapport with the patients and to form the basis for a working relationship with them. For highly stigmatized forms of behaviour such as addictions to illegal drugs, the offer of non-judgemental sympathy and concern is helpful. This may reduce the patient's distress, and provide relief, especially where the patient may feel hopeless, guilty, or embarrassed about his or her behaviour. Virtually all forms of psychological therapy can be affected by the relationship between therapist and patient. This involves the interest, warmth, and empathy shown by the therapist, the patient's expectations of improvement, and a range of other so-called 'non-specific' influences (Frank 1961). Such factors operate and are important during the initial assessment period. Part of the success of all forms of psychotherapy may be attributed to the therapist's ability to mobilize the patient's expectation of help. In these respects, assessment can play an important part in the treatment process and can influence both the course and response to subsequent treatment interventions. It may also, in some cases, have either an indirect or even a direct influence upon treatment outcomes.

It is useful to provide the patient with information about the structure and requirements of treatment at this stage. Ideally, patients should be given a coherent account of the nature of their problem, a rationale and description of the type of therapy, and a precise description of their own responsibilities for actively participating in treatment. For example, how many treatment sessions will there be? how long will they last? where will treatment take place? Making these issues explicit can help to increase the agreement between the therapist and patient with regard to their expectations about treatment. Providing this sort of structured and relevant information improves adherence rates (Dunbar and Stunkard 1979) and can also be used to support and build motivation and strengthen commitment for change. If the patient and therapist have different expectations this can lead to subsequent problems, increasing the probability of treatment noncompliance and possibly leading to the patient dropping out of the treatment programme.

One practical question involves the place of assessment within the clinica programme. In some programmes, patients are required to complete assess ment before seeing a therapist. As well as depriving the therapist of the oppor tunity to establish good rapport from the first session, this assessment-firs procedure gives assessment an implied low status and may lead the patient t respond carelessly or defensively. Used in this way, assessment can be an obstacl to treatment and increase the risk of premature drop-out.

It is sometimes believed that a protracted assessment process can be used t distinguish between motivated and unmotivated treatment applicants. Ther is little evidence to support this. In a comparison of treatment retention rate among patients who received an extended (1–3 day) assessment process an others who were accepted or rejected after a single assessment interview Woody *et al.* (1975) found that the patients who received the minimal assess ment procedure had better retention rates at 2 and 5 months. Similarly, in study of the time spent by out-patient staff in attempting to predict ho patients would respond to in-patient treatment, Gossop and Connell (1983 found little consistency between staff predictions, and little associatio between staff predictions and subsequent patient behaviour.

In the worst case, assessment staff assume the role of gate-keeper, and th assessment process becomes a set of obstacles that the applicants are require to negotiate before they are allowed to receive treatment.

Goals

With regard to the aims and goals of treatment, it may be more appropriate t think in terms of reaching mutual agreement (between the patient and ther apist) about goals rather than simply setting goals. It is useful to discuss and agre the goals of treatment during the assessment phase. Specifying treatment goal and negotiating the mutual agreement of these between therapist and patien delineating treatment procedures, and providing feedback about progress ar core features of effective treatments. Properly defined goals help both the the apist and the patient to be clear about the aims and purposes of treatment.

The specification of goals and of the procedures required to reach thos goals serves to identify and to avoid or reduce problems of misunderstandin and failures of communication between therapist and patient. This is espe cially relevant in the treatment of problem drug users since many differer parties are in competition for control of goal setting. Patients, therapist family, programme managers, treatment funders, criminal justice personne politicians, and other interested parties are likely to have different, and som times conflicting interests and priorities with regard to the goals of treatmen

It is now widely recognized that there may be a range of treatment goals, including:

- abstinence from all drugs;
- abstinence from the main problem drug(s);
- attainment of controlled, non-dependent, or non-problematic drug use;
- reduction of harmful or risky behaviour associated with the use of drugs (e.g. sharing injection equipment);
- reduction of psychological, social, or other problems directly attributable to drug use;
- reduction of psychological, social, or other problems not directly related to drug use.

These goals are not mutually exclusive. Treatment goals may (and often will) include the attainment of abstinence and the improvement of psychosocial functioning in areas that may not be directly related to drug use. However, the choice of treatment goals will depend upon the motivations and specific circumstances of each individual. Each patient's motivation and degree of treatment readiness must be addressed. Some patients may be at a stage of their drug-taking career where they are willing to commit themselves to a determined effort to become abstinent. Others may be unwilling to give up drugs, but may still be prepared to make changes in their behaviour (e.g. reduction in risk behaviour).

From the perspective of the treatment services, UK Department of Health (1999*b*) guidelines suggested that aims of assessment should include:

- treatment of any emergency or acute problem;
- confirmation that the patient is taking drugs (history, examination, and urine analysis);
- assessment of the degree of dependence;
- identification of complications of drug misuse and assessment of risk behaviour;
- identification of other medical, social, and mental health problems;
- providing advice on harm minimization, including, if appropriate, access to sterile needles and syringes, testing for hepatitis and HIV, and immunization against hepatitis B;
- determining the patient's expectations of treatment and the degree of motivation to change;

- ◆ assessment of the most appropriate level of expertise required to manage the patient (this may change over time), and referral/liaising appropriately with other services;
- ◆ determining the need for substitute medication.

There has been considerable controversy about the extent to which different treatment goals for drug injectors are appropriate or acceptable. This issue has always been less contentious in the UK than in many other countries (Stimson 1995). Strang (1993) described some of the efforts that were made in the UK to avoid the unnecessary and unhelpful polarization and opposition of abstinence-oriented and harm-reduction treatment approaches. During the early years after the identification of HIV, an influential national report (ACMD 1988) stated that 'the first goal . . . with drug misusers must . . . be to prevent them from acquiring or transmitting the [HIV] virus . . . . In some cases this will be achieved through abstinence. In others . . . efforts will have to focus on risk reduction.' Subsequent statements of the possibilities of working towards intermediate treatment goals have been made on many occasions (Strang 1990; Gossop 1994a). In practice, both abstinence and intermediate risk reduction outcomes are achieved by substantial numbers of drug injectors. Both outcomes confer benefits, though the benefits of abstinence are greater. Abstinence is an excellent means of achieving harm reduction (Strang 1993).

Different types of outcome may sometimes be interrelated (though there are also instances in which they are independent of each other). One of the types of behaviour that has been found to relate to other outcomes is cessation of injecting drug use. Drug users who were injectors at intake to treatment but who had stopped injecting at follow-up achieved consistently superior outcomes across a range of other problem behaviours (Gossop *et al.* 2002a). Non-injecting drug users at follow-up showed greater reductions in the use of illicit opiates, benzodiazepines, and stimulant drugs. The most marked reduction in problem behaviours was shown by those who were abstinent from drugs at follow-up. Those who were abstinent from heroin also achieved greater reductions in frequency and quantity of alcohol consumption, as well as greater improvements in their physical and psychological health problems.

These results should not be interpreted as showing that abstinence should automatically be recommended as the preferred treatment goal for all drug injectors. Drug misusers who choose abstinence or harm reduction goals differ in several important respects. For some drug misusers, long-term drug maintenance treatments may be chosen precisely because of a history of repeated attempts and failures to become abstinent. This was one of the original entry criteria for methadone maintenance specified by Dole and

Nyswander (1965). Where injectors are resistant to the idea of giving up drugs, interventions directed towards reducing the harm associated with injecting or sharing injecting equipment can be of value both to the individual and in public health terms. There are no simple rules that permit the identification of specific types of drug users for whom the different treatment goals can be recommended (Hunter *et al.* 2000). Nor are clinical staff able to predict which individual patients will do well in particular types of treatment programme (Gossop and Connell 1983).

Chapter 7

Withdrawal and detoxification

The purpose of detoxification

One intermediate treatment goal, and a preliminary phase of those treatments that are aimed at abstinence involves withdrawal from drugs or 'detoxification'.[1]

Within the US federally funded treatment programmes in the 1980s, more than 40 per cent of the heroin users who received some sort of treatment were admitted to detoxification programmes (Lipton and Maranda 1983). This compared with about a quarter (26 per cent) who were admitted to methadone maintenance programmes and about a third (36 per cent) who were admitted to drug-free treatment during the same period. A more recent estimate suggested that there were about 100 000 detoxification episodes per year in the USA (Institute of Medicine 1990a).

The reasons why detoxification is popular with users and with some treatment providers are easy to understand. Detoxification attracts drug misusers who believe (generally incorrectly) that this is all they need to get off drugs and remain drug-free, as well as those who want only short-term relief from their habit. Detoxification is also used by those for whom detoxification is a first step in a longer treatment process. Some residential rehabilitation programmes require drug users to be drug-free before they enter treatment, and some methadone maintenance programmes require clients to have made at least one attempt at detoxification before they are eligible to receive maintenance treatment.

Detoxification has been tried with various pharmacological agents and non-pharmacological interventions. It has been tried rapidly and slowly, with and without counselling or other supportive services, and in a variety of settings, including specialist in-patient drug dependence units, psychiatric hospital wards, residential rehabilitation programmes, out-patient clinics, and prisons. Each setting has advantages and disadvantages. Different settings may be suitable for

---

[1] The term 'detoxification' can be misleading. It was coined to refer to the process of ridding the body of the toxins believed to be caused by physical dependence. However, the term is so widely used that it is retained here to avoid having always to use the more cumbersome phrase 'treatment of withdrawal symptoms'.

different users with different types of circumstances and problems, or even for the same user at different stages of their addiction career.

Whatever method is used to manage withdrawal, this only has meaning within the wider context of other treatment or intervention strategies (Edwards *et al.* 1997). When withdrawal takes place at the same time as initial assessment and goal-setting, the withdrawal phase can more readily be placed within a wider context. This is easily forgotten when detoxification takes place as a crisis management response.

The importance of detoxification is often overestimated. Detoxification is not, in itself, a treatment for drug dependence, and it is not appropriate to expect detoxification on its own to produce long-term abstinence. Detoxification alone is not effective in this respect (Lipton and Maranda 1983). Among drug users who received detoxification treatment, the outcomes at 1 year showed either small and non-significant improvements or no improvements at all (Simpson and Sells 1990). Out-patient detoxification offered no more therapeutic benefit than formal intake-only procedures (i.e. without any treatment) (Simpson and Sells 1983). Other studies of out-patient detoxification found similar outcomes (Wilson *et al.* 1975) with patients achieving little benefit from detoxification alone. Detoxification may be a necessary, but is not a sufficient condition for long-term abstinence.

Nonetheless, the importance of the treatment and management of withdrawal should not be underestimated. Detoxification may act either as a barrier to recovery or as a springboard. Even though drug withdrawal is seldom medically serious, many addicts are anxious about the prospect of detoxification, and for some, their fears about withdrawal may deter them from seeking treatment (Phillips *et al.* 1986). For this reason, detoxification should be managed in a way that involves as little discomfort as possible. After starting a detoxification programme, the discomfort of withdrawal symptoms may interfere with treatment and may, in some circumstances, lead the patient to drop out of treatment.

The term detoxification covers many types of procedures that have been used to alleviate the short-term symptoms of withdrawal from dependent drug use. It does not produce, nor is it intended to lead to the psychological and behavioural changes that provide a secure foundation for sustained abstinence. Detoxification is a clearly delineated phase of treatment designed to eliminate or to reduce the severity of withdrawal symptoms when the physically dependent user stops taking drugs. The criteria by which the effectiveness of detoxification should be judged are:

- *acceptability* (is the user willing to seek and undergo the intervention);
- *availability* (is the treatment available or can it be made available through existing treatment services);

- *symptom severity* (is the treatment effective in the specific sense of reducing or eliminating the discomfort and distress of withdrawal);
- *duration of withdrawal* (does the treatment reduce the overall duration of the withdrawal syndrome);
- *side-effects* (the treatment should have no side-effects, or only side-effects that are less subjectively severe and/or less medically serious than the untreated withdrawal symptoms);
- *completion rates* (do a sufficient number of patients manage to complete the programme and achieve a drug-free state at the end of the detoxification treatment).

A regular misconception is that the effectiveness of detoxification can be judged in terms of longer-term abstinence rates. However, a detoxification treatment may be fully effective in terms of all the criteria listed above but still not touch upon the powerful psychosocial and other factors that may subsequently lead to relapse. The majority of the factors that put the ex-user at risk of relapse are different to and separate from those associated with the withdrawal symptoms and their treatment.

Withdrawal from heroin (and other opiates)

The clinical features of the heroin withdrawal syndrome are well known and their underlying mechanisms relatively well understood. Many clinical features of opiate withdrawal can be linked to increased firing of noradrenergic neurons projecting from the locus ceruleus (Aghajanian 1978). Chronic occupancy of opiate receptors within these neurons induces postreceptor neuroadaptation, and this serves to normalize neuronal firing so long as opiate receptor occupancy is maintained. However the potential hyperexcitability of these neurons is unmasked by sudden opiate abstinence, initiating what is sometimes described as a 'noradrenergic storm'. Neuronal firing rates are closely related to withdrawal responses.

The opiate withdrawal syndrome is uncomfortable and can be extremely unpleasant. A commonly drawn analogy is that it is similar to a bad case of influenza (Kleber 1981). It is very rarely associated with life-threatening problems such as may sometimes arise during unmodified alcohol or benzodiazepine withdrawal (Farrell 1994; Mattick and Hall 1996). Commonly reported heroin withdrawal symptoms are vomiting, diarrhoea, stomach cramps, restlessness, drowsiness, pain, muscular stiffness, spontaneous muscle twitches, tremor, feelings of coldness, gooseflesh, hot and cold flushes, increased sweating, runny nose, heart pounding, fatigue or tiredness, muscular aches, yawning, sneezing, runny eyes, and insomnia.

Even for heroin users who are dependent upon extremely high doses, detoxification can be straightforward, and without serious medical complications. In a study of high-dose heroin addicts in Pakistan, Gossop (1989*b*) found that heroin users dependent upon daily doses of up to 5 g of heroin could be withdrawn with relative ease using only symptomatic treatment. The heaviest user in this study reported taking up to 13 g per day (equivalent to 3900 mg when adjusted for purity). Despite their high-dose dependence, these heroin addicts returned to relatively normal levels of functioning within 10 days.

A self-completion questionnaire for the assessment of the opiate withdrawal syndrome, the Short Opiate Withdrawal Scale (SOWS), is shown in Table 7.1. This scale assesses 10 commonly reported symptoms. It is quick and easy to administer, and provides clinically useful information that is relevant to the planning and delivery of treatment programmes.

The withdrawal syndrome is similar for all of the opiates, though it tends to be less severe for less potent drugs such as codeine and propoxyphine (McKim 2000). It is widely believed that withdrawal from methadone is 'qualitatively similar to that of morphine, but it develops more slowly and is more prolonged, although usually less intense' (Jaffe 1985). It has also been suggested that methadone withdrawal symptoms are more persistent than those for heroin. There is, however, little empirical evidence to support this view, which appears to be derived from early work by Isbell, Vogel, and others (Vogel *et al.* 1948).

Table 7.1 Short Opiate Withdrawal Scale

Name:	Date:			
Please put a tick in the appropriate box if you have had any of the following during the last 24 hours.				
	None	**Mild**	**Moderate**	**Severe**
Feeling sick				
Stomach cramps				
Muscle spasms/twitching				
Feelings of coldness				
Heart pounding				
Muscular tension				
Aches and pains				
Yawning				
Runny eyes				
Insomnia/problems sleeping				

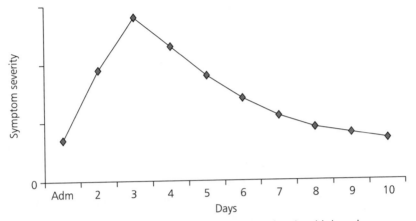

Fig. 7.1 The figure shows the severity and course of the heroin withdrawal syndrome over a 10-day period. The data were collected from a sample of high-dose heroin addicts in Pakistan who received only symptomatic treatment to manage their withdrawal symptoms. The data are from the study of Gossop (1988). 'Adm' shows withdrawal severity on day of admission.

A more recent investigation of withdrawal symptoms shown by opiate addicts who were using either heroin or methadone prior to treatment found no differences in peak withdrawal severity for heroin and methadone (Gossop and Strang 1991). Nor was there any difference in the duration of withdrawal symptoms for the heroin and methadone users.

The course of the unmodified heroin withdrawal syndrome is shown in Fig. 7.1, though the precise timing of the onset, peak, and course of the heroin withdrawal syndrome will vary from case to case, and according to other circumstances. When heroin is abruptly discontinued, the agonist effects wane over a period of 6–8 hours. After about 8 hours, and certainly after 12–15 hours, the addict will start to feel uncomfortable. During the early stages, addicts may feel drowsy and be subject to frequent bouts of yawning. After about 18 hours, they will definitely feel unwell, and withdrawal symptoms will increase in severity usually leading to a preoccupation with the discomfort and with ways of avoiding withdrawal symptoms. After about 24 hours they are anxious and restless, and find it difficult either to sleep or to rest comfortably. Glandular secretions increase: the eyes and nose run, and salivation and sweating are increased.

Withdrawal symptoms are usually at their most intense between 24 and 72 hours. The bones, muscles, and joints ache, and the addict may also suffer from stomach cramps, vomiting, and diarrhoea. Thereafter, the symptoms will gradually lessen in intensity, though it may be more than a week or even 10 days before the addicts start to feel well again.

Some heroin addicts manage their own detoxification without using drugs, especially if they have sufficient psychological and social resources to help support them through withdrawal. More often addicts self-treat their withdrawal by using tranquillizers (Gossop *et al.* 1991*b*). Tranquillizers may also be used as part of medically supervised withdrawal treatments (Drummond *et al.* 1989).

In most heroin detoxification programmes, the withdrawal syndrome is treated by various sorts of drugs to make it less uncomfortable. In a review of 218 research studies, Gowing *et al.* (2000) identified a wide range of opiate detoxification procedures. These included tapered methadone, tapered methadone plus adjunctive medication, other opioid agonists, clonidine, lofexidine, other adrenergic agonists, buprenorphine, opioid antagonists alone or with miscellaneous adjunctive treatment, opioid antagonists following or combined with buprenorphine, opioid antagonists combined with clonidine, opioid antagonists administered under anaesthesia or sedation, hypnotic or anxiolytic drugs, antidepressant or antipsychotic drugs, drugs to modify receptor activity, symptomatic medications, and electrostimulation or acupuncture.

Detoxification using methadone

One of the most widely used methods to manage withdrawal from opiates involves gradually reducing doses of an opiate agonist, usually oral methadone (Kleber *et al.* 1980), and methadone has been described as having been shown to be the most effective pharmacotherapeutic agent currently used in short-term detoxification treatment (Kreek 2000).

Where users are dependent upon heroin, methadone is substituted for the heroin prior to withdrawal. Typically, detoxification takes place with gradually reducing doses of methadone over periods of 10–28 days (Gossop *et al.* 1984, 1989*d*), and most treatments use a linear reduction schedule with regular, equal dose decrements from an individually tailored starting dose to zero (Strang and Gossop 1990).

This form of 'tapering' treatment has also been used as a self-detoxification treatment by heroin addicts. In his novel, *Junkie*, William Burroughs (1953, p. 72) wrote 'I had one sixteenth of an ounce of junk with me. I figured this was enough to taper off, and I had a reduction schedule carefully worked out. It was supposed to take 12 days. I had the junk in solution, and in another bottle distilled water. Every time I took a dropper of solution out to use it, I put the same amount of distilled water in the junk solution bottle. Eventually I would be shooting plain water. This method is well known to all junkies.'

Although slower detoxification schedules are sometimes believed to be less stressful, there is little evidence to support this view. Indeed, it is possible that the more protracted the schedule the lower the success rate because of patients dropping out prior to completing detoxification. Addicts are not alone in finding it difficult to tolerate prolonged physical and psychological discomfort. Few of us would thank the dentist who offered to extract a tooth slowly. In many ways, the quicker the detoxification process can be completed the better. Certainly, the less discomfort it entails the better.

One drawback of gradual methadone withdrawal is that it leads to a protracted residual withdrawal response, with withdrawal symptoms persisting well beyond the last methadone dose (Gossop *et al.* 1986, 1989*b*). Residual withdrawal symptoms may continue for as long as the original detoxification procedure. When given over a 21-day period, patients are not fully recovered until 40 days after the beginning of withdrawal (Gossop *et al* 1989*b*). The same residual withdrawal effect can be seen for 10-day reductions with symptoms persisting for about 20 days (Gossop and Strang 1991). The period around the end of the methadone reduction schedule is generally associated with the greatest levels of discomfort. This can cause clinical problems since many patients expect the last methadone dose to coincide with the last day of withdrawal discomfort, and the continued presence and relatively high severity of the residual withdrawal symptoms may be unsettling.

Attempts have been made to identify more rapid and more effective methadone detoxification procedures. One attempt to improve the efficacy of methadone detoxification has involved modification of the slope of the reduction curve with proportionate (exponential) dose reductions rather than a fixed (linear) dose reduction schedule. It was hoped that a more rapid decrease in the earlier stages coupled with a more gradual reduction during the later stages would reduce withdrawal severity and/or reduce the duration of residual withdrawal symptoms.

In a randomized, double-blind study, and for low-dose addicts, an exponential reduction resulted in more rapid passage of the opiate withdrawal syndrome without any significant increase in withdrawal severity or drop out (Gossop and Strang 1991). However, for high-dose addicts, the exponential curve resulted in higher levels of withdrawal distress during the acute phase of the withdrawal syndrome without any reduction in symptom severity at a later stage nor a more rapid resolution. There was no effect of treatment condition upon treatment retention and, for both conditions, there was still evidence of protracted, residual withdrawal symptoms.

The cheapest but often the most difficult option is out-patient/community detoxification. The majority of detoxification programmes for people who are dependent upon opiates are likely to occur on an out-patient basis. In the treatment of people with alcohol problems it is generally accepted that it is preferable for detoxification to be carried out while the person continues to live and function in their own home (Edwards *et al.* 1997). This view is sometimes uncritically applied to the treatment of opiate addicts. However, there appear to be marked differences in the outcomes of drug-dependent and alcohol-dependent patients when detoxified in out-patient settings.

Consistently low completion rates have been reported for opiate-dependent patients detoxified in out-patient programmes (Maddux *et al.* 1980). The percentage of users treated as out-patients who achieve abstinence from opiates for even as little as 24 hours after treatment has been found to be between 17 and 28 per cent (Gossop *et al.* 1986; Dawe *et al.* 1991). This compares with abstinence rates for in-patient detoxification of 80–85 per cent (Gossop *et al.* 1986; Gossop and Strang 1991). The poor completion rates for out-patient detoxification may be largely due to problems of drug availability and exposure to drug-related cues that are associated with daily contact with other users and with neighbourhoods where drug use is prevalent. Such pressures put very high demands upon the patient.

Another factor that may increase successful completion of detoxification is the extent to which patients are involved in deciding their own withdrawal rate. Banks and Waller (1988) suggest that it is best to respond to a patient's own determination and time-scale to withdraw from drugs, and that the doctor should adjust the rate of withdrawal accordingly. There has been considerable enthusiasm for adopting a more flexible and negotiable approach to clinical work with drug users including the management of detoxification (ACMD 1988), and it was hoped that the introduction of flexible detoxification schedules would be an improvement upon existing 'fixed' detoxification procedures.

Dawe *et al.* (1991) randomly allocated out-patient opiate addicts to either a fixed rate methadone reduction over a 6-week period, or a flexible, negotiable programme that allowed subjects to regulate the rate of their reduction within a 10-week period. As in other studies (Unnithan *et al.* 1992), relatively few patients completed out-patient detoxification. It was disappointing that opiate users receiving the negotiable detoxification extended the period of time over which their withdrawal took place, but fewer of them completed the programme. There was no difference in retention rates between the fixed and negotiable groups.

The many problems that are associated with the delivery of effective detoxification programmes in out-patient settings raise questions about the continued reliance upon this type of treatment provision within national treatment systems, both in Britain and in other countries.

Detoxification using clonidine and lofexidine

Centrally acting alpha-2 adrenergic agonists such as clonidine and lofexidine reduce noradrenergic neuronal firing and noradrenaline (norepinephrine) turnover, and these drugs have been used in detoxification treatments.

Although first introduced as a nasal decongestant, clonidine has been used in medicine principally for its antihypertensive effects. The drug also has the capacity to reduce or suppress opiate withdrawal symptoms. Clonidine appears to affect opiate withdrawal symptoms by binding presynaptically to alpha-2 receptors and decreasing central nervous system noradrenergic activity. Opiates and clonidine both act at the locus ceruleus to decrease central noradrenergic function but, whereas opiates bind to opioid receptors and are antagonized by naloxone, clonidine's actions are mediated by alpha-adrenergic receptors and are not antagonized by opioid antagonists.

In the first clinical study of clonidine's effects on withdrawal five opioid addicts were given either clonidine followed by placebo or placebo followed by clonidine. A single dose of clonidine was found to produce a rapid and substantial reduction in observed withdrawal symptoms. Similar reductions were noted in subjective distress ratings and in systolic and diastolic blood pressure (Gold *et al.* 1978*a*). This paper was immediately followed by others with samples of methadone (Gold *et al.* 1978*b*) and heroin addicts (Gold *et al.* 1979), and they showed that clonidine produced 'a rapid, prolonged and significant reduction of opiate signs and symptoms' (Gold *et al.* 1979).

In both open and double-blind trials clonidine has been found to produce a rapid and prolonged reduction of withdrawal symptoms (Gossop 1988). This reduction in symptoms is sufficiently acceptable to addicts for many to complete detoxification. However, although clonidine reduces withdrawal severity, it does not completely eliminate symptoms and, in many studies, patients have been given additional medication (usually hypnotics) to modify residual symptoms. When compared to existing methadone withdrawal procedures, clonidine and methadone produce broadly similar levels of overall reductions in withdrawal symptom severity. There are, however, differences in the pattern of withdrawal response to the two drugs. Patients experience more withdrawal symptoms in the first few days of clonidine treatment, whereas methadone patients experience more discomfort at a later stage.

The hypotensive effects of clonidine may restrict the manner in which it can be used, though there is some disagreement about the extent and severity of these effects. Some studies suggest that the hypotensive effects are either unimportant or can be easily managed. Others have reported marked difficulties in some patients. To achieve a balance between adequate suppression of withdrawal symptoms and an avoidance of sedation or hypotensive side-effects, treatment requires relatively close medical supervision. This may limit the treatment settings in which clonidine can be safely used.

Lofexidine is a more recently available alpha-2 agonist. It has comparable clinical efficacy to clonidine, but fewer side-effects, particularly with regard to postural hypotension (Buntwal *et al.* 2000). In a randomized double-blind study, Carnwath and Hardman (1998) compared the clinical response of 50 low-dose opiate addicts to lofexidine and clonidine in the out-patient treatment of opiate withdrawal. More than half (58 per cent) of those starting treatment completed detoxification and were opiate-free at 4 weeks. More patients completed withdrawal in the lofexidine group, but the difference was not significant. Clonidine produced more hypotensive effects and more home visits were required by medical staff. There were no other significant differences in side-effects, and the authors suggested that both drugs could be used successfully for out-patient detoxification, but that treatment with clonidine requires more input in terms of staff time. Detoxification with lofexidine can also be achieved over periods as short as 5 days (Bearn *et al.* 1998). Encouraging results regarding the effectiveness of lofexidine are now available from a number of studies, including double-blind, controlled clinical trials (Strang *et al.* 1999c) and, within the past decade, lofexidine has been increasingly widely used in detoxification programmes across the UK.

Use of antagonists in detoxification

A number of attempts have been made to develop rapid opiate detoxification regimens. One of the main pharmacological strategies for promoting rapid withdrawal from opiates involves the administration of opiate antagonists (naloxone and/or naltrexone) to precipitate an acute withdrawal state, which may then be attenuated by concurrent treatment with an alpha-2 agonist such as clonidine and/or benzodiazepine-induced sedation (Bearn *et al.* 1999). Opiate antagonists bind to opiate receptors but without producing opiate effects and compete with opiate agonists such as heroin to block the receptor sites.

It has been known for some time that patients could be withdrawn rapidly from opiates using opiate antagonists. Blachly *et al.* (1975) described the detoxification of a series of 32 patients who were given naloxone by injection at a rate determined by the speed of resolution of withdrawal symptoms after each dose. The patients received naloxone until they no longer showed withdrawal responses, usually after 2 days. Patients experienced severe withdrawal symptoms after the initial injection, which subsided within 1 hour. Subsequent naloxone injections precipitated progressively milder withdrawal responses.

Resnick *et al.* (1977) gave steadily increasing doses of naloxone to opiate addicts whose methadone supply was suddenly terminated. No other drugs were administered apart from low to moderate doses of hypnosedatives. Naloxone provoked an immediate severe withdrawal response, but the severity of withdrawal symptoms decreased progressively with further naloxone doses. Kleber *et al.* (1987) described a procedure in which clonidine and naltrexone were used in combination to detoxify heroin addicts over a period of 5 days in an out-patient setting. In a similar procedure in the UK, heroin addicts were detoxified with clonidine, naltrexone, and diazepam over a 48–72 hour period (Brewer *et al.* 1988).

Rapid detoxification treatments may be carried out within periods of between several days and just a few hours. In the more dramatic instances, detoxification has been attempted over a few hours while the patient is anaesthetized and mechanically ventilated (Loimer *et al.* 1991; Brewer 1997; Strang *et al.* 1997*a*). During the past few years, there has been considerable international interest in the use of antagonists during anaesthesia to detoxify opiate addicts. In certain respects, this has its origins in earlier clinical practices. Schlomer (1955) described the use of prolonged sleep therapy with opiate addicts to permit the abrupt discontinuation of morphine. Sleep therapies and deep narcosis were once popular in treatment of various psychiatric conditions but these have not recently been used in any widespread or sanctioned manner. Gossop and Strang (1997) suggested that between 5000 and 10 000 heroin addicts may have been treated with antagonist-precipitated detoxification under anaesthesia. Despite this there has been very little controlled research or coverage of the procedure in scientific journals.

In Vienna, Loimer *et al.* (1989, 1991, 1992) described a rapid detoxification procedure in which various approaches were used to administer an antagonist in conjunction with general anaesthesia. Opiate addicts were sedated with a 30 mg injection of midazolam into a peripheral vein. Within 10 minutes, 4 mg of naloxone diluted in 200 ml of 0.9 per cent saline was administered by means of a constant perfusion pump. Sedation was maintained as necessary with further midazolam. During detoxification, heart rate and blood pressure were monitored. Benzodiazepine sedation was reversed with flumazenil (Loimer *et al.* 1991). These early studies were conducted on patients without comorbidity or dependence upon other drugs.

Some patients may be attracted to an ultrarapid detoxification during which they are anaesthetized as part of the procedure. The potential benefit of a rapid detoxification treatment includes a briefer, less uncomfortable transition from dependence to abstinence. Addicts may also be drawn to an apparently revolutionary new treatment, the claims for absence of withdrawal distress, and the speed of recovery.

Advocates of this new treatment claim that there is no withdrawal discomfort (i.e. the withdrawal syndrome occurs while they are asleep) and no residual withdrawal effects (though there may be some fatigue or other side-effects of the general anaesthesia). Such treatments may reduce the user's anxieties about detoxification. It may also useful for patients to feel that they have recovered from withdrawal as quickly as possible, especially if drug-free and symptom-free functioning is required for some subsequent phase of treatment. Family and employers may be attracted to a technique that offers less interference with family and work. Health-care purchasers and health insurance companies may be attracted to a technique that may result in a substantial reduction in the cost of a completed course of treatment, even if the *per diem* costs are greater. However, much of this perceived advantage may relate to the novelty of the procedure and to claims of effectiveness that are, at present, unsubstantiated. In animal studies the use of opiate antagonists to provoke withdrawal responses has been found to prolong withdrawal symptoms (Spanagel *et al.* 1998).

Any evaluation of rapid detoxification treatments should take account of the intrinsically benign course of opiate withdrawal under conventional management (Bearn *et al.* 1999). There are serious concerns about the possible dangers of these sorts of radical detoxification procedures. Patients are exposed to the hazards of a general anaesthetic over several hours. The risks of anaesthetic detoxification might be greater if this were attempted within existing addiction treatment services unless there was retraining and recruitment of new personnel to ensure that appropriate skills were provided during both the anaesthetic and recovery periods.

Even in healthy individuals, general anaesthesia for routine procedures carries a (low) risk of mortality (Utting 1989). Many drug misusers have physical problems (including cardiovascular disease, liver disease (chronic infection and cirrhosis), and chronic obstructive airways disease) that increase the risk of complications during general anaesthesia. Withdrawal treatments using opiate antagonists should not be offered to patients with a history of head injury or seizures (Bearn *et al.* 1999) and, where patients are co-dependent upon alcohol or benzodiazepines, there will be an increased risk of seizures.

Naltrexone has been shown to produce dose-related increases in transaminase levels and a serious potential side-effect is its hepatotoxicity (Maggio *et al.* 1985; Pfohl *et al.* 1986). Such effects may be of particular significance since many addicts have liver disease associated with viral hepatitis infections. Rates of hepatitis C infection were found among 86 per cent of patients attending a London methadone clinic (Best *et al.* 1999*b*). It is recommended that opiate addicts with liver failure should not be treated with naltrexone.

Caution should also apply to the use of general anaesthesia during withdrawal and especially to the use of such high doses of opiate antagonists. Deaths have occurred from cardiac arrest during detoxification involving naltrexone given under benzodiazepine-induced sedation (Brewer 1993) and subsequent to the use of naloxone to reverse opiate effects in non-addicts (Andree 1980). Life-threatening atypical reactions to the high doses of antagonists given in this treatment have also been reported (San *et al.* 1995). At present, it is questionable whether the uncertain benefits of the procedure justify its use other than in a research setting (Strang *et al.* 1997*a*).

Detoxification from benzodiazepines and sedatives

Dependence upon sedative hypnotics may be found as part of a pattern of polydrug use (often with co-dependence upon heroin or other opiates). Typically, dependent users take very high doses of sedative hypnotics. During the 1970s, barbiturates and methaqualone were the drugs of choice for many addicts seeking treatment (Gossop and Connell 1975). Barbiturate dependence is currently seen only infrequently, but benzodiazepines are widely used by many drug users who present to treatment (Fountain *et al.* 1999).

Among the clients in NTORS (National Treatment Outcome Research Study), 33–43 per cent (depending on treatment modality) were regular users of benzodiazepines (Gossop *et al.* 1998*b*). In a survey of drug users from clinics in seven British cities, Strang *et al.* (1994*a*) found that temazepam and diazepam were the most frequently used benzodiazepines, with temazepam capsules being the most likely forms of the drug to be used by injection. In a study of opiate-dependent drug users admitted to an in-patient treatment unit, Davison and Gossop (1996) found that almost half (42 per cent) were also co-dependent upon benzodiazepines.

Benzodiazepines and barbiturates work at receptor sites and enhance the inhibitory effects of the neurotransmitter GABA (gamma-aminobutyric acid) throughout all parts of the CNS. Both types of drugs have complex neuro-physiological effects, and other neurotransmitters and neuromodulators may be involved. Both types of drugs are readily absorbed after oral or parenteral administration, and both can produce euphoric effects.

Barbiturate withdrawal was first described in 1905, 2 years after barbiturates were introduced into medical practice. Withdrawal may begin within 12–24 hours after the final dose, though withdrawal symptoms may appear later with longer-acting barbiturates. The symptoms are similar to those of alcohol withdrawal and include anxiety, tremors, insomnia, delirium, and seizures.

Detoxification from sedative-hypnotics is generally best conducted in an in-patient setting. Ghodse (1995) suggested that out-patient detoxification is seldom appropriate for these patients, who are unlikely to comply with out-patient programmes, and who are at risk of suffering serious withdrawal phenomena such as convulsions or toxic confusional states. The greatest concern with barbiturate withdrawal is often to prevent grand mal seizures. Substitution and gradual reduction of phenobarbitone has been widely used for many years in the management of detoxification among barbiturate-dependent patients (Blachly 1964). If convulsions occur during (or subsequent to) sedative detoxification, this may indicate that prescribed doses are too low, or that the rate of withdrawal is too rapid. In such cases, intramuscular injection of sodium amylobarbitone may be given (Ghodse 1995).

Patients receiving detoxification from barbiturates (or other other hypnotic sedatives) should be discouraged from discharging themselves during any phase of sedative withdrawal. A minimum period of 2–3 days observation in hospital is generally recommended before the patient is discharged after detoxification from sedatives in case there are delayed withdrawal responses.

The clinical manifestations of the benzodiazepine abstinence syndrome are also similar to those of other sedatives including barbiturates and alcohol, though there are some differences in time course and symptom severity. Early descriptions of benzodiazepine withdrawal were given by Tyrer *et al.* (1981) and Petursson and Lader (1984).

For many benzodiazepines, the half-life is substantially longer than for the majority of sedatives, the reduction of the drug in blood levels is more gradual, and the abstinence syndrome tends to appear around the third to the sixth day after discontinuation of the drug. For benzodiazepines such as lorazepam that are rapidly eliminated from the body, withdrawal symptoms appear at an earlier stage.

In its most minor form, benzodiazepine-dependent patients may experience little more than anxiety, apprehension, dizziness, and insomnia during withdrawal. These symptoms were found among virtually all of the patients studied by Petursson and Lader (1984). Where patients present with low-dose benzodiazepine dependence, no special treatment is required, and it is likely that most will experience only mild to moderate withdrawal symptoms, which disappear after a few days to weeks. During early abstinence, patients should be given support and reassurance that the withdrawal effects are common and that they will soon reduce or disappear.

Among more severely dependent benzodiazepine users, withdrawal may include anxiety-related psychological, physiological, and perceptual symptoms (Marks 1985*a*). Psychological and physiological manifestations of anxiety are found in the majority of patients during detoxification, with hyperacuity and other physical disturbances in about half the patients: perceptual distortions are found in less than a quarter of the withdrawal responses (Petursson and Lader 1984).

Psychological symptoms may include irritability, feelings of tension, agitation, restlessness, difficulties of concentration, feelings of foreboding, or panic attacks. Physiological symptoms may include tremor, shakiness, headache, muscle twitching, muscle aches, profuse sweating, palpitations, and insomnia. Benzodiazepine withdrawal may also include perceptual distortions such as hyperacuity to light, sound, touch, and smell. In some cases the person may have impaired memory, and feelings of depersonalization and derealization, or even psychotic reactions with hallucinations and paranoid ideation. In its most severe form the benzodiazepine abstinence syndrome may include seizures (Hallstrom and Lader 1981; Tyrer *et al.* 1981).

Four strategies are often used to withdraw dependent users from sedative–hypnotics. The choice of withdrawal method is likely to reflect the particular drug of dependence, the co-occurrence of other dependent drug use, and the clinical setting in which treatment is provided. The four strategies are:

◆ gradually tapering doses of the drug of dependence;

◆ substitution and gradual reduction of phenobarbitone or some other long-acting barbiturate;

◆ substitution with a long-acting benzodiazepine, such as chlordiazepoxide, which is then reduced over 1–2 weeks;

◆ treatment of withdrawal with valproate or carbamazepine.

Phenobarbitone substitution is widely used in the management of withdrawal from many sedative–hypnotic drugs, including benzodiazepines. The pharmacological rationale for phenobarbitone substitution is that phenobarbitone is long-acting and blood levels of phenobarbitone do not change greatly between doses, allowing the safe use of gradually reducing daily doses (Smith and Wesson 1999). Signs of toxicity (such as ataxia, slurred speech, and sustained nystagmus) are easily observed, and lethal doses are many times higher than toxic doses. Since phenobarbitone is excreted primarily by the kidneys and is not toxic to the liver, it can used with patients who have liver disease.

Although withdrawal from sedative–hypnotics has been treated with antipsychotic drugs (e.g. phenothiazines) in low doses or with tricyclic antidepressants, such drugs lower the threshold for convulsions and are best avoided.

Detoxification from stimulants

Unquestionably, some users can become seriously dependent upon stimulants in the sense that they may experience strong, and sometimes overpowering urges to use these drugs, which is reflected in an impaired capacity to control their drug-taking behaviour. There continues to be some uncertainty about whether stimulant drugs such as cocaine and amphetamines should be regarded as having a true withdrawal syndrome.

Some authors have offered extensive and florid descriptions of amphetamine withdrawal (Russo 1968). Others state that psychostimulant drugs such as the amphetamines do not produce stereotyped withdrawal symptoms (Morgan 1981). Smith (1969) states that 'high dose amphetamine use . . . can produce a moderate degree of physical dependence and classic withdrawal reactions lasting two to four days', but *Meyler's side effects of drugs* states merely that 'signs of physical dependence are not considered to occur' (Nir 1980). Amphetamine withdrawal has been described as painful and even as potentially life-threatening by some authors (Russo 1969), but as 'mild' by others (Jones and Jones 1977). There is no shortage of opinion, and confident, if contradictory assertions on this subject. As is often the case, this is due, at least partly to the scarcity of empirical evidence about stimulant withdrawal.

One view is that, although some stimulant withdrawal responses occur, these are not serious and do not require treatment with medication. Connell (1958) described amphetamine withdrawal symptoms as being 'few and mainly of little moment but the most important is depression'. Washton (1987) suggested that, although some regular cocaine users may experience a generalized dysphoria coupled with sleep and appetite disturbance for several days after stopping cocaine, 'unlike the heroin addict or severe alcoholic, the cocaine abuser generally requires no substitute medication and no gradual withdrawal regime.'

Long-term and regular stimulant use may lead to neuroadaptive changes and to subsequent withdrawal responses on discontinuation of stimulant use. Because of the failure of many patients to respond adequately to psychological treatments, clinicians and researchers have tried a number of pharmacological agents, including lithium, tricyclic antidepressants, stimulants, and dopamine agonists and neurotransmitter precursors (Gawin and Kleber 1984; Kosten 1992).

The rationale for using tricyclic antidepressants (TCAs) such as desipramine is that, since dopamine appears to mediate the acute euphoric effects of cocaine, the dysphoria after long-term cocaine use could be due to homeostatic adaptations in the dopaminergic system that might be reversed by these drugs. Desipramine affects both dopamine and catecholamine receptors and has fewer anticholinergic side-effects than other drugs with similar receptor effects (Kosten 1992). In both open and double-blind trials, cocaine-dependent patients have achieved abstinence from cocaine and shown reduced craving after high doses (starting at 50 mg and increasing to as high as 200 mg by the fourth day) of desipramine (Gawin *et al.*1989). As would be expected with desipramine, some effects were delayed, with the drug usually taking full effect after the second or third week. However, studies of the efficacy of desipramine have yielded mixed results (Kosten 1992). Where TCAs are used, blood pressure and cardiac rhythm should be carefully monitored.

When the regular user stops taking amphetamines, several withdrawal responses may occur. Some of these appear to be rebound-type effects that are opposite to the drug effects, such as lethargy, tiredness and depression. It has also been suggested that the changes in sleep patterns following withdrawal of amphetamines may be explained in terms of tiredness or exhaustion after prolonged stimulant abuse (Gawin and Kleber 1986).

However, although hypersomnia (excessive sleeping) is often reported as a withdrawal symptom after giving up regular stimulant use, abstinence after regular use of amphetamines can lead to more complex and prolonged disruption of sleep patterns. In a study of withdrawal responses among amphetamine misusers, Gossop *et al.* (1982*a*) monitored sleep patterns during a 20-day period. Although there was an initial period of oversleeping, this was not followed by a return to a normal sleep pattern. Instead there followed a period during which the total amount of sleep time was reduced. Typically this involved day-time drowsiness and night-time wakefulness. It was not clear how long this phase of reduced sleep lasted, since it was still evident on the twentieth night with no signs of a return to normal levels of sleep when data collection ceased.

Sleep difficulties are one of the more distressing symptoms of drug withdrawal and may aggravate other problems, such as depressed mood. Where drug users are bothered by sleep difficulties after discontinuation of stimulant use, there may be some merit in considering the prescription of night-time sedation, especially where detoxification occurs in a residential or supervised setting.

A survey of physician members of the American Society of Addiction Medicine asked for views about the usefulness of pharmacotherapies for cocaine treatment (Halikas *et al.* 1993). Five hundred and two physicians reported using medications with approximately 80 000 patients for cocaine detoxification, and with about 37 000 patients for abstinence-oriented treatment. For both types of treatment, the four most commonly prescribed medications were amantadine, bromocriptine, desipramine, and l-tryptophan.

Dopamine (DA) neurotransmission plays an important role in the development and maintenance of stimulant dependence (Gold and Miller 1992), and the early phase of psychostimulant withdrawal is characterized by a depressive state that includes fatigue, depressed mood, anhedonia, and psychomotor retardation.

These symptoms are consistent with DA hypoactivity within the mesolimbic system (Imperato *et al.* 1992; Rossetti *et al.* 1992; Weiss *et al.* 1992). Dopamine agonists such as amantadine and bromocriptine have been used to treat stimulant withdrawal and have been found to reduce cocaine use and craving (Tennant and Sagherian 1987). Other clinical trials with dopamine agonists and antagonists have found that such agents have only limited efficacy (Withers *et al.* 1995). At this time, no pharmacotherapies have established themselves as of proven value for the effective treatment of stimulant withdrawal.

Other non-pharmacological detoxification treatments for stimulants have been tried, though with little research to support their effectiveness. Some services provide auricular (ear) acupuncture as a treatment for stimulant withdrawal. In a single-blind placebo study, 150 individuals seeking treatment for cocaine/crack abuse were randomly allocated to receive either experimental or placebo acupuncture treatments (Lipton *et al.* 1994). Treatments were provided in an out-patient setting over a 1-month period. Both groups showed reduced cocaine consumption and treatment retention was similar for both groups. Those who received 'active' acupuncture achieved better outcomes as shown by urinalysis results.

Multiple drug detoxification

It is common for drug users seeking treatment to present with dependencies upon several drugs that require some sort of clinical detoxification. The most common multiple dependencies that require clinical management during withdrawal involve combinations of two or more of the opiates, benzo-diazepines, alcohol, and stimulants. This issue of multiple dependencies and multiple detoxification treatments is one that confronts clinicians every day, but there is little in the literature to indicate how these problems such be treated nor whether such treatments should be delivered simultaneously or consecutively. In view of the importance of these questions, it is surprising that the topic has received little research attention.

Unless there are good reasons to do otherwise, a good general principle is to withdraw the less problematic drug(s) first, and subsequently to tackle the more problematic drug. Where it is necessary to provide some detoxification treatment for stimulant co-dependence, this can generally be done first. Similarly, where a heroin addict is co-dependent upon alcohol, it has been our clinical practice (in an in-patient setting) first to withdraw them from alcohol (with chlordiazepoxide over about 7 days) and then from opiates. Where a heroin addict is co-dependent upon benzodiazepines he or she is generally withdrawn first from opiates and then from benzodiazepines. Where patients are co-dependent upon extremely high doses of benzodiazepines (e.g. dose equivalents of 60 mg or more of diazepam) this may be reduced on a schedule of up to 21 days. In those cases where a withdrawal from opiates, alcohol, and benzodiazepines is required, the drugs are withdrawn in the order, alcohol, then opiates, then benzodiazepines.

Where patients are dependent upon both cocaine and opiates and require pharmacological management of withdrawal responses to both types of drugs, this may create problems due to the opposing pharmacological effects of tricyclic antidepressants and the alpha-2 adrenergic agonists (such as lofexidine and clonidine). These medications have opposite effects upon the noradrenergic system that may interfere with, or even cancel, the effectiveness of either or both drugs (Keaney *et al.* 2002).

Many drug addicts are also heavy and often excessive drinkers, and co-dependence upon alcohol is a common clinical issue (Gossop *et al.* 2002*c*). Where drug misusers are physically dependent upon alcohol, they will experience significant physiological disturbance when they stop drinking. As with other substances, alcohol dependence and rebound withdrawal are distributed along a continuum. Some drinkers will show mild or moderate degrees of dependence and will experience only moderate discomfort during withdrawal, which can be managed in a straightforward manner. This may entail out-patient treatment and relatively low levels of medication. In some cases, no medication may be required. Edwards *et al.* (1997) suggest that few patients with a primary dependence upon alcohol require medication with a benzodiazepine for more than 2 days, and that withdrawal regimes of longer than 7–10 days are rarely if ever necessary for uncomplicated alcohol withdrawal. However, where the individual is dually (or multiply) dependent upon alcohol and upon other drugs, it is unlikely that withdrawal will be uncomplicated.

Where individuals present with high levels of dependence upon alcohol, stopping drinking may precipitate severe withdrawal symptoms. In extreme cases, alcohol withdrawal can precipitate forms of life-threatening disturbance.

Trembling is one of the most common alcohol withdrawal symptoms and may occur after a drinking bout lasting a few days. In a mild form it often occurs among chronic drinkers in the morning before the first drink of the day. In more severe cases, increasing tremor appears 12–24 hours after the last drink, and is often accompanied by restlessness, agitation, and insomnia. The tremor is promptly relieved by further drinking. Auditory hallucinations ('hearing voices') sometimes occur within a few days of alcohol abstinence, though these are uncommon and are usually associated with severe withdrawal. Sounds that start as buzzing or ringing in the ears can evolve into delusional voices often saying unpleasant or accusatory things.

The most severe form of alcohol withdrawal is delirium tremens. The complete syndrome is a serious condition that develops 2–5 days after alcohol abstinence. Its onset is often abrupt, but may be preceded by increasing restlessness and feelings of apprehension, and nightmares. Its onset is often at night. Once the condition is established, it tends to be associated with restlessness and agitation, fear increasing to panic, confusion, disorientation, and hallucinations. Delirium tremens usually subsides in 2–3 days but has a significant morbidity and mortality due to injuries sustained during periods of confusion, and from dehydration, hypothermia, and pneumonia (Royal College of Physicians 1987).

A number of different drugs can be used to manage alcohol withdrawal. Minor tranquillizers such as the benzodiazepines (and especially chlordiazepoxide) and chlormethiazole are among the most widely used. In severe cases of alcohol withdrawal, it may be necessary to use substantial doses. For example, doses of 40–60 mg of chlordiazepoxide, three or four times a day (or possibly even more than this), may be required (Edwards *et al.* 1997). Where there is an immediate need to bring severe symptoms under control, drugs such as lorazepam may be given by intramuscular injection, or diazepam by slow intravenous injection.

Where a drug-dependent patient presents with a co-dependence upon benzodiazepines and alcohol, detoxification can be managed by means of substitution and gradually reducing doses of a long-acting benzodiazepine such as chlordiazepoxide. For patients who are dependent upon both benzodiazepines and alcohol, withdrawal responses tend to differ from those of a simple alcohol dependence and are more similar to those of benzodiazepine dependence (Benzer and Cushman 1980). Where patients are co-dependent upon benzodiazepines and alcohol, this affects the prescribing of benzodiazepines as a withdrawal treatment, not least because of the increased levels of tolerance to the benzodiazepines themselves. In such cases, phenobarbitone substitution can also be used to withdraw those who are dependent on multiple sedative–hypnotics, including alcohol.

Withdrawal seizures constitute one of the most severe physical problems that can occur during alcohol withdrawal. These are usually encountered 12–48 hours after alcohol abstinence and are sometimes a portent of delirium tremens. Where the user is dependent upon alcohol and upon other drugs, and particularly upon benzodiazepines or related drugs, the risk of seizures is increased and will also be more difficult to manage. Where such patients present in acute and severe withdrawal, or if they have had or are judged to be at risk of withdrawal seizures, an intramuscular injection of phenobarbitone may be administered (Smith and Wesson 1999).

Where drug users are dependent upon more than one substance that requires treatment for the associated withdrawal syndromes, there are advantages to providing treatment in an in-patient setting. This helps to provide a suitable setting for the medically safe treatment of complicated withdrawal states where there are multiple dependencies. Treatment in an in-patient setting allows more intensive medical supervision and control of withdrawal symptoms. It also is more likely to lead to abstinence (Gossop *et al.* 1986), not only for the 'main' drug of dependence, but also for other drugs (including alcohol) upon which the patient may dependent. It can also provide a useful first phase of an integrated treatment programme in which patients are returned to out-patient care in a drug-free state and ready for relapse prevention treatments (Chutuape *et al.* 1999).

Psychological components of withdrawal

Drug withdrawal syndromes are powerfully influenced by neurophysiological and neurochemical processes, and physiological symptoms such as abdominal cramps, diarrhoea, and muscle spasms are a prominent feature of the (opiate) withdrawal syndrome. In addition, detoxification often involves the administration of drugs. Partly for these reasons, detoxification is often seen primarily in physical terms, and treatment has been seen primarily as a 'medical' procedure.

Detoxification should not be seen as merely a 'physical' treatment. There is considerable evidence of the impact that social and psychological factors have upon the withdrawal syndrome. Physiologically based withdrawal symptoms also have psychological effects. Insomnia is a common symptom of withdrawal from many types of drugs. Gossop *et al.* (1982) described the prolonged sleep disruption that followed discontinuation of amphetamines with reductions in total sleep time and increases in night-time waking (Gossop and Bradley 1984). Lack of sleep is distressing for most people and, at times of particular stress such as during detoxification, it may sap the individual's motivation to change and commitment to treatment.

The manner in which an addict responds to drug withdrawal is powerfully influenced by psychological factors. Many addicts report feeling frightened of the prospect of withdrawal, and the anxieties and expectations of the addict have been found to be important determinants of the severity of the withdrawal symptoms that the addict experiences during detoxification. This finding has direct clinical implications. Anxiety-related factors, for example, increase the severity of the withdrawal response, and can have a more powerful influence upon withdrawal symptoms than the dose of heroin upon which the addict was dependent prior to detoxification (Phillips *et al.* 1986). It has been found that telling people what sensations they can expect during painful stimulation can reduce the distress that is experienced (Johnson 1973). Providing information about dental treatment to reduce uncertainty or false expectations has been found to be useful in reducing anxieties about dental treatment (Lindsay 1983).

Psychological interventions can play a valuable role even during such an apparently 'medical' or 'physical' phase of treatment as detoxification. Psychological procedures that reduce fears and anxieties about withdrawal could be expected to reduce withdrawal symptomatology. Providing addicts with accurate but reassuring information about withdrawal can alter the nature of the withdrawal response (Green and Gossop 1988). Opiate addicts who had been informed of the nature and severity of their probable responses to detoxification experienced lower peak withdrawal scores, and showed lower levels of residual withdrawal symptoms after a methadone reduction schedule than a non-informed group of heroin addicts. In addition, the informed group was more likely to complete the detoxification programme.

Chapter 8

Psychological treatments

A range of treatments based upon the assumptions, theories, and research traditions of psychology has been developed within the general ambit of behaviour therapy or behaviour modification. Kazdin (1978) described five general characteristics that are common, if not universal, among these psychological treatments:

- a focus upon current rather than historical determinants of behaviour;
- reliance upon psychological research as a source of hypotheses about treatment and therapy techniques;
- specificity in defining, measuring, and treating the target problems;
- explicit description of treatment procedures in objective terms;
- emphasis upon overt changes in behaviour as the main criteria for treatment effectiveness.

These psychological treatments for addiction are also largely based upon research into the processes of learning. As such, they further assume that drug problems and drug dependence are substantially influenced by normal learning processes, that addictive behaviour is functional for the drug users, and that, as a learned behaviour, addictive behaviour can be modified or 'unlearned'.

Clinical behaviour therapy initially developed as a neobehaviouristic stimulus–response approach, based on the application of conditioning principles and procedures (Wolpe 1969). Within its initial formulations, cognitions were seen as being unimportant or subordinate to conditioning processes, and for many years the tension between stimulus–response and cognitive theories was an important source of disagreement among learning theorists.

Recent developments in psychological treatments for addiction (and other) problems have been profoundly influenced by the work of Bandura (1977) and others who drew attention to the importance of 'cognitive' factors in learning. Nonetheless, an important feature of social-learning theory is that, while cognitive mechanisms are increasingly used to explain the acquisition, regulation, and modification of behaviour, many of the most potent methods for therapeutic change appear to be performance-based. This is an important distinction. The earlier neglect of cognitive variables by some strict behaviourists may have restricted the scope and efficacy of their treatment interventions. The tendency of some cognitive therapists to rely unduly upon symbolic rather than behavioural methods runs the risk of returning to the type of 'talking treatment' that the introduction of behaviour therapy originally did much to improve upon (Wilson 1980). Within social learning theory, although cognitions are important, performance is paramount (Franks and Barbrack 1991).

Since its formal beginnings in the 1950s and 1960s, the range of behavioural therapies has expanded and diversified. This is reflected in the variety of different techniques that are now used, and that are variously referred to as behaviour therapy, behaviour modification, behavioural medicine, cognitive behaviour therapy, cognitive therapy, and psychosocial treatment. Despite the differing procedures (and titles), it has been suggested that these behavioural treatments do not differ in fundamental respects, but represent a set of procedures that are characterized by the application of behavioural science principles within a broadly conceived learning theory framework (Franks and Barbrack 1991).

Conditioning and deconditioning

Pavlov demonstrated that animals can acquire responses to contextual stimuli that have been previously associated with the onset of drug effects. The clinical implications of this were recognized by Abraham Wikler (1948) who provided the first explicit statement of the important role of conditioning factors in the development and maintenance of drug addiction. Animals were known to increase their rate of operant responding when this was followed by intravenous opiates, CNS stimulants, or sedatives. Wikler proposed that drug-related behaviours and objects became secondary reinforcers as a result of their repeated pairings with the primary drug-related reinforcement. It was recognized that the self-administration of heroin (or other drugs) became associated with many environmental variables, such as the sight and smell of the drug itself, the rituals surrounding drug taking, drug-using peers, dealers, and specific locations, and that these may also acquire the properties of discriminative stimuli in operant conditioning. Drug-seeking and drug-taking behaviours are powerfully reinforced on thousands of occasions during the course of a person's drug-using career.

The stimuli that are regularly associated with withdrawal symptoms can also acquire conditioned aversive properties (Kumar and Stolerman 1977). Wikler (1980) suggested that the high relapse rate among addicts could be due to incomplete extinction of both positive and negative secondary reinforcers. This is consistent with the comments of addicts who have described a craving for drugs when they visited places associated with buying or using drugs.

Another line of conditioning research led to what has been referred to as the opponent-process explanation of tolerance. This Pavlovian model suggests that conditioned responses to drugs can be opposite in direction to the unconditioned effects. When the usual cues for drug administration are presented without the drug, there is an enhancement of compensatory conditioned responses (Siegel 1983). With the gradual increase in the strength of the conditioned responses, the unconditioned drug effect decreases leading to the build-up of tolerance. Tolerance is also influenced by prior experiences related to the environment in which drug administration occurs, as well as to the drug effects. In these respects, tolerance shares many similarities with other memory or learning processes. Both tolerance and learning are retained over long periods of time and both are disrupted by electroconvulsive shock, frontal cortical stimulation, and metabolic inhibitors (Siegel 1979).

There is an apparent contradiction between these two conditioning accounts. In Wikler's theory the conditioned response is similar to the observed drug effect. In Siegel's account the conditioned response is the opposite of the drug effect. Eikelboom and Stewart (1982) suggested that these apparently contradictory predictions may be due to a misunderstanding about the unconditioned stimulus and unconditioned response in the drug conditioning paradigm. Drug administration does not necessarily serve as the unconditioned stimulus. Nor is the observed drug effect necessarily the unconditioned response. Eikelboom and Stewart suggested that a drug should be considered to be an unconditioned stimulus only when it acts on the afferent arm of the CNS, and that only those drug effects that are CNS-mediated physiological reactions should qualify as unconditioned responses.

Several attempts have been made to apply conditioning principles to the behavioural treatment of dependence disorders. These include: (1) attempts to reduce the strength of drug-related conditioned stimuli (CS) through classical extinction (repeated presentation of the CS not followed by drug administration) also commonly referred to as cue exposure; (2) counter-conditioning of other responses to the same drug-related CS.

Cue exposure and the treatment of craving

Cue exposure methods have attracted a good deal of attention in recent years and have been advocated as a potentially effective means of treating addictive behaviours (Heather and Bradley 1990). The rationale most often cited for using cue exposure to treat addictive behaviours is based on a classical conditioning model of learning, in which the drug is the unconditioned stimulus, and the drug effects are the unconditioned responses. The circumstances surrounding the use of drugs become conditioned stimuli that are capable of evoking conditioned responses that moderate or mediate drug seeking and drug consumption (Conklin and Tiffany 2002).

Drug use and relapse are often strongly cue- and context-specific (Drummond *et al.* 1995). When an addict encounters drug-related cues, such as meeting other users, seeing drugs or drug paraphernalia, or going to places or contexts in which drugs have been taken, these can produce urges to take drugs, withdrawal-like symptoms, and drug-seeking behaviour. One heroin addict (Sharples 1975) noted that, as part of his recovery, 'In practice I had to avoid the company of other addicts, for their presence and conversation was . . . the strongest stimulus of all . . . Equally there were whole areas, geographical and social, financial and cultural, which overlapped with the junk community and which I had to avoid.'

Conditioned euphoria may occur in the presence of drug-related cues (O'Brien *et al.* 1974). The abstinence syndrome can also be conditioned as a response to specific environmental stimuli in both animals and man (Wikler 1980). Both unconditioned and conditioned drug effects can act as reinforcers (Stewart *et al.* 1984). Equally, it has been found that both conditioned agonist effects and conditioned withdrawal are extinguished following repeated exposure of the conditioned stimuli in the absence of the original (unconditioned) stimulus (Siegel 1983). Cocaine addicts show significant decreases in subjective and physiological reactivity to cocaine-related stimuli following systematic non-reinforced exposure to drug cues (O'Brien *et al.* 1990), though autonomic responses have been found to show weaker levels of extinction than self-report (O'Brien *et al.* 1990).

Typically, cue-exposure treatments involve repeated unreinforced exposure to drug-related stimuli in an attempt to extinguish conditioned responses to such cues. This technique has been utilized in treatments for users of opiates, cocaine, alcohol, and nicotine. In the clinical setting, the application of cue exposure has generally involved exposing drug misusers to personally relevant drug cues that have been assessed as being likely to provoke craving and drug use. This exposure may be *in vivo* (handling drug paraphernalia). Opiate addicts have been exposed to the same drug-related cues that they would encounter in real life, such as needles and syringes and the drugs themselves (Childress *et al.* 1984, 1986; McLellan *et al.* 1986). Exposure may also involve using symbolic or cognitive cues (imagining being offered drugs, or looking at photographs or videotapes of drug taking) in the absence of drug ingestion.

In their day to day life, addicts are likely to be confronted by various stimuli that have been conditioned to different aspects of their drug-taking behaviours. These conditioned stimuli will elicit conditioned responses that in turn are likely to lead to drug seeking and drug taking (Powell *et al.* 1993) and that may be experienced by the user as 'craving'. Cue-exposure treatments have sometimes been seen specifically as treatments to reduce craving.

The term 'craving' has been criticized as being poorly defined, and has provoked considerable debate over many years. Half a century ago, a World Health Organization expert committee concluded that the term 'should not be used in the scientific literature . . . if confusion is to be avoided.' The confusion surrounding the term has been exacerbated by the lack of any agreed definition and by the way that it has been indiscriminately used to refer to different physiological, psychological, and behavioural states. Isbell (1955) suggested that it was unhelpful and, indeed, tautologous to suggest that craving may be both an integral part of the relapse to drug taking as well as a cause of that relapse. In addition, the term was criticized on the grounds that it is overloaded with connotations and assumptions from outdated theories of addiction in which the disease model and physical dependence models of addiction played a more prominent role than they do today. The WHO committee tended towards the view that craving could be seen in psychiatric terms, as a neurotic state or as one linked to an underlying personality disorder (Isbell 1955). Duchene (1955), for example, suggested that 'almost all cases of alcoholism derive from neurotic personality disturbances.'

Despite the problems that have surrounded the term, 'craving' has shown a remarkable persistence, and the issues that prompted the deliberations of 1955 expert committee on craving re-emerged more than 30 years later in a debate in the *British Journal of Addiction*. Kozlowski and Wilkinson (1987) argued that the mismatch between the current technical use of the term and its use in ordinary language was so great that it should be avoided, a position that was supported by Hughes (1987). Kozlowski and Wilkinson's concerns were similar to those of the 1955 WHO expert committee, as was their suggestion that craving should be replaced by the more cautious and prosaic phrase 'strong desire'. Mardones (1955) had previously suggested that craving could be defined as 'an urgent and overpowering desire'.

Others have been more positive about the value of the term. Marlatt (1987), for example, suggested that craving can be a useful term because it so precisely captures the essence of addiction in terms of its compulsive qualities. It also appears to be a useful concept for addicts who seem to understand what they mean by it, often report experiencing it prior to using, and during recovery, and are able to rate its strength in clinical studies (O'Brien and Childress 1991). As Stockwell (1987) pointed out, there have been no better alternatives that have proved capable of replacing 'craving'.

What is necessary is a clear and explicit separation of three different issues:

1 craving as a phenomenon in its own right;

2 the mechanisms underlying or leading to craving;

3 craving as an explanatory construct.

The failure to distinguish between these three levels of discourse has been a principal cause of confusion, and of dissatisfaction with the term. Quite apart from any question of whether they are correct or not, it is necessary to treat differently such statements as 'we can define craving for alcohol as an urgent an overpowering desire to drink' (level 1: Mardones 1955), 'the best formulation for the phenomenon of craving is a psychiatric one' (level 2: Isbell 1955), and 'craving may be equated with the tendency to relapse after a period of abstinence' (level 3: Isbell 1955).

Cue exposure has been used for the treatment of different types of drug misuse. In work with methadone-maintained opiate addicts, Childress *et al.* (1984, 1988) demonstrated habituation of subjective craving, with improved clinical outcomes at follow-up among those who received cue-exposure treatments. In other studies of drug users who were dependent upon cocaine, Childress *et al.* (1988) showed significant responses to cocaine-related cues after 28 days of cue-exposure treatment. However, such effects do not always transfer readily to a clinical setting. In a randomized clinical trial of cue-exposure treatments for heroin addicts, Dawe *et al.* (1993) found that cue exposure provided in six sessions over a period of 3 weeks produced no more improvement in outcomes than a standard treatment-as-usual condition. The cue-exposure group and the standard treatment group showed substantial but similar levels of reductions in cue reactivity after treatment.

In addition, drug- and alcohol-related cues do not reliably lead to conditioned responses. Avants *et al.* (1995) found that about one-third of their cocaine-dependent patients showed no craving response to drug-related cues, and a further 16 per cent of those who did respond to such cues showed no increase in their levels of craving. Similarly, Rohsenow *et al.* (1992) found that one-third of alcoholics did not report an increased urge to drink in a laboratory-based, cue-exposure situation. In another study, as many as 40–50 per cent of alcoholics exhibited no elicited response to alcohol cues (Litt *et al.* 1990). Subjective and physiological reactivity to drug-related cues has been found to vary both within and across studies (Modesto-Lowe and Kranzler 1999).

Another issue is whether cue reactivity predicts future substance use behaviours. In a study of cue exposure with heroin addicts, Powell *et al.* (1993) found that there was no relationship between any of the measures of craving that were taken prior to and after the cue-exposure treatment and posttreatment drug use outcomes. Drummond and Glautier (1994) found that cue exposure was more effective than relaxation training, not in preventing relapse but in reducing drinking after an initial lapse, and prolonging the time of progression to heavy drinking. Despite its sound theoretical base, the literature remains somewhat inconsistent both with regard to the extent to which cues elicit craving responses, and in the relationship of cue reactivity to subsequent substance use.

Conklin and Tiffany (2002) reviewed 18 cue-exposure addiction treatment studies. This meta-analysis provided little evidence to support the effectiveness of cue exposure for the treatment of addiction. However, its proponents suggest that cue exposure continues to have potential merit if the optimal parameters could be identified (choice of the most appropriate cues, a sufficient number of treatment sessions, its combined use with some other form of psychotherapy).

Aversion therapies

Other sorts of behaviour therapies for addiction problems have been based upon the principle of counterconditioning. One of the earliest, crudest, and probably least promising, of the behaviour therapy treatments for drug addiction involves aversive conditioning. It is, perhaps, unfortunate that this is one of the forms of behaviour therapy that is best known to the general public. Such treatments have often involved pairing incompatible or aversive consequences with specific stimuli associated with the use of drugs.

Some of the earliest counterconditioning studies attempted to establish a conditioned aversion to drugs or alcohol, or to whatever undesired behaviour the person had become addicted. Both chemical and electrical forms of aversion therapy were being used to treat alcoholics as early as the 1930s. Voegtlin (1940) used chemically induced nausea in the treatment of alcoholics and claimed an abstinence rate of more than 60 per cent after 1 year. In a later study, Wiens et al. (1976) also reported a 63 per cent abstinence rate. In contrast, however, Wallerstein (1956) found that only 4 per cent of the alcoholics treated with chemical aversion therapy achieved abstinence.

The variability in outcome rates subsequent to the use of electrically based procedures has been equally great. Vogler et al. (1975) reported an 80 per cent reduction in alcohol consumption among alcoholics in a multimodel programme who received electrical aversion compared with 41 per cent in a control condition without aversion therapy. Miller (1978), on the other hand, found no difference between the effectiveness of behavioural treatment programmes with and without an electrical aversion component. There have also been several small case studies of electrical aversion with opiate addicts (e.g. Teasdale 1973). Overall, these studies have not offered convincing evidence of its value in the treatment of drug addiction.

Although behavioural treatment approaches have sometimes been thought of as equating to the use of aversion therapies, such treatments have seldom been used in standard clinical practice, and they are extremely rare in current treatment programmes. Indeed, most clinical programmes have never used such techniques. Interest in such methods has tended to be confined largely to academic researchers. Although there was some early interest in aversion therapy methods, this initial enthusiasm declined, both for ethical reasons and because they proved to be ineffective (Rachman and Teasdale 1969; Hodgson 1972). The stressful and sometimes painful nature of these treatments, their high drop-out rates, and the lack of evidence of their effectiveness provide good reasons for not using such methods.

An alternative form of aversion therapy has involved *covert conditioning*, or *covert sensitization*, in which thoughts of the unwanted behaviour are paired in imagination with unpleasant stimuli (e.g. arrest, humiliation). Hedberg and Campbell (1974) compared covert sensitization with several other treatments in a trial with alcoholic patients. They found that electrical aversion therapy was the least effective of the treatments but that covert sensitization was also relatively ineffective and led to lower rates of improvement than either systematic desensitization or behavioural family therapy. Telch *et al.* (1984) found covert sensitization to be less effective than supportive group therapy in the treatment of alcoholics. Again, despite some early enthusiasm, this approach is also of uncertain efficacy and is not widely used.

Contingency management

The theoretical foundations for contingency management are based upon the principles of operant conditioning rather than those of classical conditioning. The principles of operant conditioning suggest that addictive behaviour, like other forms of behaviour, is maintained by environmental and other reinforcers and that it can, therefore, be changed by altering the consequences.

Contingency management provides a system of incentives and disincentives that are designed to make continued drug use less attractive and abstinence more attractive. As described by Stitzer *et al.* (1989), contingency management 'organizes treatment delivery, sets specific objective behavioural goals, and attempts to structure the [drug user's] environment in a manner that is conducive to change'.

The first clinical applications of operant techniques were used with institutionalized psychiatric patients to change psychotic behaviour, such as violent acts, psychotic talk, and inappropriate eating behaviour. Cigarettes and praise were generally used as reinforcers, and the withdrawal of attention from the patient was used as a means of extinction. Ayllon and Azrin (1968) used vouchers as reinforcers to change patients' behaviour. These could be exchanged for other rewards and privileges, and this system came to be known as a *token economy*. This work was influential because it demonstrated that this sort of intervention could be used with patients (such as those with chronic schizophrenic illnesses) who had not previously been regarded as amenable to such approaches. More recently, it has been suggested that the effectiveness of the token system may also have been due to the feedback and specific behavioural guidance about behaviour change that were given at the same time as the tokens (Hall and Baker 1986). Structured social reinforcers such as praise and attention from the therapist have sometimes been used as alternatives to tokens (Hawton *et al.* 2000).

A basic principle in all forms of contingency management is that consequences are made contingent upon the individual's behaviour. Many different types of reinforcers could be used in contingency management programmes to promote a desirable change in behaviour. However, different studies have used a relatively limited number of different parameters in association with reinforcement. In addiction treatment programmes these have most often included changes in take-home methadone privileges (Iguchi *et al.* 1996), the offer of money or vouchers with a monetary value (Hall *et al.* 1979), and increases/decreases in methadone dosage (Stitzer *et al.* 1986). In a study of patients' preferences for different reinforcers, take-home doses and increases in methadone dose were rated as the ones most preferred (Chutuape *et al.* 1998). Monetary incentives have also been used to improve treatment outcome behaviours among drug-dependent patients (Silverman *et al.* 1996*b*). Few studies have been carried out on the relative impact of different types of reinforcers, and there is, at present, little evidence to suggest that preference for reinforcers is related to the effectiveness of that reinforcer in changing behaviour.

Another potentially important parameter involves the use of positive or negative reinforcement. In contingency management, positive reinforcement techniques reward patients for favourable changes in behaviour (such as reductions in illicit drug use). A different approach might use punishment such as a methadone dose decrease, rapid detoxification, or discharge from treatment as a result of a drug-positive urine. In some contingency management studies, a combination of both positive reinforcement and punishment has been used to help promote changes in behaviour, for example, by increasing dose levels of methadone in response to a negative urine screen or decreasing doses in response to a positive urine screen. All three types of incentive systems have yielded encouraging results, and only one study (Iguchi *et al.* 1988) has made direct comparisons showing that both incentives were equally efficacious in reducing drug use, although the use of positive incentives has been found to retain drug users in treatment for longer periods.

Contingency management has been found to be useful not only for extinguishing negative or undesirable behaviours such as continued polydrug drug or failure to comply with basic treatment standards, but also as a means of encouraging positive behaviours such as engagement with treatment services or good time-keeping. Some contingency management programmes have used positive reinforcement alone. Others have used mixed positive and negative reinforcement schedules. Many contingency management interventions have been conducted with patients in methadone treatment programmes. One reason for this is that, within methadone programmes, methadone or such features of methadone provision as dose level, dosing frequency, or the take-home option lend themselves readily for use as reinforcers.

Robles *et al.* (1999) suggest that the key features of a contingency management intervention include:

♦ the target behaviour that the treatment programme seeks to change (e.g. attending counselling sessions, producing drug-free urine specimens);

♦ the conditions (or antecedents) under which the target behaviours are to occur (e.g. attendance every Monday at a stated time with no reminders from programme staff);

♦ the reinforcer (e.g. one bus token);

♦ the contingency—specifies the rules according to which reinforcers are earned for producing the target behaviour (e.g. one bus token for each counselling session attended).

An extended programme of research into contingency management has been conducted by Stitzer and others at the Johns Hopkins University School of Medicine in Baltimore. This research has shown that contingency management techniques can be effective in reducing continued drug misuse among methadone patients (Strain *et al.* 1999), including their use of cocaine (Kidorf and Stitzer 1993; Silverman *et al.* 1996b), and benzodiazepines (Stitzer *et al.* 1982).

Incentives have been found to be effective in leading to increased attendance at counselling sessions. Methadone maintenance patients attended more counselling sessions when take-home methadone doses were contingent upon attendance than when they were offered non-contingently (Stitzer *et al.* 1977) or when none were offered (Kidorf *et al.* 1994). This may be a useful option where treatment attendance is of special importance. Jones *et al.* (2001) showed that a short-term contingency management programme led to increased full-day treatment attendance and abstinence from cocaine use among pregnant women in methadone programmes.

Vouchers have been found to be effective in reinforcing abstinence from cocaine among primary cocaine-dependent out-patients (Higgins *et al.* 1994). Patients were randomly assigned to a behavioural programme with, or without an added abstinence reinforcement component. The reinforcement programme provided vouchers that could be redeemed for goods and services contingent upon drug-free urines. The value of the initial vouchers was low (US$2.50) but this increased with consecutive cocaine-free urines. Patients in the voucher treatment group achieved more consecutive weeks of cocaine abstinence than the no-voucher group, and more of them remained in treatment. In a study in which cocaine-abusing methadone patients were randomly assigned to receive voucher reinforcement contingent on cocaine abstinence or to a control group, patients receiving contingent vouchers stayed abstinent from cocaine for longer than patients in the control group (Silverman *et al.* 1996*b*).

Contingency management has been found to be particularly useful as a treatment intervention for 'non-responsive' patients. For many years, addiction treatment services have been concerned about those patients who do not appear to get better as a result of their contact with treatment. Although methadone maintenance is effective for many patients in leading to reductions in illicit drug use, their use of illicit drugs is often not completely extinguished, and polydrug use is frequently found among many patients in such programmes. Other problems of non-responsiveness may also include criminality or continued use of risky injecting practices such as sharing needles or syringes. All programmes tend to have a number of patients who continue to be involved in these sorts of undesirable behaviours and for whom standard treatment components appear not to be effective.

A common response of treatment programmes has often been to use punitive measures, such as reducing methadone dosage, which tends to increase the dissatisfaction of the patient, and which may lead to a continuation or even an escalation of illicit drug use (Iguchi *et al.* 1988). All of which tends to increase the chances of the patient dropping out of treatment or even being discharged from treatment by the programme staff. The use of contingent rewards offers a more promising alternative. Even with otherwise unmotivated patients, a substantial number can be helped to give up drugs when the reward value is sufficiently increased. For example, Robles *et al.* (2000) found that combining a high-magnitude reinforcer (vouchers with a value of US$100) and a low response requirement (2 days of abstinence) yielded cocaine abstinence initiation in approximately 80 per cent of the patients.

In a meta-analysis of 30 studies, Griffith *et al.* (2000) concluded that contingency management with drug users tended to be more effective under certain conditions. Some of the studies that showed the clearest treatment effects involved increases in methadone dose and methadone take-home privileges. These appeared to be among the most effective reinforcers for behaviour change. The length of time before the delivery of reinforcement was also an important factor. Immediate and mixed (both immediate and delayed) intervals were found to lead to a greater treatment response than when rewards were delayed. Contingency management interventions were most effective when directed towards changing the use of a single illicit drug than when they were targeted towards reducing multiple drug use. Another factor related to the effectiveness of contingency management was the level of monitoring of the targeted behaviour. Where interventions were based upon illicit drug use as monitored by the results of urine screening, the collection of three specimens per week was more effective than the collection of fewer weekly urine specimens.

It could not be determined if contingency management procedures worked better as a stand-alone technique or as part of a multimodal treatment programme, and the role of counselling and social support services in relation to contingency management interventions was also unclear. Many studies did not indicate if those patients who received contingency management also attended counselling and, where counselling was mentioned, there was seldom a description of its intensity of type (e.g. individual and group). Many studies also failed to report whether or to what extent other social support services were provided or made accessible. An important issue that requires further investigation is how contingency management might most effectively be incorporated with other psychosocial or pharmacological treatments.

Cognitive–behavioural therapies and psychosocial treatments

The basic tenets of the cognitive–behavioural treatments are that people respond primarily to cognitive representations of their environments rather than to the environments *per se*, that most human learning is cognitively mediated, that thoughts, feelings, and behaviours are causally interrelated, and that expectancies, attributions, self-talk, and other cognitions are central to producing, predicting, and understanding problem behaviours and the effects of therapeutic interventions (Kendall *et al.* 1991).

Beck and Ellis were among the first to use cognitive–behavioural therapies (*cognitive therapy* and *rational emotive therapy*, respectively). More recently, there has been considerable interest in cognitive–behavioural models of change and in the therapies based upon such models. This is currently one of the most popular approaches to the treatment of drug misuse problems as well as for a wide range of other disorders. The application of cognitive–behavioural theories to the treatment of drug addiction is a relatively recent occurrence.

With regard to the treatment of drug problems, Liese and Najavits (1997) suggested that cognitive–behavioural theories tended to make the following assumptions.

- Drug misuse is mediated both by cognitive and behavioural processes.
- Drug misuse and its associated cognitive–behavioural processes are, to a large extent, learned.
- Drug misuse and associated cognitive–behavioural processes can be modified.
- A major goal of cognitive–behavioural treatment for drug misuse is to facilitate the acquisition of coping skills for resisting drug taking and for reducing drug-related problems.
- Cognitive–behavioural therapies require comprehensive and individualized case conceptualizations to select and guide specific cognitive–behavioural techniques.

Motivational interviewing

One form of treatment intervention that has been popular and clinically influential in recent years is motivational interviewing (MI). Miller's original account of motivational interviewing described its application with problem drinkers (Miller 1983), but it has also been applied to the treatment of a broad range of substance use disorders, including illicit drug misuse (Saunders *et al.* 1995).

The concept of motivation has a somewhat dubious history in the addictions. It has often been regarded as something fixed that the drug misuser brings to treatment. Within motivational interviewing, however, it is seen as a changeable property and as a specific target for intervention in its own right. Motivation is seen as 'a state of readiness . . . to change, which may fluctuate from one time or situation to another. This state is one that can be influenced' (Miller and Rollnick 1991). In this respect, motivational interviewing challenges the idea of 'denial' as a characteristic of people with drug problems. This approach also challenges treatment interventions that use forms of aggressive confrontation. Denial, for example, is seen not as an attitude or personality characteristic of the drug user, but as a product of the way in which the counsellor interacts with the patient. The strongest assertion of this view states that 'Client resistance is a therapist problem' (Miller and Rollnick 1991).

One limitation of many treatments for drug addiction is that they presume a prior commitment to change on the part of the drug user. This commitment is often somewhat shaky and in some drug misusers may be almost entirely hidden. Motivational interviewing assumes that the drug user in treatment is characterized by an ambivalence about their drug-taking behaviour and sees itself as 'an approach designed to help clients build commitment and reach a decision to change' (Miller and Rollnick 1991). Motivational interviewing differs from some other treatment approaches in that it avoids trying to persuade or convince the patient to do something about their drug use, but seeks to supervise a process of decision-making in which the patient makes the decisions. Motivational interviewing has been found to be a useful tool in many stages of treatment but it has been particularly useful in helping people who are still at an early stage of committing themselves to treatment or to changing their behaviour.

Motivation itself is conceptualized as the product of an interpersonal process in which the behaviour of the therapist has considerable influence on the subsequent attributions and behaviour of the patient. Motivational interviewing is used to help explore and resolve ambivalence about change. Its aim is to increase levels of cognitive dissonance until sufficient motivation is generated for the patient to begin to consider the options and interventions for change. Motivational enhancement methods have often been closely linked to stages of change models (Prochaska and Diclemente 1982; Prochaska *et al.* 1992).

Motives do not translate directly into outcomes, and motivation alone is unlikely to be sufficient for change or the maintenance of change among the long-term, highly problematic users of drugs who seek treatment in most addiction services. The majority of these drug users will already have committed themselves to change on repeated occasions, and will have made several serious attempts to change their drug-taking behaviours. More than three-quarters of the drug misusers admitted to the NTORS (National Treatment Outcome Research Study) treatment programmes had attended a drug treatment service on at least one occasion in the previous 2 years (Gossop *et al.* 1998*b*). Treatment processes can also, to some extent, affect outcomes regardless of the user's initial motives (Institute of Medicine 1990*a*). Nevertheless, the user's motivation to seek treatment is likely to influence their engagement with the treatment services offered, as well as the probability of them remaining in treatment long enough to benefit from exposure to the therapeutic process.

Unlike some other behavioural therapies, motivational interviewing is specifically concerned with the nature of the patient–therapist interaction. Motivational interviewing is seen primarily as a counselling style rather than a technique to be applied (Rollnick 2001). Miller (1983) recommended that the therapist initially adopt an empathetic stance and suggested using techniques similar to those operationalized by Carl Rogers. This process is, however, modified. Rogerian reflective listening is used selectively to reinforce statements of concern and elicit self-motivational statements. The therapist is not just being reflective but is subtly steering the patient towards change.

One of the main purposes behind the apparently Rogerian stance is to encourage the active involvement of the patient. The therapeutic style is not truly reflective, as the patient's comments are fed back in a modified form and are selected so as to increase dissonance. This selection must be a clandestine operation and the therapist should include doubts expressed by the patient so as to preserve the credibility of the procedure. The patient's own terminology should be used as far as possible. As Miller says 'the counsellor should not put words in the client's mouth, because this will be easily detected as a ploy'. There is a real concern that this could lead to resistance if the individual realizes they are being directed and then becomes more likely to follow an opposite course of action. The internal attribution of this moulded feedback generates dissonance that can be directed in an appropriate direction. The therapist should not discuss treatment options or alternatives until this critical mass of motivation is reached and, even then, the alternative intervention options should include self-directed change strategies as well as traditional treatment options. The therapist assists the patient in identification of appropriate goals and in the implementation of strategies to achieve these changes.

The patient is steered to construct his or her own inventory of drug-related problems, to express concern, and to identify possible options for change. Miller and Rollnick (1991) stated that a wholly non-directive Rogerian approach can leave the patient confused and directionless. The role of the therapist is to encourage the active involvement of the patient in the identification of the problem and in the analysis of the various available options for continued drug taking or change according to the 'pros' and cons' or costs and benefits of the different courses of action (Janis and Mann 1977; Powell *et al.* 1993). The approach is intended to enhance the importance of personal responsibility and the internal attribution of choice and control.

Promising results have been obtained in a series of treatment evaluation studies with different types of patient groups. In a comparison of a standard assessment versus an enhanced assessment-plus-motivational interviewing session, those drug users who received MI were more likely to attend subsequent treatment sessions (Carroll *et al.* 2001). When opiate addicts attending a methadone clinic were allocated to either a motivational interview or a control group, the motivational group showed more commitment to treatment goals, more compliance with treatment requirements, and reported fewer opiate-related problems and fewer relapses (Saunders *et al.* 1995).

Daley *et al.* (1998) found that cocaine-dependent out-patients with depression were more likely to remain in treatment, complete the programme, and have fewer posttreatment psychiatric problems than a 'treatment as usual' condition. Baker *et al.* (2001) randomly assigned amphetamine misusers to a cognitive–behavioural treatment (CBT; MI plus skills training) or to a control (self-help booklet) group. Those in the CBT condition were more likely to become abstinent or to show greater reductions in drug use. Adults seeking treatment for cannabis problems showed greater reductions in drug use and drug-related problems after MI than in a delayed treatment control condition (Stephens *et al.* 2000). In a study of drug misusers who received court orders to undergo treatment, Lincourt *et al.* (2002) found that those who received MI were more likely to attend treatment sessions and to complete the programme. In a systematic review of 29 randomized trials of MI interventions applied to four behavioural domains—substance abuse (drugs and alcohol), smoking, HIV risk behaviours, and diet/exercise—Dunn *et al.* (2001) found improvements in at least one behavioural outcome domain in 60 per cent of these studies. When used with substance misusers, nearly three-quarters of the studies (11/15) showed significantly improved outcomes.

Relapse and its treatment

An important aspect of social-learning approaches (Bandura 1977) is the separation of initial change and the maintenance of change. The factors and procedures that are most effective in inducing behaviour change may not be the most effective for producing generalization and maintenance of treatment effects.

The problem of relapse is an important characteristic of all of the addictive disorders. A large proportion of people who have been treated for addictive behaviour problems tends to return to that behaviour within a short time of leaving treatment. This has been found for alcoholics, cigarette smokers, and heroin addicts (Hunt *et al.* 1971; Marlatt and Gordon 1985; Litman *et al.* 1979; Gossop *et al.* 1989*a*). Even for the heavily dependent drug user it can be relatively easy to stop taking drugs. The greater difficulty is in remaining drug-free. The problem of relapse is how to maintain habit change. As such, an understanding of the processes of relapse and how to prevent or manage relapse is central to our capacity to treat addiction.

Relapse prevention (RP) has been an important and influential form of psychosocial treatment (Marlatt and Gordon 1985). Marlatt (1985, p. 3) described RP as

> . . . a self-management program designed to enhance the maintenance stage of the habit-change process. The goal of RP is to teach individuals who are trying to change their behavior how to anticipate and cope with the problem of relapse. In a very general sense, relapse refers to a breakdown or setback in a person's attempt to change or modify any target behavior. Based on the principles of social-learning theory, RP is a self-control program that combines behavioral skill training, cognitive interventions, and lifestyle change procedures. Because the RP model includes both behavioral

and cognitive components, it is similar to other cognitive behavioral approaches that have been developed in recent years as an outgrowth and extension of more traditional behavior therapy programs.

The primary goal of relapse prevention is to teach drug users who are trying to change their drug taking behaviour how to identify, anticipate, and cope with the pressures and problems that may lead towards a relapse. The key components of relapse prevention are:

◆ identifying high-risk situations for relapse;

◆ instruction in and rehearsal of coping strategies;

◆ self-monitoring and behavioural analysis of substance use;

◆ planning for emergencies and lapses.

Of these, the two essential features are the identification of high-risk situations that put the individual at increased risk of relapse, and the development and strengthening of appropriate and effective coping responses. High-risk situations may be situations, events, objects, cognitions, or mood states that have become associated with drug use and/or relapse. Risk factors often occur together, either in clusters or in sequence (Bradley *et al.* 1989), and they may operate in an additive or interactive manner (Shiffman 1989).

Relapse among opiate addicts has been investigated both in terms of lapses from abstinence (Gossop *et al.* 1989*a*), and lapses to illicit drug use within methadone treatment programmes (Chaney *et al.* 1982). In a study of opiate-dependent out-patients in a methadone detoxification programme, Unnithan *et al.* (1992) found that lapses to illicit opiate use were common. Almost half (40 per cent) had lapsed to illicit opiate use within the first 2 weeks of starting the withdrawal programme and after only a small dose reduction had been achieved.

Various factors have been found to be associated with the event of lapse. Most lapses have been found to be related to negative emotional states, social pressure, and interpersonal conflicts (Cummings *et al.* 1980). Social context, and particularly interpersonal difficulties such as arguments and loss of socially supportive relationships, also increase the chances of relapse. The majority of lapses among heroin addicts occur in the company of drug takers or in a social context related to drug taking (Gossop *et al.* 1989*b*). The three most common factors found to be associated with relapse were cognitions, negative mood states, and external (including interpersonal) events (Bradley *et al.* 1989). Antecedents to lapse may also include subjective experiences of 'urge' (sudden impulse to engage in an act) and 'craving' (subjective desire to experience effects of a given act) (Heather and Stallard 1989).

Opiate addicts who take illicit drugs during treatment were found to have been exposed more frequently to drug-related cues, to have had more contact with other drug users, and to have experienced strong urges to use drugs. Unnithan *et al.* (1992) showed the extent to which drug misusers are exposed to drug-related cues. More than three-quarters (79 per cent) of the opiate addicts in an out-patient methadone reduction programme had met other drug users during the previous week, and 21 per cent had met drug users every day. Nearly two-thirds (62 per cent) of them had been offered drugs on at least one occasion during the previous week and 14 per cent had been offered drugs every day. Under such circumstances, the likelihood of a lapse to drug taking must be massively increased for even the most strongly motivated patient. But the study pointed to further pressures towards relapse. Approximately half of the sample reported persistent feelings of depression, boredom, and anxiety. Negative mood states are themselves often associated with relapse (Cummings *et al.* 1980; Bradley *et al.* 1989; Heather and Stallard 1989).

A study of opiate addicts who had been successfully withdrawn from drugs in an in-patient treatment programme showed that the first few weeks after discharge were a critical period in terms of the individual's chances of staying off drugs (Gossop *et al.* 1989a). Within 1 week of leaving the unit, nearly half of the sample had used opiates on at least one occasion and, within 6 weeks of discharge, almost three-quarters of them had used opiates.

However, this initial lapse to opiate use did not herald a full-blown relapse to addiction. The study also showed a 'recovery-after-lapse' effect that is not shown in those studies that have used the initial lapse to drug taking as an indicator of a failed outcome. The RP model explicitly distinguishes between lapses and relapses (Marlatt and Gordon 1985). In the 6 months after leaving treatment there was a gradual increase in the number of people who were abstinent from opiates, which included many of those who had used drugs immediately after treatment. Six months after discharge, about half of the sample were abstinent with no signs of having substituted other forms of drug taking for their prior opiate dependence. One of the strongest predictors of good outcome was the number of protective factors in the person's environment, and this included people, activities, or social structures that were identified by the individual as being helpful to them in their efforts to stay off drugs (Gossop *et al.* 1990).

The provision of treatment within a relapse prevention framework involves an individualized assessment of drug-taking behaviour within what are, for each drug user, individually relevant high-risk situations for relapse. Global measures of personality or cognitive functioning are not generally useful as predictors of particular behaviours. Instead, situationally specific measures of behaviours and specific drug-taking situations must be assessed for each individual. Annis (1986) also suggests that assessment should take account of cognitive appraisals of past successes and failures in relation to these same drug-taking situations. Bradley *et al.* (1992) found that opiate addicts who attributed to themselves greater responsibility for negative outcomes and who saw relapse episodes as being more amenable to their personal control were more likely to remain abstinent from opiates or to be able to contain the effects of a lapse into opiate use after in-patient treatment.

What is needed in treatment, therefore, is a microanalysis of each high-risk drug-taking situation for each patient in terms of their social and environmental circumstances, their cognitive appraisal of those situations, and their expectations regarding the options for and effectiveness of coping behaviours that they could use in such situations. The effective delivery of relapse prevention requires close attention to the interrelationship between assessment and treatment planning. Assessment of high-risk situations and the availability of coping skills forms the basis for designing and rehearsing homework assignments or tasks for the drug user in treatment.

Patients are taught to recognize the particular factors that increase the risk of their returning to the problematic behaviour(s), and to avoid or to cope with these factors. To support the maintenance of change, RP requires the development of specific coping strategies to deal with high-risk situations. These may include skills training and the development or strengthening of more global coping strategies that address issues of lifestyle imbalance and antecedents of relapse.

Positive expectancies may engender feelings of hope and optimism that facilitate treatment effectiveness, and self-efficacy beliefs also play an important role in RP. The role of self-efficacy in therapeutic change has been discussed at length by Bandura (1977, 1997). There is, for example, an important conceptual distinction between outcome expectations, that is, the individual's belief that a specific action will result in a particular outcome, and efficacy expectations—the individual's belief that they are capable of performing the behaviour necessary to produce the desired outcome (Bandura 1977). Efficacy expectations are reflective of the individual's sense of personal control and influence, whether they are likely to initiate coping behaviour, what degree of effort will be devoted to that behaviour, and how long it will be maintained in the face of obstacles.

Within the RP model, self-efficacy refers to the person's judgements or expectations about their capacity to cope with specific high-risk situations. It is concerned with perceived ability to perform a coping response, and not with the general ability to exercise will power to resist temptation (Marlatt and Gordon 1985). In the absence of high-risk situations, there is little threat to this perception of control, since urges and temptations are minimal or absent.

In the presence of a high-risk situation, a conflict of motives occurs between a desire to avoid and the temptation to take drugs.

Bandura (1997) suggested that, where a coping response is successfully performed, self-efficacy beliefs will be strengthened, and repeated experiences of success will reduce the risk of future lapses or relapse in such situations. Conversely, where individuals fail to cope with a high-risk situation, their belief about their own capacity to cope with the situation is further undermined and the probability of relapse increases. This loss of confidence may be particularly pronounced among those who rely upon will power alone as a way of dealing with risk situations, since there is nothing they can 'do' to cope. This reinforces the sense of failure, helplessness, and lack of control.

Annis has given particular emphasis to the importance of self-efficacy beliefs and outcomes (Annis and Davis 1988), and has stressed the specificity of self-efficacy beliefs. These may apply to the development of addictive behaviour, choice of treatment goals, and the maintenance of addictive behaviour change during recovery (Sklar *et al.* 1997). Relapse prevention was found to be useful as part of an aftercare programme for substance abusers who had just completed an intensive treatment intervention (Brown *et al.* 2002).

Relapse prevention procedures may be applied to anticipate and prevent the occurrence of a relapse after the initiation of a habit change attempt (e.g. to prevent a heroin addict from returning to dependent heroin use after they have achieved abstinence) and to help the individual recover from a 'slip' or lapse before it escalates into a full-blown relapse. In principle, such RP procedures can be used regardless of the theoretical orientation of the therapist or the intervention methods applied during the initial treatment phase. Once a heroin addict has stopped using drugs, for example, RP methods can be used to support continued abstinence, regardless of the methods used to initiate abstinence (e.g. attending 12-step meetings, psychotherapy, or voluntary cessation) (Marlatt 1985).

Marlatt and Gordon's (1985) relapse prevention model is important for several reasons. It was the first major cognitive–behavioural approach in the treatment of substance use disorders, and it provides a straightforward conceptual model for understanding drug misuse problems (Liese and Najavits 1997). Relapse prevention has altered earlier views of relapse as merely a poor outcome, and redirected attention to relapse as a process that can be understood, anticipated, and avoided. It identifies practical, flexible interventions that can be applied by clinicians with a range of backgrounds and skills, it has given direction and purpose to treatment in day-to-day clinical settings by showing how assessment should be targeted at key problem areas, and it can be used adjunctively with other treatments.

Chapter 9

Narcotics Anonymous, twelve-step programmes, and rehabilitation treatments

This chapter looks at a number of treatments, which, although they differ in several respects, also share many common features. All owe their origins, to a greater or lesser extent, to Alcoholics Anonymous (AA), and they all share a common focus upon abstinence as the overriding goal of treatment. These treatments see recovery from addiction as requiring a profound restructuring of thinking, personality, and lifestyle, and involving more than just giving up drug-taking behaviour. Drug addicts tend to be seen as people with a particular kind of problem personality. This is reflected in anxiety and self-doubt, the need to convince themselves and others of a success that isn't real, and an inability to risk close, honest relationships, which leads to impulsive self-centred lives and a lack of awareness of other people except when they can be used to meet the addict's own needs (Kennard 1998).

Narcotics Anonymous

The origins of Alcoholics Anonymous are usually traced back to 10 June 1935, the day on which Dr Bob Smith, a surgeon from Akron, Ohio who co-founded AA with Bill Wilson, had his last drink. Since then, and for more than 6 decades AA has influenced the treatment of alcoholism and has gained increasing international popularity. AA has been estimated to have as many as two million members world-wide (Makela 1993). Its philosophy is based on mutual help, group affiliation, and identification, and it is widely believed to be an effective intervention for alcoholism (Miller and McCrady 1993). Since its inception, AA has subsequently been adapted for a variety of other addictive behaviour problems.

Narcotics Anonymous (NA) is a direct descendant of Alcoholics Anonymous. One of the earliest forerunners of NA may have been a group that was established in 1947 at the Public Health Services Hospital in Lexington (Brown *et al.* 2001). However, it is more often believed that NA was started in

Sun Valley, California, in 1953 by a group of AA members who did not see the AA fellowship as meeting their special needs as drug abusers (Galanter *et al.* 1993; Nurco and Makofsky 1981). A different version of the same story involves a group of heroin addicts being acrimoniously ejected from their local AA meeting.

Both AA and NA have flourished in many countries throughout the world. The international expansion of NA led to a reported 26 000 NA groups in 64 countries in 1993 (DuPont and McGovern 1994). By the early 1990s, it was estimated that there were more than 3000 AA meetings and around 300 NA meetings each week in the UK, with over 100 NA meetings and approximately 500 AA meetings in London alone (Wells 1994). NA may have a larger population of drug abusers involved in its programme than any other drug recovery initiative (Brown *et al.* 2001).

There are also further groups such as Cocaine Anonymous (CA), which has been reported as having more than 1500 groups in the USA (White and Madara 1992). Methadone Anonymous represents still another twelve-step initiative. Methadone Anonymous was organized in 1991 in Baltimore, Maryland, as an alternative to NA after methadone patients reported feeling unwelcome at NA meetings and in conflict with NA's philosophy of total abstinence from all drugs.

NA/AA is a fellowship of people who want to do something about their drug/drink problems and who meet on equal and friendly terms. The primary purpose of members is to stay sober and help others to achieve sobriety. The fellowship is open to all men and women and is non-professional, self-supporting, non-denominational, apolitical, and multiracial. The first 100 members collectively wrote the *NA big book*, the twelve steps, and the twelve traditions of AA.[1]

The programme consists of studying and following the twelve steps. This programme is presented, described, and discussed in AA meetings. NA retains the steps in their original form as written by the early AA members, since these 'had stood the test of time and should therefore not be altered' (Wells 1994). NA (1988) states that the twelve steps are 'the principles that made our recovery possible' and the twelve steps are seen as building upon each other.

The twelve steps (Table 9.1) are the essential principles and ingredients of the recovery process (Emrick 1999). Progression through the steps is seen as

---

[1] The twelve steps are the central element for the NA groups. These differ from the twelve traditions. The traditions define the policy and regulations that govern each fellowship, emphasize the responsibility of the fellowship to the individual member, and proscribe financial, political, or any other associations with other organizations.

Table 9.1 The twelve steps

1	We admitted that we were powerless over our addiction, that our lives had become unmanageable.
2	We came to believe that a Power greater than ourselves could restore us to sanity.
3	We made a decision to turn our will and our lives over to the care of God as we understood Him.
4	We made a searching and fearless moral inventory of ourselves.
5	We admitted to God, to ourselves, and to another human being the exact nature of our wrongs.
6	We were entirely ready to have God remove all these defects of character.
7	We humbly asked Him to remove our shortcomings.
8	We made a list of all persons we had harmed, and became willing to make amends to them all.
9	We made direct amends to such people wherever possible, except when to do so would injure them or others.
10	We continued to take personal inventory and when we were wrong promptly admitted it.
11	We sought through prayer and meditation to improve our conscious contact with God as we understood Him, praying only for knowledge of His will for us and the power to carry that out.
12	Having had a spiritual awakening as a result of these steps, we tried to carry this message to addicts, and to practise these principles in our affairs.

essential for achieving and maintaining abstinence. It is the responsibility of each NA member to involve himself or herself in 'working the steps'. This involves studying the written materials made available through the fellowship, monitoring his or her own functioning, praying for guidance and support, and trying to stay abstinent 1 day at a time. This leads from an initial recognition of helplessness in the face of their addiction, through a personal commitment to change with the help of Higher Power, and ultimately to a responsibility for positively influencing the lives of others.

The steps emphasize two general themes:

- *spirituality*: belief in a 'Higher Power,' which is defined by each individual and which represents faith and hope for recovery;
- *pragmatism*: belief in doing 'whatever works' for the individual, meaning doing whatever it takes in order to avoid taking the first drink/drug.

The group meetings are one of the best known aspects of NA. Meetings, which may be 'open' or 'closed', are held weekly and usually last for an hour.

The 'closed' meetings are only for those members who are willing to describe themselves as 'addicts', and in these groups, members are encouraged to share their experiences, achievements, their fears, and their failures with peers who provide support and advice. In open meetings, non-addicts and outsiders with concerns about friends or family are permitted to attend. In speaker meetings, members tell their 'stories'. They describe their experiences with drugs and alcohol and talk about their recovery. Step meetings usually are closed meetings and consist of a discussion of the meaning and ramifications of the twelve steps.

When individuals join NA, they are usually encouraged to attend more than one meeting a week and a target of attending 90 meetings in 90 days is often set (DuPont and McGovern 1994). For individuals who have a dual addiction to drugs and alcohol, this can involve attendance at separate NA and AA meetings (Krupka and Blume 1980; Nurco et al. 1983). As members achieve sustained abstinence they may attend meetings less often, although it is recommended that they continue to attend meetings at least once a week, and more often if they feel vulnerable to relapse.

NA/AA has been seen as the paradigm of the self-help movement for recovery from addiction (Dumont 1974), though many of the members tend to dislike the self-help label and prefer to see the fellowship as providing mutual support. Reliance upon the fellowship is seen as one of the primary therapeutic agents that sets NA/AA apart from other forms of treatment. In standard addiction treatments, the professional relationship is seen as setting a boundary between doctor and patient, and the intervention is more easily seen in terms of the application of the skills and techniques of the clinician.

NA/AA has sometimes been non-professional or even anti-professional in its attitudes and style. Some groups have deliberately avoided reliance on professionals, believing that professionals do not understand their particular problems or needs. More recently, however, many groups have moved towards a greater willingness to work in alliance with professionals, and many groups are currently linked to or operate with close working links with professional organizations.

Brown et al. (2001) identified several essential characteristics of initiatives such as NA that differentiate them from other interventions. Firstly, they involve the individual acting in collaboration with others who share the same problems, to provide mutual support for each other's recovery. NA suggested that 'a meeting happens when two or more addicts gather to help each other stay clean' (Narcotics Anonymous 1988). This element of mutual support is seen as a key dynamic for change. It occurs both through the involvement of members of the fellowship who share common problems and through the specific support that can be offered by the sponsor.

The twelfth step can involve sponsoring another member, and sponsorship is also seen as an important component of recovery. Each person who joins the fellowship is encouraged to find as a sponsor another member who is willing to offer support and guidance in working the programme. Sponsors are expected to provide support, information, and advice. They should be stably abstinent and they must be of the same sex as the individual being sponsored. A sponsor is expected to be someone who has achieved a substantial period of sobriety and who has studied and worked the twelve steps. Being a sponsor is not merely an act of altruism, but can also be a part of the sponsor's own recovery. Sheeren (1988) found that an important predictor of stable abstinence was acting as a sponsor to another member.

The NA/AA philosophy sees addiction as an illness that permeates all aspects of the individual's life, and that can only be controlled by life-long abstinence. This vast and daunting project is broken down into manageable parts and taken 'one day at a time'. All of the twelve-step programmes see recovery from substance abuse as a continuing process with every day involving a struggle to remain free from drugs.

The 'disease concept' of addiction has provoked opposition in some quarters. Heather and Robertson (1989) describe the NA/AA view of addiction as 'primitive' (p. 66) and criticize what they see as the implication that the intentions of the drinker or drug taker 'have nothing to do with what takes place and that the only relevant consideration is the physical impact of the drug' (p. 68). They also suggest that the twelve-step model is unhelpful in that it serves 'to absolve the alcoholic [or drug addict] from moral responsibility for his actions'.

This view is strongly rebutted by NA/AA. Paradoxically, the NA/AA disease concept is used to emphasize the need for the addicts to take responsibility for their own behaviour and to participate actively in their own recovery (Hill 1985). Wells (1994) also pointed out that, although addicts are seen as not responsible for their illness, they are certainly seen as 100 per cent responsible for their own recovery. Although family, social, and socio-economic factors are recognized as possibly having contributed to the addict's plight, it is the individual who must take responsibility for the ways in which they respond to these conditions. 'No one has to be a drug addict, so it is up to the individual to choose, and to change' (Kennard 1998).

NA/AA has also been criticized for its 'religious' orientation. Six of the twelve steps make some reference to God, and prayer and meditation are seen as important parts of the process of recovery. However, members of the fellowship are encouraged to interpret the 'higher power' in a way that is based upon their own personal understanding of a 'power greater than oneself'. Examples of this may include the power of the group, the power of nature, love, collectivity, or some force connected with truth and honesty (Wells 1994). Feelings of well-being engendered by the process of collective personal growth are often referred to as 'spiritual'. And while some members become involved with 'organized religions', others experiment with forms of meditation, martial arts, or yoga, or completely ignore the spirituality suggested by the programme.

In a study conducted with drug- and alcohol-dependent patients in standard hospital-based in-patient addiction treatment services, Best *et al.* (2001*a*) investigated attitudes towards the twelve steps. There were marked differences in attitudes towards different steps. Some steps received broad levels of acceptance (step 10), whereas others received much lower levels of agreement (step 3). There was much more willingness to accept 'personal responsibility' steps, than those that related to a 'Higher Power'.

It is not necessary to accept the whole NA philosophy to see that NA offers a number of social and psychological support systems for the recovering addict. It has been suggested that apparently dissimilar treatment interventions such as twelve-step programmes and relapse prevention may share a number of common underlying process factors (Brown *et al.* 2001). Edwards (1987) also suggested several therapeutic processes through which AA may operate. These included 'coherent flexible ideas' (an ideology), 'an action programme' (the twelve steps), 'the rewards of sobriety', and 'the possibility of recovery'. It is also possible to reinterpret many of the functions of NA in what would be regarded as more conventional academic or psychotherapeutic concepts and terms.

Positive role modelling

NA offers a peer group that can support efforts to achieve and maintain abstinence. Most people with drug addiction problems have acquired a social network consisting of other drug users (Fraser and Hawkins 1984), and continuing involvement with this drug-oriented network greatly increases their risk of relapse (Bradley *et al.* 1989; Waldorf *et al.* 1991). NA provides a peer group that shares the same problems, but which actively supports the learning of new, prosocial behaviours and is aggressively opposed to all forms of drug taking (Brown *et al.* 2001). This is a powerful asset for anyone seeking to recover from drug addiction. In a study of factors associated with recovery among heroin addicts after treatment in an in-patient hospital service, Gossop *et al.* (1990) noted that 'new social relationships may mean that the subject mixes with non-users who do not expose [them] to drugs or drug-related behaviours and whose beliefs and value systems support abstinence rather than heroin use'. The role-modelling function of NA can be further assisted by the support, mentoring, and policing offered by the sponsor.

Restructuring lifestyles

A further supportive function is that NA provides a structure for the member's free time. Many drug addicts have difficulties in finding new ways of using their leisure time. Simpson *et al.* (1981) found that involvement in prosocial leisure activities was associated with the avoidance of relapse, and the NA group, with its evening meetings, provides an activity during a high-risk time of day, which helps to support continuing abstinence.

Cognitive restructuring

Many cognitive therapists see treatment as involving the patient in learning to attend to shifts in thinking and emotions, and feel that problematic forms of behaviour will be reduced if patients are helped to think effectively and positively about life events (Patterson and Welfel 1994). The therapeutic work of Ellis (1962), Beck (1976), and Meichenbaum (1977) has been substantially based upon notions of cognitive restructuring. Ellis (1962) suggested that, when thoughts, assumptions, and expectations are inaccurate, false, or irrational, clinical interventions should redress the thought processes rather than the responses to them. Most cognitive therapies regard thinking errors as the basis for emotional upsets and inappropriate behaviours and focus on the patient's internal dialogue as a foundation for the ways in which they react to life events.

Several general principles underlie the therapeutic procedure for cognitive restructuring (Goldfried 1988). These include: (1) helping the patient to see that thoughts affect emotional responses; (2) helping the patient to identify unrealistic beliefs and to offer alternatives to those beliefs; (3) helping the patient to re-evaluate their beliefs, and to provide guidelines and practice for change to more effective options.

With the progression of alcohol addiction, certain changes in cognitions occur, which form what has sometimes been referred to as 'alcoholic thinking.' These are ways of thinking and rationalizations that are also accompanied by characteristics of 'grandiosity, omnipotence, and low frustration tolerance' (Brown 1985). These cognitive changes grow with the addiction and create a pattern of emotional immaturity, self-centredness, and irresponsibility.

Twelve-step programmes can help to tackle the faulty beliefs and maladaptive cognitions that need to be identified and changed in recovery (DiClemente 1993). As such, they provide a form of cognitive restructuring therapy (Steigerwald and Stone 1999). NA/AA meetings encourage members to admit and explore their own selfish, self-seeking, and self-centred thinking (Khantzian and Mack 1994). Henman and Henman (1990) suggested that addiction can be seen as a thought disorder, and offered a model of counselling for alcoholics that encouraged participation in a twelve-step programme with a therapy based on cognitive–behavioural modification. This was designed to help the client cognitively to restructure the old faulty alcoholic assumptions, beliefs, attitudes, perceptual filters, internal dialogue, and unconscious patterns of processing information. The twelve steps formulate the basis for cognitive restructuring and abstinence, and the sponsors as mentors and teachers also support the development of new ways of thinking about problems and solutions.

Aftercare

The importance of posttreatment aftercare is widely accepted (Ouimette *et al.* 1998). The period immediately after leaving treatment has been described as 'one of massively high risk . . . there is . . . every reason to provide the best possible support for the patient during this immediate post-discharge phase . . . it is extremely important that the hard-won gains of [treatment] should not be lost through the absence of adequate support at the point of leaving treatment' (Gossop *et al.* 1989*a*). However, only a small minority of programmes have sufficient resources to provide any form of aftercare (Hubbard *et al.* 1989). Because of its self-supporting nature, NA provides a form of aftercare at no cost to existing treatment services. Treatment programmes can make use of NA as an aftercare resource merely by recommending participation and encouraging their clients to attend meetings.

Twelve-step facilitation programmes

The influence of twelve-step programmes now extends beyond the NA/AA meetings themselves, and many treatment programmes provide forms of treatment based upon twelve-step principles. Some of these treatment programmes are directly and substantially based upon the twelve steps. Many other services supplement their programmes by recommending NA/AA attendance as an aftercare resource. In some programmes, the twelve steps have been formally incorporated as a major part of a structured, professionally delivered treatment package.

One such form of treatment can be provided within the framework of standard out-patient programmes. One of the most clearly described examples is the twelve-step facilitation (TSF) treatment programme within Project MATCH. This TSF treatment was explicitly based on the twelve-step model and was one of three forms of treatment in the study (Project MATCH Research Group 1997, 1998). The TSF programme was provided in an out-patient treatment setting and was of 12 weeks duration. The programme was highly structured. Each session had a specific agenda and followed a prescribed pattern. Sessions included specific 'recovery tasks', and patients were also asked to keep a personal journal. A central component of the TSF programme was the strong encouragement given to the patient to attend several AA meetings each week and to read the *Big Book* (Alcoholics Anonymous) as well as other AA publications throughout the course of treatment.

Research into twelve-step treatments

Despite the popularity of twelve-step treatments, research has been limited in methodological range and inconsistent in conclusions. Compared to many other addiction treatments, there are relatively few systematic evaluations of the effectiveness of twelve-step treatments in general, and of NA in particular. Much that has been written about NA is descriptive and anecdotal. In recent years, a greater interest has been shown, both within twelve-step programmes and among academic researchers, in the application of structured evaluation methods to these types of treatment.

Project MATCH was a study of people with alcohol rather than drug problems. It is included in the present discussion since its treatment protocols provide one of the clearest and most explicit statements of how twelve-step facilitation can be delivered within a treatment service. However, although the study provides good outcome data, its findings relate directly only to the treatment of people with alcohol problems.

The TSF programme consisted of 12 sessions. These were:

♦ 12 individual sessions with unmarried patients; or

♦ 10 individual sessions plus 2 conjoint sessions with patients and their partners if they were in a stable relationship.

In addition, a maximum of two individual emergency sessions could be provided if these were needed. The full programme was designed to be delivered within a 12-week period.

During the 12 weekly TSF sessions the therapist introduced patients to the first five of the twelve steps of Alcoholics Anonymous, and encouraged them to become involved in AA. Although the TSF programme was based upon the twelve steps, it differed in that it was a professionally delivered, individual therapy, and in this respect it differed in an important way from the peer support system of normal AA meetings. This form of treatment was not intended either to duplicate or to substitute for the traditional form of AA.

The main conclusions from Project MATCH were that all three of the study treatments were effective. Those who received the TSF treatment had slightly fewer drinking days than those who received either of the other treatments. For patients who were more severely dependent upon alcohol, TSF led to greater improvement in drinking behaviour than cognitive behavioural treatments (Project MATCH Research Group 1998).

Other research into NA/AA has investigated engagement and affiliation as mediators of outcome. Johnsen and Herringer (1993) reported a relationship between frequency of NA/AA attendance and abstinence, and Christo and Sutton (1994) found that length of time in NA was related to abstinence from illicit drugs. Fiorentine (1999) and Christo and Franey (1995) also found an inverse association between NA attendance and drug-using outcomes.

While weekly or more regular NA/AA attendance has been found to be associated with favourable substance use outcomes, less than weekly NA/AA attendance appears to be no more effective than non-attendance (Fiorentine 1999; Fiorentine and Hillhouse 2000). Irregular attendance appeared to lead to a poorer prognosis than either regular or non-attendance, suggesting that 'mis-affiliation' or incomplete affiliation may be associated with poorer treatment outcome (McLatchie and Lomp 1988). Favourable outcomes may be less dependent on attendance at meetings than upon the extent to which those at the meetings embrace the philosophy (Morgenstern et al. 1997; Montgomery et al. 1995).

The benefits of NA/AA have been demonstrated not only in comparison with other forms of substance misuse treatments, but also as a complementary intervention. Fiorentine and Hillhouse (2000) reported that, contrary to the beliefs of some professionals, the clients themselves frequently use both twelve-step and other types of drug treatment programmes as integrated services rather than as alternatives. Some studies have found favourable outcomes for those who attend AA following other types of treatment (Fiorentine 1999; Ouimette et al. 1998; Emrick 1987) while others found no significant relationships between AA attendance and favourable outcomes (Miller et al. 1992). Ouimette et al. (1998) investigated the impact of aftercare among substance abuse patients who chose to attend one of three types of aftercare groups (twelve-step groups only, out-patient treatment only, and out-patient treatment plus twelve-step groups) and among patients who did not participate in aftercare. The patients who received no aftercare had the poorest outcomes. Patients who participated in the out-patient treatment plus twelve-step groups achieved the best outcomes at follow-up. In terms of the amount of intervention received, patients who had more out-patient mental health treatment, who attended twelve-step groups more frequently, or were more involved in twelve-step activities had better outcomes.

Fiorentine and Hillhouse (2000) found that, when initial treatment motivation was controlled for, patients enrolled in other forms of treatment who also attended twelve-step programmes had better outcomes than those who had the other treatment alone. Such findings suggest that twelve-step programmes may be effective not only as interventions in their own right but also as supplements to other forms of treatment in order to maximize the benefits accrued by patients. Not surprisingly, it was found that substance abusers with attitudes that were congruent with the twelve-step philosophy were more likely to participate in twelve-step activities during treatment (Ouimette *et al.* 2001).

The extent to which NA/AA and the twelve-step programmes have come to permeate current addiction treatment provision was shown by Best *et al.* (2001*a*). More than three-quarters (77 per cent) of the patients who were recruited from a standard hospital-based health service treatment facility were found to have previously attended NA/AA meetings. Patients admitted to the drug dependence service were twice as likely as those in the alcohol treatment service to have previously attended both AA and NA groups. There was considerable variation in the amount of previous involvement with the fellowship, with about one in five having only ever attended one meeting. On the other hand, many of both the drug misusers and the drinkers had an extensive involvement (having attended, on average, more than 50 meetings). More than half of these patients had been referred to NA/AA by their GP, a specialist substance misuse service, or some other statutory NHS treatment service. Those patients with drug problems were more likely than those with alcohol problems to have been introduced to the fellowship through a treatment service.

It is widely believed that twelve-step treatments are not acceptable to all drug users and that many drug users who are not actively involved with NA or twelve-step programmes are reluctant or even resistant to this approach. Although the drug takers and drinkers in the study of Best *et al.* had similar levels of involvement with the fellowship, the drug users were more likely to express positive views about it. Among the drug users more than three-quarters (78 per cent) felt that NA/AA was at least partly suited to their current treatment needs compared with less than a third (31 per cent) of the drinkers. Similarly, more of the drinkers expressed negative views about the fellowship. More than one-third of the drinkers (42 per cent) were definitely resistant to the ideas and methods of the fellowship and the possibility of their own involvement with it, compared to only about one in five of the drug takers. These attitudes translated into a greater willingness of the drug users to have some future involvement with the fellowship.

Residential rehabilitation programmes and therapeutic communities

In many countries, residential rehabilitation programmes are one of the longest established forms of treatment. In some countries, they are still one of the dominant treatment modalities. This continues to be the situation, for example, in the Scandinavian countries, such as Sweden (Bergmark 1998).

In the UK, two of the main types of residential treatment programmes are those that are largely based upon the provision of twelve-step treatments and those that are based upon the principles of the therapeutic communities (TCs). The TCs may also use twelve-step principles in varying degrees. Therapeutic communities are also sometimes known as concept-based communities. The concepts include those that explain the nature of the addict's problems, those that demonstrate how therapy works, and those that underline how they ought (and ought not) to conduct themselves in the community. Other types of residential services in the UK include those that have been classified as 'Christian houses' and 'general houses' (Stewart *et al.* 2000*b*).

Many residential programmes require addicts to be drug-free on admission, though some provide their own in-house detoxification programmes. Treatment length varies from short-term with aftercare, to long-term programmes of more than 1-year duration. In the UK, residential programmes vary in length from several weeks to 6 months or more. At one time, treatments were much longer and, in some countries, they are still provided over longer periods. Of the American residential treatment programmes in TOPS (Treatment Outcome Prospective Study), the facilities ranged in size from 26 to 126 beds with an average capacity of 64 (Hubbard *et al.* 1989). The UK residential rehabilitation services studied by NTORS (National Treatment Outcome Research Study) ranged in size from 12 to 58 beds (Stewart *et al.* 2000*b*).

Some residential programmes divide their treatment programme into three main phases (Kennard 1998):

◆ induction/orientation;

◆ treatment;

◆ re-entry.

The phase one induction/orientation phase may last for a few weeks or up to 2 months. The core, treatment delivery period involves the resident living, working, and relating to others exclusively in the community, and progressing through the community hierarchy. This may often last for periods of about 12 months. In the re-entry phase, the residents have passes to go out while still living in the community, which enables them to look for work and accommodation. This phase may last for 6–12 months. Some agencies also operate 'half-way' houses with patients living in semi-independent houses after completing the main programme.

Residential programmes almost always have an explicit commitment to abstinence as their treatment goal, though they may vary in other aspects of their treatment philosophies. They typically provide a planned and structured programme of counselling and support services designed to facilitate major changes in the individual's lifestyle and to achieve long-term recovery. In the UK, many residential programmes are located away from inner city areas in order to provide a clear change of setting. With two exceptions, the TOPS residential programmes were in urban areas close to addict populations.

The term 'therapeutic community' was first used to describe the TCs that were introduced in psychiatric hospitals by Maxwell Jones and others in Britain during the 1940s. These psychiatric TCs represented a shift from treatment by individual therapists to a more social approach based upon social interaction, group methods, and milieu therapy (Kennard 1998). The therapeutic community within the psychiatric hospital was 'organized as a community in which all are expected to contribute to the shared goals of creating a social organization with healing properties' (Rapaport 1960). It is not clear to what extent these influenced the addiction TCs other than by passing on the name.

Synanon was one therapeutic community that had an important influence on residential addiction treatment services (Kennard 1998). It was set up in 1958 in Santa Monica, California by Chuck Dederich. It grew out of and was loosely based on the philosophical principles of AA. Dederich was a recovering alcoholic who applied his experiences of AA to launch and develop the Synanon programme. With several AA companions, Dederich started a series of weekly 'free association' groups in his apartment. These turned into encounter groups and within a year the weekly meetings had evolved into a residential community. In August 1959 Synanon was officially founded to treat any type of substance abuser.

Synanon was followed in the 1960s by other therapeutic communities, such as Phoenix House, Daytop Village, Odyssey House, and Gateway Foundation. These were set up by 'graduates' of one of the 'parent' programmes, who carried forward many common elements of the philosophy, social organization, and practices from the original programmes. In 1970, three graduates of Phoenix House came to Britain from the USA and founded a community in London. However, while Synanon emphasized permanent participation in its programme and the rejection of life outside the therapeutic community, the later therapeutic communities tended to work more towards a re-entry into society. By 1979 there were more than 300 therapeutic communities across the USA (De Leon and Rosenthal 1979).

The therapeutic community has been described as 'fundamentally a self-help approach [that] evolved primarily outside of mainstream psychiatry, psychology, and medicine' (De Leon 2000). Similarly,

> The quintessential element of the therapeutic community (TC) approach is community. Community is both the context and method in the change process. It is the element of community that distinguishes the TC from all other treatment or rehabilitative approaches to substance abuse and related disorders. (De Leon 2000, p. 85).

In this respect, TCs differ from other forms of addiction treatment interventions in that the continuing interaction between the individual and the community is itself seen as the treatment process.

De Leon (2000) has described the clients of therapeutic communities as 'a diverse group . . . individuals whose drug histories consist of an ever-expanding menu of drugs and who, in addition to chemical abuse, often present complex social and psychological problems.' TCs believe that recovery requires changes in all aspects of lifestyle, attitudes, and behaviour associated with drug abuse. De Leon and Rosenthal (1979) suggested that the basic goal for problem drug users in therapeutic communities in particular (but also in residential treatment programmes in general) is to undergo a complete change in lifestyle involving abstinence from drugs, avoidance of antisocial behaviour, the development of prosocial skills, and personal honesty. The specific objective of the TCs has been described as to treat individual disorders, 'but their larger purpose is to transform lifestyles and personal identities' (De Leon 2000).

Addiction treatment processes can be conceptualized in terms of the treatment ingredients (the interventions or services delivered to produce change), the ways in which the individual changes, and the mechanisms or principles that link treatment ingredients to individual changes. The treatment ingredients are described as the programme structure, the people in the TC, and the daily activities and social interactions in the TC. The process of change is described as being sometimes gradual and incremental, but sometimes as being erratic and 'punctuated by distinctive moments of personal change involving a "total" experience' (De Leon 2000). Such moments may provide critical, therapeutic experiences in leading to change.

In a description of the psychological principles underlying the processes of change within TCs, De Leon (2000) suggested that the three important principles are social role training, vicarious learning, and efficacy training. The resident positions within the TC hierarchy provide experience of work roles and, as individuals learn their various social roles in the community, they undergo a wide range of social and psychological changes. Changing the social roles of individuals is seen as an effective way of facilitating learning across a much wider range of behaviours, attitudes, emotions, and values. The purpose of role training is to build new behaviours, skills, and attitudes that are socially and psychologically supportive to the individual in their recovery. The principle of vicarious learning is also seen as an important feature of community life, with peers and staff providing role models for appropriate behaviours and attitudes. Meeting community expectations in performance, responsibility, self-examination, and autonomy leads to increased self-efficacy and self-esteem.

A system of privileges and sanctions is typically used to motivate and direct behaviour within residential programmes (Brook and Whitehead 1980). This may include the offer or withdrawal of the sorts of privileges and sanctions (such as permission to write and receive letters, to make and receive telephone calls, or to go out alone) that would be regarded as a behaviour modification programme if provided by professional staff in a conventional psychiatric setting. Despite their use of rewards and punishments, these terms are seldom used within TCs. Measures such as 'shooting someone down the hierarchy' are seen not as punishments but as opportunities for greater self-awareness. Promotion in the hierarchy is seen less as a reward than as an opportunity to acquire skills and self-confidence.

Role modelling within the TC also includes practising a broader range of behaviours and attitudes that reflect the values and expectations of the community. The expectations include those of student, apprentice, teacher, and leader, and these describe the changing relationship of the individual to the community. As the individual successfully learns their various social roles in the community, they undergo a range of social and psychological changes. More importantly, De Leon (2000) suggests that the residents' performance of various day-to-day jobs in the TC provides experience of the work roles that are required in the working environment of the outside world.

There is a broad consistency of philosophies and approaches across most residential programmes and TCs. As in the twelve-step programmes, addiction is often seen as an 'illness' or a disorder that cannot be cured but can only be put in remission by reliance on self-help and support from other addicts (Yablonsky 1965). Within US residential programmes, abstinence has been ranked most highly as a treatment goal, followed by self-understanding, self-esteem, and coping skills. Physical health and social functioning were given less priority (Hubbard *et al.* 1989). However, the overall aim of treatment was seen as changing dysfunctional behaviour to an effective and productive lifestyle.

General houses typically have a more cognitive–behavioural approach to treatment, and provide support through individual and group sessions. Each resident usually has a key worker or counsellor with whom they meet regularly to plan their care. These types of programmes are generally less overtly challenging and confrontational than other types of residential services. Other residential programmes using this type of eclectic approach are the Christian houses, which also tend to use individual counselling and house meetings rather than confrontational groups, but in addition believe that residents need a Christian philosophy in order to combat drug and alcohol problems.

Residential programmes differ in terms of the provision of specific therapies and activities. However, individual and group counselling provide the common therapeutic methods. Clients in US residential programmes have been found to spend about 3 hours per day in therapy of some kind (Brook and Whitehead 1980). Holland (1982) found that about 12 hours per week were spent in group or individual counselling, 13 hours a week in re-entry activities (vocational counselling and use of community resources), and about 8 hours in interpersonal activities. Counselling was mostly delivered in groups, but individual counselling (usually at least once a week) was also available in all programmes (Hubbard *et al.* 1989). The duration of counselling sessions varied from 90 minutes to 3 hours. The 24-hour community experience is regarded as a fundamental element of the residential treatment programmes (De Leon 1995).

There are similarities between the methods and practices of residential rehabilitation programmes and TCs. The primary staff members in many residential programmes are often former offenders or recovering drug abusers who have themselves been rehabilitated in therapeutic communities. Ex-addict counsellors are often the most numerous members of staff and provide the most counselling input. In a study of 32 long-term residential programmes, Holland (1982) reported that about 40 per cent of the staff were recovering substance abusers. In the larger programmes these staff are often supported by professional staff with specific areas of expertise. Hubbard *et al.* (1989) noted that, despite their use in TCs, there have been few studies of the impact of ex-addict versus non-addict professional counsellors.

Holland's (1986) survey of long-term (12 months or more) residential programmes showed that these emphasized a self-help approach and relied heavily on the use of programme graduates as peer counsellors and role models. Programmes were highly structured, with nearly every moment accounted for. Members were expected to progress through a series of clearly demarcated programme stages with successive stages carrying more responsibility, often accompanied by more personal freedom. Group counselling or therapy sessions were a key element and were usually confrontational in nature with a requirement for openness and honesty. Members were assigned to work duties within the house, with their levels of responsibility determined by their current position in the community.

Many of the longer-term residential programmes make extensive use of sanctions and privileges and emphasize peer responsibility for explaining, clarifying, and giving feedback on behaviour (Holland 1982). Most programmes use some kind of loss of privilege as a sanction (Hubbard *et al.* 1989). Peer pressure is one of the most commonly used types of influence. Hubbard *et al.* noted that the programmes tended to be non-permissive, and all programme directors reported that violation of programme rules and regulations was an important reason for dismissing clients. Programmes did, however, vary in the nature and extent of use of sanctions and privileges.

Although there tends to be broad agreement between residential programmes on the general approach to treatment, they increasingly differ in their planned duration of treatment. At one time, traditional TCs worked with planned durations of stay of 2–3 years (Cole and James 1975). Recent changes in client population and the realities of funding requirements have encouraged the development of modified residential TCs with shorter durations of stay. Traditional therapeutic communities often required at least 15 months in residence for graduation (De Leon and Rosenthal 1979). De Leon (2000) has described the tendency in recent years for some TCs to modify their traditional approach and methods by supplementing a variety of additional services related to family, education, vocational training, and medical and mental health. Modified TCs may work with a 6–9 month programme, and the short-term programmes with a 3–6 month programme (De Leon 2000). This has been accompanied by changes in the earlier balance of staff to include an increasing proportion of traditional mental health, medical, and educational professionals who work alongside the recovered paraprofessionals (Carroll and Sobel 1986; Winick 1990–1991).

Another influential recent development has been the growth of relatively short-term, residential 'chemical dependency' programmes, which are often based upon twelve steps and which are strongly focused upon recovery through abstinence. The 'Minnesota model' (sometimes also referred to as 'Hazelden' or chemical dependency) treatments grew out of hospital-based approaches to treating alcoholism in Minnesota in the 1960s. These programmes typically provide a highly structured 3–6 week package of residential care involving an intensive programme of daily lectures and group meetings designed to implement a recovery plan based upon the twelve steps.

Although the Minnesota model treatments share some structural characteristics with the TCs, there are important differences (Institute of Medicine 1990*a*). These programmes are similar to the TCs in that they are highly structured and virtually every moment of the day is accounted for. Progress through the phases is evaluated, and many of the counselling staff may have themselves been through similar programmes as part of their recovery from a drug or alcohol problem. Both during and after treatment, clients are often encouraged to attend AA/NA meetings. Among the differences are the relatively short duration of the residential component for Minnesota model programmes, less involvement of clients in routine 'housekeeping' chores, and the greater use of professional or trained staff compared to the TCs, which rely more upon staff who are themselves 'in recovery'.

The Minnesota model treatment approach has provoked criticism because of the dogmatic assertions of some of its proponents that this treatment alone has all the answers. This over-assertiveness has been compounded by the fact that the Minnesota model treatment programmes represent the predominant therapeutic approach of private sector providers in the USA (Institute of Medicine 1990a). Such programmes also have close associations with the private sector in the UK and in some other countries. These links have sometimes created an unfortunate image of an elite treatment that is available only to the privileged few. However, there are now, at least in the UK, a number of 'state-assisted' places available in such programmes (Cook 1988).

Cook's (1988) review of the evidence for the effectiveness of Minnesota model treatments suggested that, despite some extravagant claims for the success of this form of treatment, there were few sound follow-up studies. In addition, what little published work is available was often limited by methodological problems. Nonetheless, Cook concluded that the available evidence was encouraging, and suggested that as many as two-thirds of the clients treated in such programmes might achieve significant improvements after treatment.

Studies from the UK and the USA have shown improved outcomes after treatment in residential rehabilitation programmes (Bennett and Rigby 1990; Gossop et al. 1999b; De Leon and Jainchill 1982). Evaluations have been conducted with TCs with programme durations varying from short-term with aftercare, to long-term programmes of over 1-year duration. Improved outcomes were usually associated with longer periods of time spent in treatment, with episodes of at least 3 months associated with positive outcomes (Simpson 1997). The reductions in illicit drug use that have been found after residential treatment have also been shown to be relatively robust and to persist across lengthy follow-up periods (Simpson et al. 1979; De Leon 1989a).

Among the DATOS (Drug Abuse Treatment Outcome Study) clients who were treated in long-term residential and short-term in-patient treatment modalities in the USA, the drug use outcomes after 1 year were good. Regular cocaine use (the most common presenting problem) was reduced to about one-third of intake levels among clients from both the long-term and short-term programmes, as was regular use of heroin (Hubbard *et al.* 1997). Rates of abstinence from illicit drugs have also been found to improve after residential treatment. In the UK, NTORS examined outcomes after discharge from 16 residential rehabilitation programmes. About half of the clients (51 per cent) had been abstinent from heroin and other opiates throughout the 3 months prior to follow-up: rates of drug injection were also halved, and rates of needle sharing were reduced to less than a third of intake levels (Gossop *et al.* 1999*b*).

Moos *et al.* (1999) conducted a naturalistic, multisite evaluation of more than 3000 men who received twelve-step, cognitive–behavioural, or combined twelve-step plus cognitive behavioural treatments provided in 3–4 week in-patient programmes. All three treatments appeared to be equally effective in reducing substance use and psychological symptoms, and in reducing post-treatment arrests and imprisonment (Ouimette *et al.* 1997; Finney *et al.* 2001). The case-mix-adjusted outcomes showed that the patients who received twelve-step treatments were more likely to be abstinent, free of substance abuse problems, and employed at 1-year follow-up. Moos *et al.* (1999) concluded that their findings provided evidence to support the effectiveness of twelve-step treatment.

Case-mix issues are important here because residential programmes often accept the most chronic and severely problematic cases (Gossop *et al.* 1998*b*). Indeed, it is an explicit intention of stepped care treatment approaches that residential services should be used for the more difficult cases (Sobell and Sobell 1999; ASAM 2001). In some instances, residential programmes have been designed to tackle such cases. Egelko *et al.* (2002), for example, provided a residential treatment programme for homeless clients with mental illness and drug abuse problems. Their results indicated significant improvements in mental health during treatment.

However, one issue that affects many research evaluations of residential programmes is that treatment drop-out is common. Typically, studies have reported that many patients leave treatment prematurely. De Leon (1985) reported that a quarter of TC clients left within 2 weeks and 40 per cent within 3 months. In common with outcomes from other treatment modalities, those clients who completed residential programmes achieved better outcomes on drug use, crime, employment, and other social functioning measures (De Leon *et al.* 1982; Hubbard *et al.* 1989).

Some of the strongest criticisms of the twelve-step programmes and the TCs have been based not upon empirical evidence about their effectiveness (or otherwise), but upon theoretical, aesthetic, or ethical objections. In addition to criticisms of their religious or spiritual emphasis and of the 'disease concept' of addiction (see above), there have been objections that some of the concept-based residential communities and TCs demand too great a level of conformity. They apply what amounts to a complete handbook of behaviour, attitudes, and values that applies to all aspects of community life.

There has also been criticism of the sanctions used in some TCs for inducing conformity and commitment. Their ways of dealing with serious transgressions of the community's norms, such as stealing or using drugs, have sometimes been regarded as excessive. Among the sanctions that have aroused the disquiet of professionals and others are shaving men's heads (women wear stocking caps) or having offenders wear a placard declaring misbehaviour (such as 'I steal things'). In a caring environment, such measures may be intended to be constructive and corrective, but it is easy to see how they might also be used aggressively as forms of punishment and humiliation. Many communities have given up such sanctions in favour of less severe or less controversial measures.

Others have criticized the confrontational interventions used in the communities. Miller and Rollnick (1991) suggested that the use of strong confrontational methods such as those used in TC encounter groups would be regarded as 'ludicrous and unprofessional' if used in the treatment of other psychological or medical problems. They go on to state that confrontational strategies of this kind have not been supported by clinical outcome studies, and that therapist behaviours associated with this approach have been shown to predict treatment failure, whereas empathic approaches are more likely to be therapeutically effective.

However, Miller and Rollnick (1991) do not completely deny the uses of confrontation, which they describe as being a goal of all forms of counselling and psychotherapy. In a general sense, the purpose of confrontation is to help the client to see and accept reality, so that they can make appropriate changes. The experience of being confronted by a disquieting image of oneself may be the precipitating force for many sorts of behavioural changes (Orford 1985).

It has also been suggested that some communities operate as 'cults'. This criticism was made of Synanon. Kennard (1998) noted that there were similarities between cults and TCs. Both are often started and run by a charismatic leader, both claim to help people who feel psychologically and socially inadequate, both seek a high level of commitment to the community, and both operate, to some extent, in isolation from the outside world. The differences between cults and TCs are in the aims of the community, what is offered to and expected from members, and in the way in which control is exercised. Whereas cults often seek to establish an ideal lifestyle and to convert others to this way of life, the therapeutic community should seek to provide a culture in which individual change is possible. In a cult, leadership and decisions about the community are usually not openly discussed, and may often be determined by an individual or small group whose authority is not open to question. In a therapeutic community, decisions may be freely discussed and challenged in group meetings.

Chapter 10

Methadone treatments

A brief background and history

The origins of methadone are generally traced back to the Second World War when the drug was synthesized as a substitute for morphine by German chemists at I.G. Farben. After the war, in 1947, methadone was used as a medication for pain relief or as a cough suppressant. Soon afterwards, during the late 1940s, studies of its pharmacological effects identified the abuse liability of methadone.

The best known and most influential early work on methadone as a treatment for opiate dependence was that of Vincent Dole and Marie Nyswander in the 1960s at Rockefeller University, New York. Dole and Nyswander are generally regarded as the innovators of methadone treatment for opiate dependence. However, others were also experimenting with methadone as a treatment for opiate addiction and had been doing so before Dole and Nyswander. One of the first evaluations of methadone's effects in humans was carried out in Lexington, Kentucky. In this study, 15 former morphine addicts were given methadone by injection four times a day, with some receiving daily doses as high as 600–800 mg per day (Isbell *et al.* 1948). Not surprisingly, at such high doses, signs of toxicity appeared and the highest doses were reduced to 200–400 mg per day.

Work on the potential application of methadone as a short-term treatment for opiate addicts had also taken place in Vancouver as early as 1959 (Williams 1971), where the Narcotic Addiction Foundation of British Columbia had used methadone in 12-day detoxification programmes. In 1963, the Canadian programme was expanded to include a more prolonged period of out-patient methadone treatment. The average methadone dose used in the Vancouver programme was 40 mg per day.

After a series of trials in late 1963 that examined the potential efficacy of morphine maintenance, Dole and Nyswander began treating opiate addicts with methadone at an in-patient unit at Rockefeller University. In the initial studies, addicts were admitted to an in-patient service to be evaluated and stabilized on a daily dose of oral methadone before transfer to an out-patient clinic for continued treatment. Subsequently, it was decided that treatment could be provided in an out-patient setting without the need for the preliminary in-patient phase of treatment.

This early work with methadone was highly controversial and that of Dole and Nyswander, in particular, aroused fierce opposition. The most concentrated attack came from the US Federal Bureau on Narcotics. Indeed, the early methadone treatments were only able to continue through the defence of Dole and Nyswander mounted by Rockefeller University and its lawyers.

Early papers on outcomes after methadone maintenance treatment reported encouraging results. There were good rates of patient retention, reduced criminality, and improved social rehabilitation (Dole and Nyswander 1965; Dole *et al.* 1966, 1968). These studies attracted considerable attention, both in the USA and in other countries. Soon afterwards, there was a rapid expansion of methadone treatment. In 1969 in New York City, almost 2000 patients were in methadone treatment. By 1970 this had increased to 20 000. During the 1970s, methadone maintenance treatment was greatly expanded in New York City and established throughout much of the USA. In 1989, there were 667 methadone maintenance programmes in the USA. Most programmes were located in large, and often east-coast, cities.

However, by the 1980s, the expansion of methadone maintenance treatment in the USA had ceased, and there followed a period of stability or retrenchment. No new treatment facilities were opened in New York City during a 10-year period. Most existing programmes were underfunded. There were cutbacks in treatment and rehabilitative services, staff turnover was high, and the quality of care declined. There were approximately the same numbers of patients in methadone maintenance treatment in the USA in 1997 as there were in 1977 (Kreek 2000). The number of patients in treatment was limited primarily by the available treatment places. These were limited both because of funding constraints and the unwillingness of community groups and others to have treatment programmes located in their neighbourhoods or business areas.

By the mid-1990s there were probably about 250 000 patients in methadone treatment worldwide, with the USA continuing to have the largest population of methadone patients. A single-day survey in 1994 estimated that there were about 110 000 patients receiving methadone treatment in the USA (SAMHSA 1996). The most recent estimates suggest that there may currently be about 179 000 patients receiving methadone maintenance in the USA (Kreek and Vocci 2002).

In many countries, the introduction and development of methadone maintenance programmes led to ideological battles and controversy. This was often largely due to a negative moral view of methadone treatment as merely switching the drug misuser's dependence to a legally available opioid, with many patients continuing to use heroin and other drugs and to commit crimes. This led to a situation in which methadone maintenance programmes were described as working 'under stress with little recognition, underfunded, over-regulated, misunderstood in their communities, often vilified by special interest groups' (foreword by Dole, in Ball and Ross 1991). Nonetheless, almost all countries that are confronted by a substantial opiate addiction problem have introduced methadone clinics for the treatment of drug addicts.

Methadone maintenance treatment (MMT)

Various rationales have been given for prescribing methadone maintenance. It has been suggested that methadone acts by preventing withdrawal, which enables addicts who are maintained on the drug to be freed from the need to seek and use illicit heroin. Whereas this may apply to some addicts, we know from self-administration studies of laboratory animals that physical dependence is not necessary for self-administration of opiates. Non-dependent animals will self-administer opiates at a high rate because of the positively reinforcing effects of these drugs even though they have never experienced withdrawal.

It has also been suggested that, by occupying opiate receptor sites, methadone prevents craving and that, if the user takes any heroin, the methadone blocks the euphoric effects of the heroin. The consumption of heroin is associated with sharp rises and falls in the drug level in the blood with peak concentrations reaching opioid receptors in the brain for only a few hours. In order to achieve the desired effect, frequent administration of heroin is necessary. Unlike heroin and the natural opiates, methadone is orally efficacious (with a bioavailability in excess of 90 per cent) but it is also, for most patients, long-acting (Tennant 1987; Wolff *et al.* 1997) and can thus be prescribed only once daily.

Another rationale is the pragmatic one, namely, that giving methadone in a clinical setting enables opiate addicts to be assessed and supported in tackling a range of behavioural, social, and health problems. The evidence from a huge number of studies suggests that it can be effective in this respect.

The US Institute of Medicine report (1990*a*, pp. 12–13) provides a definition of the aims and methods of methadone maintenance that states:

> Methadone maintenance is a treatment for extended dependence on opiate drugs (usually heroin). A sufficient daily oral dose of methadone hydrochloride, which is a relatively long-acting narcotic analgesic, yields a very stable metabolic level of the drug. Once a newly admitted client has reached a stable, comfortable, noneuphoric state, without the psychophysiological cues that precipitate opiate craving, he or she is

amenable to counseling, environmental changes, and other social services that can help shift his or her orientation and lifestyle away from drug seeking and related crime toward more socially acceptable behaviors.

Methadone programs are nearly always ambulatory [i.e. out-patient], with daily visits to swallow the methadone dose under observation in the clinic, except for traditional Sunday take-home doses. After several months in the program with a 'clean' drug testing record and good compliance with other program requirements, one or more daily doses may be regularly taken home between less-than-daily visits; however, this convenience is a revocable privilege. Some methadone clients voluntarily reduce their doses to abstinence and conclude treatment after some time, whereas others remain on methadone indefinitely, particularly if earlier attempts to leave methadone have ended in relapse.

Programme diversity

In practice, methadone treatments are extremely diverse. All involve the prescription of the same pharmacological agent, methadone hydrochloride.[1]

But apart from this common element, they differ in many fundamental respects. As a consequence of the expansion in services that took place in the USA during the late 1960s and the 1970s, methadone maintenance changed from a medically supervised treatment for a designated population of heroin addicts to a more diversified programme of services and interventions provided to unselected addict patients. The new programmes differed in terms of the number of patients treated (from a few dozen to many hundreds), the qualifications of the director (psychiatrist; physician, social worker, ex-addict, administrator), type and qualifications of staff, the amount and type of counselling and medical services provided, methadone dose commonly prescribed (from less than 30 mg to over 100 mg), and policies about urine testing, take-home methadone, and many other aspects of treatment.

In a study of six methadone maintenance programmes in three US cities, Ball and Ross (1991) described differences between the structures, procedures, and practices of these methadone treatment programmes. The programmes differed in fundamental ways, including the doses prescribed to patients, provision of counselling services, treatment policies, and, not least, in drug use outcomes. Stewart *et al.* (2000*b*) reported similar sorts of differences between 31 methadone programmes in England.

Such differences have been found both within and between countries. A World Health Organization study of methadone treatment in six countries

---

[1] Even in this respect there is some variation. In contrast to other countries, two forms of methadone have been used in Germany (Gerlach 2000). These forms are laevomethadone, otherwise known as polamidon, which is not used elsewhere, and the racemic mixture (D, L-methadone), which has been available for use in Germany since 1 February 1994.

(Gossop and Grant 1990) found marked variability in the content and structure of programmes. The variation included issues of direct relevance to the nature and probable effectiveness of the interventions. Programmes differed in dose levels, programme entry criteria, time limits for prescribing, frequency of clinic attendance, the manner of dispensing (supervised or unsupervised), and, in some countries including the UK, the formulation of the drug used (syrup, tablets, or ampoules). A survey of methadone prescribing in England and Wales in 1995 showed that, whereas 80 per cent of methadone prescriptions were for oral formulations, 11 per cent were for methadone tablets, and 9 per cent were for injectable methadone ampoules (Strang and Sheridan 1998).

It is difficult to understand why methadone tablets continue to be prescribed by British methadone programmes to this extent. Methadone tablets are often crushed and injected by patients. The injection of such an unsuitable preparation is clearly unsatisfactory and carries a number of health risks. National Guidelines (Department of Health 1991) that were circulated to all doctors in England, Wales, and Scotland, stated that there were 'no grounds whatsoever for the prescribing of methadone tablets in the treatment of opiate addiction' because of the frequency with which they were crushed and injected by the patient or re-sold on the black market to be crushed and injected by others. It is possible that prescribing doctors were either unaware of the guidelines or that many of them chose to ignore the guidelines. The potential problems associated with this prescribing practice are increased by the further finding that four times as many tablet prescriptions were for daily doses in excess of 100 mg compared with prescriptions for oral methadone (Strang and Sheridan 1998).

Such marked variation in the provision of methadone treatments is of considerable clinical importance. Whereas many patients respond well to methadone maintenance and show improvements in their illicit drug use and/or in other problem behaviours, about one in four patients treated in methadone programmes tend not to respond well to treatment (Institute of Medicine 1990a). This was also found by Gossop et al. (2000a) who found marked reductions in illicit drug use among 59 per cent of their sample, and a poor response in terms of continued and unchanged use of illicit drugs among 18 per cent. The treatment response profiles of the treatment groups are shown in Fig. 10.1. Patient responses may be related to the variation in treatment procedures. An important clinical question, therefore, is how to achieve a more precise understanding of the ways in which patients respond to different procedures and interventions provided in methadone treatment.

It is possible to argue both for the advantages and for the disadvantages associated with the variations in methadone treatment programmes and services.

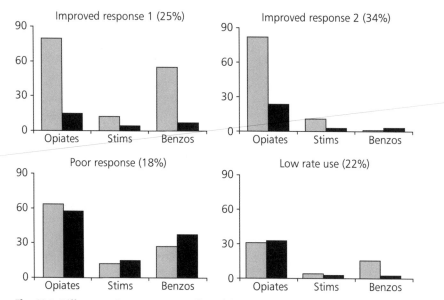

Fig. 10.1 Different patient response profiles while receiving treatment with methadone. The majority of patients (profiles 1 and 2) showed substantial reductions in illicit drug use. Group 3 showed a poor response to methadone treatment with no significant reductions in illicit drug use. Patients in group 4 were characterized by relatively low rates of illicit drug misuse at the time of treatment intake, and by little change during treatment. The data are from the study of Gossop *et al.* (2000*a*).

It now seems increasingly implausible to argue that any single uniform treatment response will be appropriate to the needs of all addict patients, and this is not a viable objective to pursue. The needs of different patient populations are likely to require several types of methadone maintenance treatment packages. Clients with serious psychological or psychiatric problems will require different treatment input to those without such problems. The need for vocational and rehabilitative counselling will be different in a programme where most of the patients are already employed at admission to that in a programme where few patients are employed. Similarly, programmes in which the patient group includes a large proportion of mothers with young children or pregnant women should provide different treatment components to meet the special needs of these individuals.

The provision of methadone treatments to opiate addicts in the UK has a different history to that in other countries. Methadone treatment became established as an important part of the national response during the early 1970s. But unlike in the USA where methadone treatments were introduced with specific protocols and often with stringent controls, in the UK they have been subject to only the most general controls. As a consequence, the clinical delivery of methadone treatment has been extremely variable. The reasons for this variation have rarely been made explicit, but are sometimes justified in terms of the need to provide an 'individualized' response to meet the needs of each patient.

The disadvantage of having diverse treatment services provided by methadone maintenance programmes is that mere diversity is not conducive to the improvement of treatment, especially if the diversity is due to the whims of staff, or worse, is a result of programmes being compelled to remove, reduce, or alter services because of lack of funding and other resource cut-backs.

Dose

After decades of clinical experience and research with methadone as a treatment for opiate dependence, the question of appropriate dosing remains controversial. Clinics vary greatly in the average dose of methadone prescribed, with some clinics prescribing low doses and others using high doses. In NTORS (National Treatment Outcome Research Study), the average initial daily dose of the patients in the methadone treatment programmes across England was 48 mg. Two-thirds received methadone in doses of 30–60 mg; 20 per cent received doses of 60 mg or more, and 13 per cent received doses of 30 mg or less (Gossop *et al.* 2001*a*). Similar evidence of variations in dosing practices has been reported in the USA (Strain 1998, 1999).

In a randomized double-blind trial of moderate versus high-dose methadone (Fig. 10.2), Strain *et al.* (1999) found that patients receiving doses

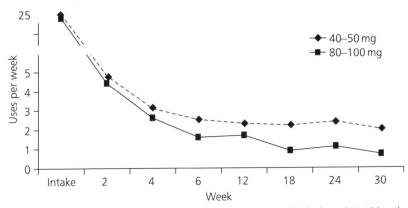

Fig. 10.2 The responses of methadone maintenance patients to high doses (80–100 mg) or moderate doses (40–50 mg) of methadone over a 30-week period. The use of illicit opiates was significantly reduced in both groups, but with a better outcome among the high-dose patients. The data are from the study of Strain *et al.* (1999).

of 80–100 mg showed greater reductions in illicit heroin use than the moderate dose group who received doses of 40–50 mg. Both groups showed substantial and significant reductions in illicit drug use compared to pretreatment levels. There were no differences in treatment retention between the high- and moderate-dose groups.

A slightly different perspective on this issue was offered by Kreek (1997*b*) who suggested that steady doses of methadone are essential for both normalization of physiology and for the effective reduction or elimination of drug craving, thus preventing relapse to illicit opiate use. Kreek suggested that the interactions that take place between drugs as a result of multiple drug use may interfere with attempts to maintain the delivery of a steady dose, and that drug–disease interactions that occur during methadone treatment may also disrupt steady-state plasma levels.

Comprehensive reviews of the research literature on the relationship between methadone dose and treatment outcome were conducted by Cooper *et al.* (1983) and Ward *et al.* (1992, 1998). These reviews concluded that treatment outcomes are improved when doses of 50 mg or more are used, when compared to lower doses. They also concluded that there was no evidence to suggest that routine dosing at levels in excess of 100 mg per day results in any benefit for the majority of patients, though relatively few studies of high-dose treatment have been carried out. Ward *et al.* (1998) suggested that the evidence both from randomized controlled trials and from observational studies showed better outcomes for patients in programmes where the majority of patients are maintained in the range of 50–100 mg per day. However, it is possible that some patients may be successfully maintained on lower doses, especially if they are more highly motivated to change and more psychologically stable (Schut *et al.* 1973; Williams 1971).

Studies of the effects of different methadone doses usually involve studies of the doses used in treatment settings or controlled clinical trials. In observational studies, the results are typically taken under normal clinical circumstances in which patients and staff are aware of the doses used, doses are individualized based on each patient's clinical response, and the effectiveness of the prescribed dose is likely to be influenced by other non-pharmacological treatment interventions. The controlled clinical trials, on the other hand, tend to provide a more focused but restricted assessment of the effects of medication and the results may not be completely transferable to the clinical setting.

Strain (1999, p. 75) cautioned that:

> Extrapolating from well-designed and well-conducted clinical trials to actual clinical use should be done with extreme caution. Outcomes certainly can be improved when features of a clinical trial such as double-blind dosing are not present, more intensive

non-pharmacologic treatments are used, and dosing is adjusted based on the purity and quantity of heroin being used by a particular patient. Thus, results from these double-blind studies represent treatment outcomes that are obtained under artificial circumstances, and it should be possible to achieve even better treatment results in a community methadone clinic that provides more individualized treatment for each patient.

Where clinical problems arise in establishing an effective dose level for methadone, it should be borne in mind that there are individual differences in the metabolism of methadone (Wolff and Strang 1999). Therapeutic drug monitoring may be used to measure methadone concentrations in the blood since the blood concentration of methadone provides a better measure of the amount of methadone available to the opiate receptors than the ingested dose. Dole (1989) suggested that the correct dose of methadone for the patient is the amount that sustains the plasma concentration above a critical minimum needed for continuous opioid receptor occupancy for the complete dosing interval.

In most cases, there is a satisfactory relationship between oral dose ingested and methadone plasma concentrations (Wolff et al. 1991). Therapeutic drug monitoring may, however, be useful where there is concern about the dangers of toxicity at doses near to upper therapeutic ranges, or where there is wide variation in the disposition of the drug across individuals or across time.

Supplementary treatments

In practice, the provision of methadone treatments is rarely restricted merely to the provision of methadone pharmacotherapy. Dole and Nyswander's original treatment regimen provided comprehensive medical and rehabilitative services, and it has been suggested that the label 'methadone treatment' may be misleading because it gives undue emphasis to the pharmacological aspects of treatment (Strain and Stoller 1999). The treatment also includes, and is a combination of, both pharmacological and non-pharmacological therapies. Optimal outcomes are obtained when both are provided. For the majority of patients, improved clinical outcomes are seldom achieved simply by ingesting a daily dose of methadone. This was emphatically stated by Dole (quoted in Courtwright et al. 1989, p. 338):

> Some people became overly converted. They felt, without reading our reports carefully, that all they had to do was give methadone and then there was no more problem with the addict. . . . I urged that physicians should see that the problem was one of rehabilitating people with a very complicated mixture of social problems on top of a specific medical problem, and that they ought to tailor their programs to the kinds of problems they were dealing with. . . . The stupidity of thinking that just giving methadone will solve a complicated social problem seems to me beyond comprehension.

These non-pharmacological aspects of methadone treatment can include individual counselling, group therapy, couples counselling, urine testing, contingency contracting, HIV testing and counselling, primary medical care services, and psychiatric assessments and treatment of comorbid disorders. The methadone clinic may be best viewed as a site for the comprehensive treatment of patients.

Nonetheless, there is some evidence that even the provision of a methadone-only intervention may help some patients. For example, a study by Yancovitz *et al.* (1991) in an 'interim methadone clinic' found that the provision of methadone alone, without counselling or other services, produced significant reductions in opiate use when compared to the patients' pretreatment levels of drug use and also when compared to patients on a waiting list comparison group.

In an interesting study, McLellan *et al.* (1993) investigated whether the addition of counselling, medical care, and psychosocial services improved the efficacy of methadone treatment programmes. Patients were randomly assigned to one of three treatment groups for a 6-month clinical trial. The three conditions were: (1) minimum methadone services (MMS)—methadone alone (a minimum of 60 mg/day) with no other services; (2) standard methadone services (SMS)—the same dose of methadone plus counselling; and (3) enhanced methadone services (EMS)—the same dose of methadone plus counselling and medical/psychiatric and family therapy.

The MMS treatment procedure was designed to provide the lowest level of acceptable clinical care. Methadone was the only therapeutic component provided on a regular basis. Initial methadone doses of 60 mg/day could be increased either when the patient requested an increase (e.g. because of withdrawal symptoms), or when opiate-positive urine samples were detected. The procedures for adjusting methadone doses were the same for all groups throughout the study. No ancillary medications, counselling, or other professional services were provided except in emergency circumstances.

The patients in the standard methadone group, in addition to receiving methadone, also received regular counselling. The goal of counselling (in both the SMS and EMS groups) was to change problem behaviours in relation to illegal drug use, employment status, criminal activity, and family/social relations. The counselling involved contingency contracting to achieve positive behavioural changes (as described by Stitzer *et al.* 1986). The enhanced methadone treatment was designed to provide the highest level of care using the standard components of methadone treatment and counselling, together with extended on-site medical/psychiatric, employment, and family therapy services.

The results showed that the provision of additional counselling and medical and psychosocial services produced marked improvements in the efficacy of treatment compared to that of methadone alone. Patients who received standard treatment showed reductions in their use of opiates and cocaine, with some additional changes in alcohol, legal, family, and psychiatric problem measures. There were no significant improvements in medical or employment status.

The patients receiving enhanced treatment showed improvements in employment status, decreases in alcohol and other drug use and illegal activity, improved family relations, and improved psychiatric health. The enhanced group showed better outcomes than the standard treatment condition on 14 of the 21 outcome measures, with significantly better outcomes among the EMS patients in the areas of employment, alcohol use, and legal status.

Some patients who received the minimum methadone services showed improvements, but their response to treatment was generally unsatisfactory. More than two-thirds of the patients in the MMS condition had to be 'protectively transferred' from the trial because of problems associated with their continued use of opiates or cocaine, or because of medical/psychiatric emergencies. This was much higher than among the SMS patients (41 per cent) and the EMS patients (19 per cent).

The fact that 69 per cent of the MMS subjects had to be transferred to standard treatment within the first 3 months of the trial required separate analyses for that group. After their transfer, these patients immediately received counselling and more medical attention. Their use of opiates was halved (from a weekly high of 69 per cent prior to transfer to 34 per cent following the transfer), with similar reductions in cocaine use. These patients also reported some decreases in alcohol use and an increase in the number of days in employment following the transfer. These improvements after transfer to a more intensive treatment programme are also impressive since these patients had demonstrated at least 8 weeks of virtually continuous drug misuse and poor social adjustment during the study.

McLellan *et al.* (1993) concluded that patients who received the same dose of methadone but also received contingency-based counselling (the SMS group) showed more improvements and faster and greater improvements than the methadone-only patients. The inclusion of psychosocial services in addition to the counselling (the EMS condition) produced more improvements than standard treatment in employment, alcohol use, criminal activity, and psychiatric status.

Overview of methadone maintenance treatment

Methadone maintenance has been extensively studied in different countries, with different treatment groups, and over a period of 4 decades. It is the most thoroughly evaluated form of treatment for drug dependence. In a meta-analysis of methadone maintenance studies, Marsch (1998) reported consistent, statistically significant associations between MMT and reductions in illicit opiate use, HIV risk behaviours, and drug and property crimes.

In its summary of the evidence for methadone maintenance, the US Institute of Medicine report (1990a, pp. 13–14) concluded:

> Methadone maintenance has been the most rigorously studied modality and has yielded the most positive results for those who seek it . . . . Regarding behaviour and treatment, the extensive evaluation literature on methadone maintenance yields firm conclusions as follows:

- There is strong evidence from clinical trials and similar study designs that opiate-dependent individuals have better outcomes on average in terms of illicit drug consumption and other criminal behavior when maintained on methadone than when not treated at all, when simply detoxified and released, or when methadone is tapered down and terminated as a result of client request, program expulsion, or program closure.

- Methadone clinics have significantly higher retention rates for opiate-dependent populations than do other treatment modalities for similar clients.

- Although methadone dosages need to be clinically monitored and individually optimized, clients have better outcomes when stabilized on higher rather than lower doses within the typical ranges currently prescribed (30 to 100 milligrams per day).

- Following discharge from methadone treatment, clients who stayed in treatment longer have better outcomes than clients with shorter treatment courses.

Methadone reduction treatment (MRT)

One issue that is of considerable importance to our understanding of methadone treatment programmes concerns the treatment goal. A World Health Organization report (Gossop *et al.* 1989c) noted that 'insufficient attention has been paid to the manner in which the effectiveness of methadone treatment . . . might be maximised . . . there remains considerable confusion both about the identification of goals for the treatment and management of opioid dependence and also about how such goals are related to treatment methods.' In the UK and in other countries there is a tension between the use of methadone as a treatment that is intended to meet a goal of harm reduction (elimination or reduction of illegal drug use, injecting, needle sharing, criminal behaviour, etc.) and the use of methadone as a device or as an intermediate phase of treatment in which complete abstinence from drugs, including prescribed drugs, is the goal.

Methadone maintenance treatment (MMT) is such a widely used and well-known treatment that it may seem unnecessary to require definition. However, it is worth explicitly stating that two of its essential features are:

◆ MMT involves the provision of methadone in stable doses;

◆ MMT is intended to reduce problematic behaviours associated with illicit drug use (but is not, in itself, an abstinence-oriented treatment, and entails continuing use of prescribed methadone).

These features differentiate MMT in important respects from methadone reduction. A basic feature of methadone maintenance is that the drug is prescribed on a stable-dose, non-reducing basis and, following stabilization at a suitable dose level, the patient may be maintained for either a fixed or for an indefinite period.

Methadone reduction treatment (MRT) has been widely used in the UK for many years. Seivewright (2000) commented that 'it would be impossible to overstate the importance of this form of methadone prescribing in the UK'. Typically, MRT involves prescribing methadone over relatively long periods of time, with the expectation that the dose will gradually be reduced and that the patient will eventually be withdrawn from the drug and become abstinent from opiates. Although the objectives of methadone reduction treatment are seldom stated, its practice generally involves providing the lowest dose at which the discomfort of withdrawal can be prevented.

The policy of 'reduction' was formulated soon after the establishment of the British clinic system. The prescription of opiates was seen as a 'lure' to attract drug misusers into the treatment services so that 'regular contact between the addict and the doctor . . . gives the opportunity for a relationship to be built up that may eventually lead to the addict requesting to be taken off the drug' (Connell 1969). The role of the clinic was 'not for the continuing handouts of drugs, but for treatment: the patient may not initially be motivated to accept withdrawal but . . . motivation will gradually be built [and] dosage gradually reduced' (Edwards 1969). From the 1970s, clinic policy moved towards 'an attempt to replace indefinite prescribing' and 'a limited stabilisation period was followed by reducing prescriptions' (Mitcheson 1994). This contrasted with the situation in the USA at that time when many methadone programmes tended to actively discourage their clients from attempting to detoxify themselves from methadone (Glasscote *et al.* 1972).

Although not directly comparable, MRT as delivered in the UK has certain similarities to methadone programmes in other countries. There are some similarities, for example, with the gradual methadone detoxification programmes (Senay *et al.* 1977), and with the 90- and 180-day detoxification programmes that have been implemented in the USA (Iguchi and Stitzer 1991;

Reilly *et al.* 1995; Sees *et al.* 2000). The 180-day methadone programmes were made available after federal guidelines were revised in 1989 to provide this modality as an 'intermediate' form of treatment between short-term 21-day detoxification and long-term maintenance. In the USA methadone reduction is sometimes provided in what are referred to as 'maintenance-to-abstinence' or 'methadone-to-abstinence' programmes.

It is misleading to regard methadone reduction simply as a detoxification procedure. It is a less well-defined and, in practice, more complicated procedure. In principle, out-patient methadone reduction programmes provide a form of medium-term, abstinence-oriented substitution treatment. In practice, however, the parameters of methadone reduction programmes are frequently not clearly stated, and such programmes are implemented in a variety of ways. Reduction programmes may vary in duration from several weeks to many months, and possibly even years. Reduction schedules may be fixed (i.e. set by the prescribing agency without the patient having any involvement in the duration of the treatment or the timing or rate of reduction), or they may be negotiable with the patient having some involvement in decisions about how dose reductions are being made. Even where reduction schedules are fixed, alterations may be made to the timing of dose reductions or the duration of the treatment because of changed circumstances or crises presented by the patient. In reduction programmes, methadone is usually provided by means of prescriptions that are filled by retail pharmacists with the drug being taken away and consumed without supervision.

In contrast to methadone maintenance, relatively little research has been done with methadone reduction treatments. Strang *et al.* (1997*b*) compared outcomes of patients randomly allocated to methadone maintenance or methadone reduction treatments, and found improvements in a range of substance use and other problem behaviours during the first month of treatment, but with no differences between the two methadone conditions. In the study of Strang *et al.* (1997*b*), no data were available about the treatment interventions actually provided, and it is possible that their failure to demonstrate any differences between methadone maintenance and reduction may reflect a treatment 'cross-over' effect, with many reduction patients actually receiving some *de facto* form of maintenance. This 'drift into maintenance' was also noted by Seivewright (2000). Studies of shorter-term out-patient reduction programmes have found generally poor outcomes with high drop-out rates, and few patients achieving even short-term abstinence at the end of the treatment regime (Gossop *et al.* 1986; Dawe *et al.* 1991; Unnithan *et al.* 1992).

Gossop *et al.* (2000*a*) also found that patients who sought treatment in the methadone maintenance and the methadone reduction programmes achieved substantial improvements at 1-year follow-up. It seems surprising that patients recruited to two such different treatment modalities apparently achieved such similar outcomes. However, there were variations in treatment delivery within each modality. There were also similarities between the modalities in the treatments received by patients (e.g. in methadone doses and in treatment retention rates). For these reasons, the authors suggested that it was unsafe to interpret the findings as showing that methadone maintenance and reduction treatments led to similar outcomes. The apparent similarity in outcomes was provisionally regarded as reflective of exposure to some general methadone substitution treatment (probably including *de facto* forms of methadone maintenance).

In a further investigation of the methadone treatments actually received by each patient, it was shown that MRT was frequently not delivered as intended (Gossop *et al.* 2001*a*). Whereas the majority (70 per cent) of the patients allocated to methadone maintenance received maintenance doses, only about a third (36 per cent) of the patients allocated to MRT received reducing doses. Many patients who failed to receive MRT as intended appeared to have received some form of maintenance. The NTORS findings raise other troubling questions about the effectiveness of MRT.

For the methadone maintenance patients, reductions in illicit heroin use were associated with higher methadone doses and retention in treatment. For the patients who received MRT, the more reducing doses they received, the worse their outcomes. In particular, the more rapidly the methadone was reduced, the worse the heroin use outcomes. This suggests that, where MRT patients achieved improved outcomes after treatment, this may have occurred because of some generic treatment effect conferred by receiving a medically prescribed supply of methadone or, alternatively, because many of them actually received some form of maintenance. Where MRT was delivered as intended, it was associated with poor outcomes. Capelhorn *et al.* (1994) also found worse outcomes for patients receiving abstinence-oriented rather than indefinite maintenance.

Supervised versus unsupervised consumption

In the USA and in many other countries, it is standard practice in methadone maintenance programmes for patients to be required to attend the programme on a daily basis and to consume their dose of oral methadone on the premises and under supervision. Within this system, the option of take-home methadone is regarded as a privilege that is granted to those patients who have demonstrated their ability to avoid the use of illegal drugs, and/or to achieve other improved outcomes. As a clinic builds up a stable group of patients who are doing well, such patients may be given take-home doses of medication for several days each week as a special privilege. Such patients may sometimes be transferred to a specialized methadone programme that provides methadone-only treatment after they have demonstrated good social functioning and absence of illicit drug use over a sustained period.

In the UK, there is a widespread practice of issuing prescriptions for methadone to be consumed without supervision. This has its origins in tradition and practice rather than any theoretically based foundation, and can be traced back to the medical history of prescribing opiates and opioid drugs for maintenance purposes in Britain. Prescribing maintenance drugs that are taken without any form of supervision was standard practice in the UK during the first half of the twentieth century and the practice was perpetuated after the establishment of the drug dependence clinics in the late 1960s. This stands in marked contrast to virtually all other countries where maintenance drugs are usually (or always) consumed under direct supervision.

One consequence of issuing methadone to be consumed without supervision is that there is an established illicit market involving the diversion and sale of methadone. Non-prescribed methadone is relatively easily available on the streets and may either be sold or traded for other drugs. Estimates of the proportion of drug users in methadone treatment who sell their prescribed drugs range from 5 to 34 per cent, with oral methadone mixture selling for about UK£10/100 mg (at 1995–96 prices) compared to about £5 for a single 10 mg ampoule of injectable methadone or a single 10 mg diamorphine/heroin ampoule (Fountain *et al.* 2000*a*). Almost half of the drug users approaching the NTORS methadone programmes reported having used non-prescribed methadone in the 90 days prior to admission to treatment (Gossop *et al.* 1998*b*).

The diversion of methadone has been a cause for considerable concern, not least among opponents of methadone treatment. The issue often emerges as a focus of attention, for example, when a child or someone who is not dependent on opiates (and hence not tolerant to their effects) is found to have used diverted methadone or, worse, to have taken an overdose. There have also been times in Britain, for example during the mid-1970s, when diverted methadone was so widely available that many of the addicts seeking treatment were dependent upon non-prescribed methadone as their most frequently used and main problem drug. Other uses of diverted methadone may be less obviously problematic, such as its use in self-detoxification attempts by dependent opiate users who are not in contact with treatment services (Gossop *et al.* 1991*b*).

A further aspect of British clinical practice is the issuing of prescriptions for the unsupervised consumption of more than 1 day's supply of methadone. Prescriptions are often given for the dispensing of as much as 1 week's supply of methadone, which may be taken away by the patient. The dispensing of methadone in single daily doses has been found to vary markedly across the UK (Strang and Sheridan 1998). This variation may be partly influenced by cost considerations, since each issue of methadone attracts a dispensing fee that is paid to the dispensing pharmacist by the prescribing hospital or agency. Less frequent dispensing may also occur in rural areas because of difficulties of access to the pharmacy. Nonetheless, the extent of the variation seems unsatisfactory. The choice of treatment procedures on any grounds other than clinical effectiveness does a disservice to the patient. Strang and Sheridan (1998) referred to 'The seemingly laissez-faire approach to . . . dispensing [with its] seemingly arbitrary geographical distribution . . . . It seems far-fetched to describe this variability of practice as evidence of commendable individual tailoring of treatment; rather it would seem to be an indication of chaos, and lack of clarity and consistency in the understanding of good practice'.

Where methadone is prescribed to addicts by GPs, fewer GPs than clinics were found to prescribe methadone to be dispensed on a daily basis (Gossop *et al.* 1999*a*). GPs were also less likely to use supervised dispensing procedures, either on site or under the supervision of a retail pharmacist. GPs and clinics also differed in the forms of methadone prescribed to patients. Almost all patients in the clinics received oral liquid methadone. Among those being treated by GPs, about one in six received methadone in tablet form. Interestingly, methadone tablets appear to have been used without any reported difficulties by employed, highly stable, high functioning patients in methadone maintenance programmes (King *et al.* 2002).

In recent years, there has been a rethinking of British prescribing practices. Department of Health guidelines (1999*b*, p. 28), whilst allowing for exceptions, state that 'Supervised dispensing is recommended for new prescriptions for a minimum of three months.' A stronger statement from the ACMD (2000, p. 65) recommended that 'methadone should be taken under daily supervision for at least 6 months and often longer. . . . The bigger the dose of methadone that is being prescribed, the greater will be the need for supervision.' There is some movement towards increased reliance upon supervised dispensing for new patients, and several of the more recently established methadone clinics have adopted supervised dispensing as the established practice. Nonetheless, despite these trends, and because of the autonomy granted to British doctors, the recommendations included in the guidelines continue to be widely disregarded.

Injectable methadone

The prescribing of injectable forms of methadone to opiate addicts within the UK is a longstanding characteristic of the 'British system' of drug treatment (Strang *et al.* 1994*b*). This practice is virtually unknown outside the UK. The exceptions include experimental studies in the Netherlands and Switzerland and a few remaining patients from the 27 heroin addicts who were started on injectable methadone in Queensland, Australia in 1977. In the Dutch experience, the Amsterdam Municipal Health Service, prescribed this form of methadone in 1990, for intravenous self-injection to 30 non-manageable, long-term, and severely addicted AIDS patients who were in a very poor condition. The intervention was not regarded as being particularly successful and the prescription was terminated for half of the patients because they failed to comply with treatment requirements. Several of those who continued taking the injectable methadone were subsequently reported to have died (cited in van den Brink *et al.* 2002). Among others who continued to receive injectable methadone, the therapeutic relationship was described as having improved, and their use of illicit heroin decreased though it was not eliminated.

There are no legal restrictions in the UK to prevent doctors prescribing methadone in either its oral or injectable form, though the prescription of injectable methadone for the treatment of addiction is controversial, and there is little research evidence to provide guidance about patient selection, patient responses, and outcomes. It has been suggested that there may be a small number of long-term injectors who can benefit from such prescribing, (Department of Health 1999*b*), though the same guidelines also stated that there is only 'a very limited clinical place for prescribing injectable methadone'. There are currently no clear criteria to guide clinical decisions about which patients might be suitable for such treatment, but repeated failure to engage with or respond to standard treatment regimens is one of the most commonly cited reasons for consideration of the use of injectable medication. Among the factors that have been cited as contraindications for injectable prescribing are signs or history of deep vein thrombosis and related pathologies, and recent or current failure to act in accordance with the principles of safe injecting.

The prescribing of injectable methadone dates back to the earliest years of the British drug clinic system. Indeed, at one time during the mid-1970s, injectable methadone was the most frequently prescribed form of methadone within British addiction clinics (Mitcheson 1994). A 1995 national survey (Strang and Sheridan 1998) found that 10 per cent of all methadone prescriptions to addicts were for injectable methadone ampoules. This was found to vary between 4 and 23 per cent across regions. Injectable methadone appeared to be rarely, if ever, prescribed in Scotland, Wales, or Northern Ireland. The prescribing of injectable ampoules of methadone appeared to be as common in the practice of GPs as it was amongst hospital-based specialists (Strang *et al.* 1996*a*).

Sell *et al.* (2001) suggest a number of reasons (or rationalizations) that are sometimes given for the use of injectable methadone. One is that, in comparison with other opiates such as heroin or morphine, methadone ampoules need only to be injected once daily while heroin administration is required at least 2–3 times daily to achieve any sort of maintenance effect. There is also good evidence to support the effectiveness of methadone as a treatment, albeit in its oral form. Also, injectable methadone preparations are not as costly as injectable heroin. The cost of maintaining a patient on injectable methadone has been estimated to be about a quarter of that for injectable diamorphine (Brewer 1995). Although it is often assumed that opiate addicts would prefer to be prescribed heroin rather than methadone, Metrebian *et al.* (1998) found that over one-third of their patients, when given the choice, preferred injectable methadone to injectable diamorphine.

A study by Battersby *et al.* (1992) looked at a group of London opiate addicts presenting to a drug clinic who received prescriptions for injectable opiates (either injectable heroin or injectable methadone) as part of their treatment programme. All of these addicts had long histories of dependence upon injected opiates. None was willing to comply with a treatment programme that did not initially include a prescribed supply of injectable opiates. It was hoped that there might be a reduction in HIV risk-taking behaviour such as frequency of injecting and the sharing of injecting equipment that would be promoted by this prescribing approach.

The results suggested that, although patients were satisfactorily retained in treatment, there was little evidence of changes in injecting behaviour. Several patients continued to use extremely risky injecting practices, such as injecting drugs into the femoral vein at the inguinal site. This is a highly undesirable and dangerous practice. In addition, the stability of the lives of 20 per cent of the sample had deteriorated. During the prescribing period, one patient developed a life-threatening illness (cervical spine osteomyelitis) and survived. The near-death of this patient pointed to the high-risk nature of this prescribing practice, where short-term benefit and consumer satisfaction may need to be balanced against the possibility of adverse consequences in the longer term.

The study also reported some positive outcomes. More than a third of the sample were rated as having made positive life changes during the study period. Almost one-quarter of the patients requested admission to an in-patient treatment unit, and became drug-free during their admission. Among those who continued to receive prescribed opioids, the mean dosage prescribed, in methadone equivalents, had reduced from 70 to 50 mg. Overall the results did not provide conclusive evidence of either benefit or harm as a result of this intervention.

Sell *et al.* (2001) reported an open clinical study of 125 long-term opiate-dependent patients who had been referred to a specialist clinic by local drug services as a result of their failure to benefit from standard treatment, usually oral methadone. The majority of these patients (86 per cent) were prescribed injectable methadone. An important treatment goal was identified as the reduction of injecting risk behaviours, and the authors reported low levels of self-reported injecting and sexual risk behaviour during treatment. A troubling observation from this study was that, because most of the patients no longer had accessible veins in their arms or hands, the most common site for injection of their prescribed drug was a femoral vein (groin injecting), and most patients did not rotate injecting sites. Groin injecting is a risky practice because of the proximity of the femoral artery and nerve, and the potentially serious consequences of femoral vein thrombosis. The interpretation of this behaviour is complicated by the fact that patients were recruited to the study because of their seriously problematic drug-taking behaviours and because of their non-responsiveness to existing treatments.

In what is the first (albeit small-scale) randomized clinical trial of injectable methadone maintenance treatment for opiate addicts, Strang *et al.* (2000*b*) compared the treatment response of opiate-dependent out-patients to supervised oral versus supervised injectable methadone maintenance treatment conditions. The two (randomly assigned) treatment groups were well matched in terms of pretreatment demographic characteristics and clinical problems. Treatment outcome was assessed at 6-month follow-up for illicit heroin use, illicit injecting, use of other opiate/opioids, crack cocaine, and benzodiazepines, as well as for drinking outcomes, health, and crime.

Patients in both the injectable and oral methadone treatment groups showed significant reductions in problem behaviours at follow-up. Major health gains were found across a number of dimensions for patients in both treatment conditions, and outcomes among the patients in the injectable methadone condition were directly comparable, in terms of drug taking and other problem areas, to those found among patients receiving oral methadone. One of the few differences to emerge was that the patients who received injectable methadone maintenance reported higher levels of treatment satisfaction than the oral maintenance patients. There was some suggestion that patients with poorer physical health and poorer psychological health at intake showed greater reductions in illicit heroin use if they had been assigned to the injectable methadone condition. One clear difference between the two treatments concerned their cost. The study estimated that the direct operational costs of providing injectable methadone were about five times greater than those for oral methadone.

Chapter 11

Other drug treatments

Maintenance with prescribed heroin

The prescribing of heroin/diamorphine to addicts is sometimes, mistakenly, regarded as a key feature of the 'British system'. The misconception that heroin is widely used in Britain is partly due to a failure to distinguish between the uses of diamorphine to treat medical conditions and its uses in the treatment and management of addiction. Heroin is not a prohibited medicine in the UK. Any doctor can prescribe it for medical conditions other than addiction. In general medical practice, the use of heroin is not regarded as either radical or controversial. For example, heroin is commonly used both by family doctors and by hospital physicians in the treatment of pain and other medical conditions. With regard to the treatment of acute myocardial infarction, for example, the *Oxford Textbook of Medicine* (Sleight 1996) recommends that 'The most immediate practical procedure...is to relieve the patient's pain with an adequate dose of intravenous morphine or diamorphine.'

This is in contrast to the prescription of heroin for the treatment and management of addiction where a Home Office licence is required to allow the doctor to prescribe heroin. Such licences are entirely the preserve of addiction specialists. Except for a short period after the establishment of the clinic system in the late 1960s, heroin prescribing has not been widely used in the UK. The swing away from heroin prescribing occurred during the early 1970s. This was not due to any change in policy but reflected a broadly based but only vaguely articulated consensus view of the doctors and staff working within the drug clinics (Gossop 1994).

By 1992, less than 1 per cent (only 117) of British opiate addicts were receiving a prescription for injectable heroin compared to about 98 per cent who were receiving prescribed methadone. There have been a few advocates of heroin prescribing in the UK (Marks 1985*b*) and some local enthusiasm for an expansion of heroin maintenance, but few signs of any major change in practice. In a survey of 105 doctors in drug treatment services, Sell *et al.* (1997) found that, of the 46 doctors who had applied for a licence to prescribe heroin, 44 (91 per cent) held a current licence. Among those who held a licence, most prescribed heroin to only a small number of patients (on average, each was seeing only seven such patients). They expressed no strong resistance to heroin prescribing but the majority felt that, although it was appropriate in at least some cases, such cases were infrequent.

For some time, British policy has reflected a lack of enthusiasm for any expansion of heroin prescribing. The Department of Health (1999*b*) guidelines devoted only a single brief paragraph to this issue and stated that, as a treatment for opiate addiction, 'there is very little clinical indication for prescribed [heroin]'.

The results of the few studies that have been conducted in the UK (e.g. Hartnoll *et al.* 1980; Gossop *et al.* 1982*b*; Battersby *et al.* 1992; Metrebian *et al.* 1998) have shown no clear or consistent effect. For many addicts, heroin may be regarded as a more desirable treatment option than methadone and, as such, heroin could be expected to attract more addicts into treatment and to hold them there. Hartnoll *et al.* (1980) reported that, 1 year after entering treatment, 74 per cent of those receiving heroin were still in treatment compared to only 29 per cent of those receiving oral methadone. However, even this result needs to be interpreted with caution. At the time of their study, the prescribing of heroin and of injectable methadone was still relatively widely available within London clinics, and oral methadone was very definitely seen by most addicts as a new and 'second-class' option. This may have influenced patient attitudes and responses to the two treatments. The retention rates should also take account of the finding that many of those offered oral methadone (40 per cent) had given up regular use of opiates at follow-up. Those receiving heroin maintenance were also more likely to have continued injecting drugs. The authors concluded that 'the results do not indicate a clear overall superiority of either approach. Both treatments have advantages in some areas but at the expense of disadvantages in other areas.' The available UK research studies into heroin prescribing can be interpreted as indicating some modest benefits for some patients.

The use of heroin as a maintenance drug is contrary to several of the principles of maintenance therapy (Kreek 1997*b*), namely, that a maintenance drug should have:

- a slow onset of action to prevent positive reinforcing effects;
- a slow decay of action to prevent negative reinforcement;
- a long duration of action to allow normalization of physiological function and permit infrequent dosing;
- be orally effective.

Heroin meets none of these requirements. It is not orally effective, has a rapid onset of action, and a short duration of action.

In recent years, the greatest interest in heroin prescribing has been found in Switzerland, the Netherlands, and Germany where clinical trials have been (or are currently being) carried out.

In the Swiss trial, the admission criteria stipulated a minimum age of 20 years, a history of heroin dependence of at least 2 years, a history of failed participation in other treatments on several occasions, and adverse affects of drug use upon health and/or social functioning (Uchtenhagen *et al.* 1999). Patients were stabilized on (average) doses of 500–600 mg heroin daily, though heroin was prescribed in conjunction with an offer to prescribe oral methadone if the user was not able to, or did not wish to attend the clinic to take their heroin. Data have also been presented for a selected subsample of patients ($n = 237$) who were retained in treatment for a period of at least 18 months (Rehm *et al.* 2001). In this subsample, the average daily dose was 474 mg with administration occurring on a mean of 2.6 occasions each day. The injections of prescribed heroin were administered under supervision, and could not be taken home (in contrast to the British practice of prescribing heroin or injectable methadone). In addition to injectable heroin, the treatment intervention package involved the provision of counselling and other forms of psychosocial care.

Patient recruitment, treatment retention, and treatment compliance were better among the patients receiving injectable heroin than for those on oral methadone. The retention rates of 89 per cent at 6 months and 69 per cent at 18 months were described as being above average compared with those of other treatment programmes (Uchtenhagen *et al.* 1999).

The results showed reductions in the use of illicit heroin and cocaine among those receiving prescribed heroin. Reductions in the use of other illicit drugs were less marked. The use of non-prescribed benzodiazepines decreased only slowly, and alcohol and cannabis consumption hardly declined at all. There were reductions in criminal activity. Income derived from illegal and semi-legal activities decreased from 59 to 10 per cent, and both the number of offenders and the number of criminal offences decreased by about 60 per cent during the first 6 months of treatment. There was also a fall in the number of court convictions. In some cases, these improvements occurred very soon after the beginning of treatment. In other cases, improvements were not seen until after several months of treatment. The mortality rate of the patients in the trial was 1 per cent per year. This is comparable to mortality rates for treatment samples of drug users in other studies (Joe *et al.* 1982; Gossop *et al.* 2002*b*).

Uchtenhagen *et al.* (1999) concluded that heroin-assisted treatment was useful for the designated target group. The authors also concluded that heroin prescribing could be carried out with 'sufficient safety' for the participants and others by establishing appropriate supervisory measures. Whereas many observers of this trial have focused exclusively upon the prescription of injectable heroin as the treatment agent, the authors note that the prescription of heroin was only one part of a comprehensive programme of patient education and therapy. Also, in terms of pharmacotherapy, the study was not strictly a heroin-only treatment study since the patients were permitted to miss heroin doses and to take methadone instead. In practice, heroin alone was prescribed on only about half of the consumption days (Uchtenhagen *et al.* 1999).

One interesting feature of the Swiss trial has received surprisingly little attention. There was less demand from drug misusers than had been anticipated. In some programmes not all available places were filled. In the Geneva programme, for example, although 80 treatment slots were planned, only 73 heroin users applied for treatment, of whom only 57 were eligible (Perneger *et al.* 1998). At the end of the experimental phase, only 9 patients from the methadone control condition took up the offer of heroin maintenance. Although the prescription of injectable heroin was seen as attractive, the full programme package (possibly the requirement that injections could be taken only in the clinic setting and under supervision three times each day) was less attractive than might have been expected.

A more recent controlled clinical trial was conducted in the Netherlands (van den Brink *et al.* 2002). Its primary objective was to evaluate the effects of 12 months' maintenance treatment with oral methadone and co-prescribed heroin, compared with standard maintenance treatment with oral methadone alone.

The study population comprised chronic, treatment-resistant heroin addicts who were currently enrolled in methadone maintenance programmes. Inclusion criteria were:

♦ a history of heroin dependence of at least 5 years;

♦ a minimum dose level of 50 mg (for those in the heroin injecting condition) or 60 mg (heroin inhaling condition) of methadone per day for an uninterrupted period of at least 4 weeks in the previous 5 years;

♦ registered in a methadone programme in the previous year, and in regular contact with the methadone programme during the previous 6 months;

♦ unsuccessful response to methadone maintenance treatment;

♦ daily or near-daily use of illicit heroin;

♦ poor physical and/or mental and/or social functioning.

Heroin is widely used by chasing as well as injecting in the Netherlands, and the primary study question was investigated separately for the prescription of injectable and inhalable forms of heroin. Patients were randomly allocated to the injectable ($n = 174$) and the inhalable conditions ($n = 375$). Treatment outcomes were evaluated in terms of a composite measure of clinical improvement assessed in terms of changes in physical and mental health, social integration and social functioning, and illicit drug use.

The patients treated with methadone-plus-heroin did better than those treated with methadone alone on most measures of outcome. This effect was found irrespective of route of administration, population in the analysis (intention-to-treat, treatment completers), and outcome parameter. Patients in both trials who received supervised co-prescription of heroin showed improvements in physical health, mental status, and social functioning. The effect size for the main outcome measure represented a 25 per cent difference in response between the treatment conditions among injectors and a 23 per cent difference among inhalers. One exception to this was for treatment retention. Perhaps somewhat surprisingly, retention rates after 12 months were higher among the methadone-only group (86 per cent) than among those receiving heroin (70 per cent).

Improvements in both the injectable and inhalable arms of the trial tended to occur relatively early in treatment, often within the first 2 months, with further improvements occurring during the course of treatment. Planned duration was not associated with improved outcomes, but a longer actual stay was related to improved outcomes. At the end of the trials, and following discontinuation of prescribed heroin, the majority (81–87 per cent) of the treatment responders in the experimental conditions deteriorated to dysfunctional levels similar to those prior to treatment.

Considering that patients were chronic, non-responders to methadone maintenance treatment, an interesting if unexpected finding was the relatively high rate of clinical improvement among patients in the control groups who continued to receive methadone (32 per cent among heroin injectors; 25 per cent among heroin inhalers). Among the possible reasons suggested for this were that their improvement may have been due to participation in a study with frequent assessments, or regression to the mean effects (van den Brink *et al.* 2002).

Even in such a well-controlled trial, there is uncertainty about the reasons for the observed findings. Since the methadone-only treatment took place in existing clinics with existing treatment staff, whereas the methadone-plus-heroin treatment took place in newly established clinics with specially recruited staff members, it is possible that location and staffing differences may have been partly responsible for the observed differences in outcome between the experimental and the control groups. Van den Brink *et al.* (2002) note that the co-prescription of heroin involved more patient–staff contact and that this may have had some influence upon the results. Also, many patients in the control condition may have used similar amounts of (illicit) heroin during the study, which suggests that the observed effects of the co-prescription of heroin could not be attributed simply to some pharmacological effect of the drug. Similarly, the trial was (necessarily) an open-label trial and it is possible that some of the differences in outcome could have been due to the influence of patient attitudes, expectations, and cognitions.

Prescribing stimulants

The medical prescription of stimulant drugs for maintenance purposes is a highly contentious procedure about which relatively little is known. During the first half of the twentieth century and for a short time after the opening of the clinics in 1968, some British doctors issued prescriptions for pharmaceutical cocaine. Within about a year of operation, a voluntary agreement was reached by the prescribing doctors in the new drug dependence clinics, who by then were the only doctors allowed to prescribe cocaine to addicts, that they would cease all further prescribing of cocaine (Connell and Strang 1994). By the end of 1969, only 81 addicts received cocaine on prescription in the UK (Spear and Mott 1993). Thereafter, the prescribing of pharmaceutical cocaine to addicts in the UK has remained extremely rare (fewer than 10 cases per year).

During the summer of 1968 London experienced a brief epidemic of methamphetamine injecting. This was largely due to several doctors who were grossly overprescribing the drug, which was being traded on the black market. Mitcheson *et al.* (1976) reported on an attempt to treat some of these users with prescribed ampoules of methamphetamine. The average daily prescribed dose was four 30-mg ampoules. This intervention was seen as 'mostly ineffectual' and a 'therapeutic failure'. A second report on amphetamine misusers treated with oral amphetamine at a clinic in London in 1968/69 concluded that such prescriptions were unlikely to be effective (Gardner and Connell 1972).

In Sweden, following a large media campaign in favour of the liberalization of drug policy, an experiment with the prescription of stimulants and opiates for injection was initiated in 1965 (Kall 1997). Its purposes were gradually to reduce the dose, to reduce drug-related crime, and to get the stimulant users off drugs. There was much diversion to the black market, few users stopped taking drugs, and the experiment was deemed a failure. It was ended after 2 years.

Although there is broad agreement that dependence upon stimulants does not constitute a suitable condition for drug replacement treatment (ACMD 1988), it remains within the authority of any doctor in the UK to prescribe amphetamines to addicts if they choose to do so. Amphetamine prescribing has been tried at two specialist centres with some monitoring of practices and outcomes (Fleming and Roberts 1994; Myles 1997). Amphetamine prescribing also sometimes occurs in general practice.

Flemming (1998) suggested that prescribing should be time-limited and restricted to primary amphetamine users with heavy and problematic use. In the UK this may mean users who take more than 1 g of street amphetamine sulphate a day. In practice heavy users may take 3 or 4 g a day, and may have taken amphetamine regularly for at least several months. Flemming suggested that prescribing can be done using dexamphetamine as an oral elixir that is dispensed on several days a week. This is said to minimize the opportunity for diversion.

McBride *et al.* (1997) compared a treatment group who received dex-amphetamine with a control group of similar drug users who attended the same service before amphetamine prescribing began. The offer of amphetamine prescribing appeared to increase treatment contact and retention. The treatment group used less illicit drugs and showed reductions in injecting activity during treatment.

In a pilot study of amphetamine substitution in Australia, patients were prescribed low, oral doses of dexamphetamine and monitored for adverse effects and psychotic symptoms (Shearer *et al.* 2001). The rate of adverse effects was reported to be low. The treatment led to satisfactory treatment retention and compliance in the experimental group. Patients receiving prescribed dex-amphetamine were more likely to attend counselling sessions, and attended twice as many sessions as the control group. When asked at follow-up whether they would continue in treatment if this option were available, the majority (80 per cent) expressed a willingness to continue. Shearer *et al.* (2001) suggested that amphetamine substitution therapy deserved further consideration as a potentially useful clinical intervention for problematic amphetamine use.

Contraindications for stimulant maintenance treatment have been described as including pregnancy, a history of hypertension, heart disease, or mental illness (Flemming 1998). The assessment of mental illness can be complicated by the paranoid feelings and psychotic episodes occasionally experienced by some heavy stimulant users. Amphetamine prescribing should be avoided if there has been a previous psychotic episode, even if this has been associated with drug use, as this may indicate a vulnerability or predisposition to the development of a schizophrenic illness.

Strang and Sheridan (1997) estimated that as many as 900–1000 patients in the UK were receiving some form of amphetamine maintenance treatment (which makes it approximately three times more prevalent than heroin prescribing). Amphetamines were often prescribed in the form of tablets of dexamphetamine. These tablets are open to abuse by users who grind them up and dissolve the powder to prepare an injectable liquid. The mean prescribed dose was about 40 mg but with doses ranging between 5 and 200 mg. The other commonly prescribed form of amphetamine was dexamphetamine as an oral liquid. In a small number of cases (3 per cent) amphetamine was prescribed in the form of methamphetamine ampoules. Strang and Sheridan (1997) described 'a disturbing lack of interval dispensing arrangements...to safeguard against diversion onto the black market'.

LAAM (leva-alpha acetyl methadol)

LAAM is a derivative of methadone, and was first developed as an analgesic. Like methadone, LAAM can ameliorate craving for heroin and prevent withdrawal symptoms. As early as 1952 it was known that LAAM could prevent opiate withdrawal symptoms for more than 72 hours. There was considerable interest in LAAM during the late 1960s and 1970s, and between 1960 and 1981 27 clinical trials were conducted with over 6000 patients.

Due to lack of funding, little research was carried out during the 1980s. The reasons for the lack of funding are themselves interesting. In general, pharmaceutical companies tend to show little interest in the development of anti-addiction medications. There are virtually no market incentives and several disincentives for pharmaceutical companies to develop such medications. The cost of bringing any new drug to market can be very great, and only a few of the potential medications eventually appear on the market. Pharmaceutical companies may also be hesitant to develop addiction medications because of the stigma that may attach to them or their drugs, especially if the drug has other medical uses.

LAAM is an opioid agonist with a relatively long duration of action. LAAM is a 'pro-drug', that is, its primary effect only occurs after it has been metabolized in the liver (Rawson et al. 1998). LAAM metabolizes to the active metabolite nor-LAAM, which in turn metabolizes to the active metabolite di-nor-LAAM. LAAM itself has a half-life of 2.6 days. The half-life for nor-LAAM is 2 days, and that for di-nor-LAAM is 4 days (Kreek 1996).

LAAM is administered orally (usually in liquid). Because of its long duration of action and unlike methadone, which requires daily dosing, LAAM is effective for up to 3 days and may be given every second day or three times a week. It has a slow elimination time with a long, slow plateau of effect.

There are a number of clinical advantages to LAAM as a maintenance drug.

♦ It reduces the need for frequent visits to the clinic without take-home doses.

♦ It frees the patient from a dependence on the clinic.

◆ It produces a more 'normal', less euphoric drug state while still blocking the effects of other opiates and preventing withdrawal (Finn and Wilcock 1997).

It also carries certain disadvantages.

◆ Adjustment to LAAM can be difficult for some patients. It can take up to 2 weeks to reach a stabilized effect on the drug.

◆ The reduced need for clinic attendance and lack of daily contact may be counterproductive for some patients who need daily support or counselling.

There are also disavantages as well as advantages to the long duration of action of LAAM. LAAM should not be administered more often than every other day because of the risks of toxicity or overdose due to accumulated doses (Kreek 1996). The long half-life of LAAM and of its metabolites can produce potential problems of toxicity, especially if LAAM is rapidly metabolized due to enhanced liver function. The potential for toxic levels of the active metabolites to build up should be noted, especially during the induction and stabilization phases of maintenance with LAAM.

In a 40-week, double-blind trial conducted at 12 sites with 430 patients, doses of 60–100 mg of LAAM, dispensed three times a week, were found to be of comparable effectiveness to 50–100 mg of methadone in reducing illicit heroin use (Ling et al. 1976). More subjects dropped out of LAAM treatment than methadone treatment in the first 4 weeks, but drop-out rates for both groups rapidly declined over time, and were in the range of 1–2 per cent per week by the third month of the study. Overall acceptability ratings and response to treatment were similar for LAAM and methadone.

When LAAM and methadone were compared with a waiting list control group, Jaffe et al. (1972) found comparable levels of improvement for the methadone and LAAM groups, and better outcomes for both the LAAM and methadone groups than for the waiting list group. When compared with low-dose daily methadone (mean = 26 mg), Freedman and Czertko (1981) found that a three times a week, low-dose LAAM regimen (mean = 24 mg) produced greater reductions in illicit drug use and better treatment retention.

High rates of patient drop-out are sometimes found during induction on to LAAM. Jones et al. (1998) found that induction with low and medium doses of LAAM can be safely and effectively achieved within 7 days. Induction with higher LAAM doses can be done over 17 days but may lead to more adverse effects and higher rates of patient drop-out. They suggest that high doses should be approached more slowly. However, in a randomized, double-blind study, Eissenberg et al. (1997) found that the clinical efficacy of LAAM is dose-related. Patients receiving high doses of LAAM showed the greatest reductions in heroin use, and patients on low doses showed the least reductions. Patients in the high-dose condition were also abstinent from heroin for longer than those in the medium- and low-dose conditions.

In a double-blind placebo trial, Walsh *et al.* (1998) found that speed of onset of drug effect was different for intravenous or oral routes of administration. Intravenous LAAM produced significant subjective and physiological effects within 5 minutes. When LAAM was orally administered, onset was slower, and effects appeared between 1 and 2 hours. The intravenous effects included agonist-type effects (subjective ratings of 'high', and 'nodding'), and the authors suggest that their results may indicate that LAAM possesses greater abuse liability than was previously believed.

A meta-analysis of trials comparing LAAM and methadone suggested that treatment with methadone produced slightly better retention and less drop-out due to side-effects (Glanz *et al.* 1997). Treatment with LAAM produced slightly (but not statistically significantly) better results in terms of reduced illicit drug use.

LAAM was approved for use in the USA in 1993. By 1999, the US Food and Drug Administration estimated that approximately 5000–6000 patients were receiving LAAM. Nonetheless, there has been considerable reluctance to use LAAM in clinical practice. Three years after its approval, only 62 of the more than 750 licensed opiate treatment programmes in the USA had patients on LAAM and only 11 clinics had more than 15 patients on LAAM (Rawson *et al.* 1998).

Buprenorphine

Buprenorphine is a mixed agonist–antagonist with unique properties that differentiate it from full opiate agonists such as heroin or methadone. Opiate agonists activate specific opiate receptors. Antagonists occupy a receptor but do not activate it (see 'Naltrexone', this chapter). Antagonists may displace agonists in a dependent drug user and provoke an immediate withdrawal syndrome (O'Brien and Cornish 1999).

Buprenorphine acts as a partial agonist at mu opioid receptor sites. Partial agonists occupy opiate receptors but activate them only in a limited way. Partial agonists may also block the occupation of receptors by full agonists, and buprenorphine also acts as an antagonist at kappa opioid receptor sites. At low doses, partial agonists can produce similar or identical effects to full agonists, but a partial agonist does not activate the receptor as much as a full agonist. Partial agonists exhibit ceiling effects and, unlike full agonists, higher doses of partial agonists do not necessarily produce greater effects. Dose increases are only effective up to a certain level.

When partial opioid agonists are given to someone who is not physically dependent on opioids, they produce agonist effects (such as mild euphoria).

When given to someone who is physically dependent, a partial agonist can act like an antagonist and even precipitate withdrawal responses, because it does not activate the receptor as much as the full agonist. There is evidence that buprenorphine can produce antagonist-like effects when a high dose is given shortly after an agonist. Strain *et al.* (1995) found evidence of mild withdrawal reactions to buprenorphine among opiate users who were maintained on methadone and given an injection of buprenorphine 2 hours after their methadone dose.

Buprenorphine has poor oral bioavailability, so it is not effective as a medication when swallowed. When used as an analgesic, it is typically given by injection. However, it is readily absorbed through mouth membranes if given sublingually, and it has been used clinically both as a sublingual solution or as sublingual tablets.

France has been the first country to make extensive use of buprenorphine in the treatment of opioid dependence. For many years, France was extremely reluctant to use maintenance treatments. As late as 1995, only two centres (in Paris) were allowed to prescribe methadone to about 50 patients in a national population of 60 million. Some clinicians prescribed codeine or buprenorphine (introduced on to the French market in 1980). From 1996, high-dosage sublingual buprenorphine was approved by the French Drug Agency as a maintenance treatment (Barrau *et al.* 2001). Despite a number of changes in policy regarding maintenance treatments, the number of authorized places in French methadone programmes remains very limited. In 1998, the total number of methadone-maintained patients in France was estimated at 7200. This was dwarfed by the estimated 57 000 patients who were being prescribed buprenorphine.

Buprenorphine is prescribed in France mainly in primary care services. One recent estimate suggests that the number of patients receiving buprenorphine maintenance in primary care settings may have increased to around 80 000 at the end of 2000 (Vignau *et al.* 2001). In this survey, 28 per cent of the physicians reported having prescribed buprenorphine, and 52 per cent of the pharmacists reported dispensing the drug at least once during the first 2 years of its availability. Thirion *et al.* (2002) found that 24 per cent of the GPs in their survey had cared for intravenous drug users and 21 per cent had prescribed buprenorphine. In a study of French GPs, Fhima *et al.* (2001) found that 101 GPs were prescribing buprenorphine to 919 patients, with the majority of these patients (71 per cent) receiving the drug on a long-term maintenance basis. Many patients (56 per cent) were retained in treatment at 2-year follow-up.

Relatively little is known about patient outcomes during and subsequent to buprenorphine treatment in France. However, it is known that there are problems associated with the diversion of the drug because of the prescription and unsupervised consumption arrangements. Buprenorphine has been reported to be readily available on the French black market (Kintz 2001). One specific problem involves the intravenous misuse of sublingual buprenorphine tablets, and this practice may be widespread among French drug users (Obadia *et al.* 2001).

Naloxone can be added to buprenorphine to minimize its abuse potential, particularly when taken by injection. Combined naloxone/buprenorphine preparations may be useful for administration in non-specialist treatment settings, and for use with treatment populations who either do not have access to methadone programmes, or for others such as adolescents who may be unsuited to them for other reasons.

There are several advantages to buprenorphine's partial agonist effects. Because its agonist effect at very high doses is less than that of a full agonist, an overdose with buprenorphine should produce less severe respiratory depression than an overdose of a full-agonist opioid. Auriacombe (2001) estimated that the annual death rate for buprenorphine is three times lower than for methadone. Kintz (2001) suggested that buprenorphine substitution programmes could be considered a success from a public health perspective since the number of fatal heroin overdoses dropped during the period of buprenorphine prescribing from about 500 cases per year to less than 100 in 1999. Nonetheless, numerous deaths have been attributed to buprenorphine. The first buprenorphine fatality was reported in August 1996, and Tracqui *et al.* (1998) reported a series of 20 fatalities among patients at five treatment centres.

The mortality risk associated with buprenorphine may be related to its combined use with other drugs (especially benzodiazepines and neuroleptics) and to the misuse of the tablets when taken by intravenous injection. Deaths have been reported due to the simultaneous injection of buprenorphine and benzodiazepines (Reynaud *et al.* 1998). The high-dose buprenorphine formulation that is widely used in France may also be a contributory factor in such fatalities. Kintz (2001) suggested that the reported deaths linked to buprenorphine challenge the supposed low risks of buprenorphine: it was also suggested that the number of buprenorphine-related fatalities in France may be substantially underestimated.

Johnson *et al.* (2000) randomly assigned 220 heroin addicts to one of four treatments: buprenorphine (16–32 mg, 3 times a week); LAAM (75–115 mg, 3 times a week); high-dose methadone (60–100 mg daily); or low-dose methadone (20 mg daily). The study showed that buprenorphine and LAAM can be as effective as high-dose methadone in the treatment of heroin addiction. All three of these medications were more effective than low-dose methadone. Drug users treated with buprenorphine, LAAM, or high-dose methadone, all reported major reductions in their use of heroin. The longest periods of abstinence from heroin were achieved by patients receiving LAAM. Retention rates were highest in the high-dose methadone group (73 per cent), with 58 per cent in the buprenorphine group, 53 per cent in the LAAM group, and 20 per cent in the low-dose methadone group.

In a review of the literature, Mattick *et al.* (1998) concluded that buprenorphine may be at least as effective as methadone as a maintenance agent in terms of reducing illicit opioid use and retaining patients in treatment. They also suggest that buprenorphine is safer than methadone in terms of the risk of overdose since it produces relatively limited respiratory depression, and is extremely well tolerated by non-dependent users.

A further potential advantage of buprenorphine is that, at least in principle, its mixed agonist–antagonist action may lead to a less severe withdrawal syndrome than that associated with pure agonists such as heroin or methadone (Kosten *et al.* 1992). Buprenorphine has been used both on its own and in combination with other drugs in the management of the opiate withdrawal syndrome. In an open-label trial in which opiate-dependent patients were allocated to receive either lofexidine or buprenorphine detoxification, it was found that the buprenorphine group reported less severe withdrawal symptoms and were more likely to complete the detoxification programme (White *et al.* 2001).

Naltrexone (and other antagonists)

Naltrexone and naloxone are relatively pure antagonists and produce little or no agonist activity at usual doses. Opiate antagonists prevent agonists from binding to the receptor and producing opiate effects.

Naltrexone was first synthesized in 1967. It is a long-acting, orally administered opioid antagonist that is absorbed rapidly from the gastrointestinal tract. It has high receptor affinity, blocking the euphoria, respiratory depression, pupillary constriction, and other effects of drugs such as heroin (Martin *et al.* 1973; O'Brien *et al.* 1975).

Naloxone is also an opioid antagonist. It differs from naltrexone in that it has poor oral bioavailability and a short half-life. Naloxone is poorly absorbed from the gut, but when given parenterally it is rapidly metabolized. One of the main uses of naloxone is for the acute reversal of opioid effects in the emergency treatment of overdoses of heroin or other opioids. Naltrexone is a structural analogue of naloxone but has much greater antagonistic potency.

Opiate antagonist drugs can be used to speed up withdrawal treatments (see Chapter 7). Antagonists can also be used to assist the diagnosis of physical dependence. If given to a dependent opioid user, an antagonist such as naloxone will produce an immediate withdrawal reaction. Of greater interest is the potential role for antagonists in helping to prevent relapse after detoxification. After taking naltrexone, and under experimental conditions, heroin addicts find that heroin is no longer rewarding and will stop self-administering it even when the drug is freely available (Mello *et al.* 1981).

Because naltrexone is so different from other available treatments for opioid dependence, its mode of action is sometimes misunderstood. It is sometimes confused with disulfiram (Antabuse), which is used in the treatment of alcoholism. The two drugs are pharmacologically different, and they have completely different modes of action. Naltrexone is used as a maintenance medication (as an 'insurance policy') in situations where there is a serious risk of relapse.

Where opiate-dependent patients are to be treated with naltrexone, it is necessary that they should have achieved a sustained period of opioid abstinence prior to the first dose of naltrexone. A minimum of 7 days without opioids (licit or illicit) is sometimes recommended (Platt 1995). If the patient is still physically dependent on opioids, the administration of a single dose of naltrexone will precipitate a withdrawal reaction. One way of ensuring that the patient is not still physically dependent before the first dose of naltrexone, is to administer a naloxone challenge by injection, followed by close monitoring of the patient for evidence of withdrawal. This can be done by clinical observation by an experienced nurse or physician. If a more precise quantitative assessment of withdrawal responses is required, a standardized instrument may be used.

If the patient is still physically dependent upon opiates, signs and symptoms of withdrawal will generally appear within 5–10 minutes after the administration of naloxone, and typically, resolve within 1–1.5 hours. Some clinicians administer a lower dose of naloxone initially, and then give a second dose after 30–60 minutes if there is no evidence of withdrawal associated with the first dose. If the naloxone challenge does not lead to a precipitated withdrawal response, it should be safe to administer the first dose of naltrexone.

In principle, naltrexone pharmacotherapy provides an almost ideal treatment for opiate addiction. Naltrexone selectively competes for opioid receptors, prevents reinforcement from opioids, and prevents a return to physical dependence. The conditioned association between heroin use and positive reinforcement should be extinguished if the individual avoids further opioid use or obtains no reinforcement from continued use. Naltrexone is orally active, and potent (with an affinity for opioid receptors 20 times greater than morphine). It can be administered on a three times weekly schedule. Because it does not produce a 'high', it has little abuse potential and raises few problems of diversion. Tolerance to the opioid antagonist effects does not appear to develop even after more than a year of regular naltrexone use (Kleber *et al.* 1985).

It generally has few side-effects at recommended doses (of 50 mg per day), though some detoxified heroin addicts report unpleasant withdrawal-like effects. The drug has some side-effects, including dysphoria (Crowley *et al.* 1985), loss of energy, depression, and gastrointestinal symptoms (Hollister *et al.* 1981). Reports of abdominal pain or discomfort have also been noted in studies of patients treated with naltrexone, although the percentage of patients with such problems is low (generally less than 5 per cent). Dysphoria has been noted less consistently, though naltrexone-induced dysphoria may be a factor that contributes to poor compliance in taking the medication.

Despite its promise, naltrexone has not lived up to its early expectations and has had little impact on the day-to-day clinical management of heroin addiction. Since naltrexone is an expensive drug its cost may be an obstacle where financial resources are limited. Perhaps more importantly, the majority of drug-dependent patients are reluctant or resistant to take naltrexone. In a survey of treatment-seeking opiate addicts, Greenstein *et al.* (1984) found that only 10–15 per cent were willing to accept treatment with a drug that 'keeps you from getting high'.

Several out-patient studies have been conducted that show the efficacy of naltrexone. One of the striking features of these studies is the problem of high drop-out rates from naltrexone treatment. Greenstein *et al.* (1981) found that, of 386 patients who expressed an interest in naltrexone treatment, 242 detoxified from opiates, remained drug-free for at least 2 days, and received at least one dose of naltrexone. Of these patients, 153 (40 per cent of the original sample) completed at least 6 days of the naltrexone induction period, and 60 (16 per cent) completed at least 2 months of naltrexone treatment. Only 3 patients (1 per cent) took naltrexone for more than 1 year. In another, large, multisite, placebo-controlled study of naltrexone, 753 patients were screened, but only 192 started on medication (naltrexone or placebo) and, of these patients, only 13 completed 8 months of treatment (National Research Council Committee on Clinical Evaluation of Narcotic Antagonists 1978). Compliance rates can sometimes be improved when naltrexone ingestion is linked to a contingency management schedule (Grabowski *et al.* 1979; Rounsaville 1995).

Naltrexone has been found to be useful in the treatment of special populations. Naltrexone has been found to work well with highly motivated patients and when used under supervision (O'Brien 1994). Several studies have found that opiate-dependent patients with good social integration and social resources tend to respond well to treatment with naltrexone (Tennant *et al.* 1984; Washton *et al.* 1984). Washton *et al.* (1984) studied 114 business executives and physicians, and reported that they preferred naltrexone to methadone. Ling and Wesson (1984) studied 60 opioid-dependent physicians and other health-care workers who were treated with naltrexone. These health-care workers preferred naltrexone, because it protected them from the impulsive use of opioids, but did not place them in a position where they might be considered to be under the influence of a drug that produces dependence.

Concern has been expressed about naltrexone's potential hepatotoxicity (Maggio *et al.* 1985). Some evidence suggests that higher-than-usual doses (e.g. 300 mg per day) can result in elevations in liver function tests (Pfohl *et al.* 1986). This finding suggests a need for caution when naltrexone is used in the treatment of addiction. However, the abnormalities in liver function tests were observed in clinical trials of the efficacy of naltrexone in the treatment of other conditions (obesity and dementia). The high doses of naltrexone (300 mg/day) used in these studies were about six times greater than those used for prevention of addiction relapse.

Age may also be a risk factor. No patients under 40 years of age who were treated with up to 200 mg per day of naltrexone developed elevations in transaminases (Pfohl *et al.* 1986). In patients who developed such abnormalities, liver function test values returned to normal when naltrexone was discontinued. Naltrexone-related transaminase elevations have not usually been observed at lower doses and with addicted patients. Several studies of the hepatic effects of naltrexone, including studies conducted with alcoholics, have found no adverse hepatic effects (Sax *et al.* 1994; Marrazzi *et al.* 1997; Croop *et al.* 1997).

Nonetheless, it remains good practice to take liver function tests (e.g. transaminase levels) prior to the initiation of naltrexone treatment, and caution is required with patients who show signs of liver disease or impaired liver function. Naltrexone should not be used with heroin (or other opioid) addicts who have advanced liver disease or serious hepatic impairment. If naltrexone is given to addicts with minor abnormalities in liver function, baseline laboratory tests should include a full battery of liver function tests, and regular retesting (O'Brien and Cornish 1999).

It is probably also prudent to monitor the results of liver function tests at regular intervals during the first 2–3 months of treatment for all patients started on naltrexone. For those patients whose test results suggest the onset of hepatic dysfunction following the initiation of treatment, continued careful evaluation is required and it may be necessary to consider the discontinuation of naltrexone treatment. However, in general, naltrexone is regarded as a safe medication with few side-effects in the typical therapeutic dose range (Platt 1995).

The mere prescription of naltrexone alone is unlikely to be effective. Naltrexone is more effective when provided as part of a broader treatment programme (Resnick *et al.* 1979; O'Brien and Cornish 1999). Although naltrexone has pharmacologically distinctive features, the fundamental requirements for effective treatment with naltrexone are no different than those for other interventions. Rounsaville (1995) suggested that, to maximize its potential clinical usefulness, naltrexone should be offered together with a package of psychosocial interventions. Rehabilitation requires a comprehensive treatment package that may include individual or group counselling, cognitive behavioural therapy, and other socially supportive measures.

Pharmacotherapies for comorbid psychiatric disorders

Where drug users have psychiatric and medical disorders as well as addiction problems, clinical services should be able to provide effective and appropriate treatment interventions for both types of disorders. These treatments may include pharmacotherapies of various sorts. This may raise difficulties where some of the medications have abuse potential, and because of interaction effects that may occur between the medications and abused drugs.

Tricyclic antidepressants (TCAs), monoamine oxidase inhibitors (MAOIs), and benzodiazepines are among the most widely used pharmacotherapies for problems of anxiety and depressed mood. Benzodiazepines have established abuse potential, and the prescribing of these drugs to people with drug abuse problems is generally contraindicated, except for very specific purposes and on a time-limited basis. The side-effects of antidepressants, their potential for abuse, additive effects if taken with opiates, and the risk of overdose must also be taken into account. The anticonvulsants, and particularly carbamazepine, can greatly enhance the metabolism of methadone. Patients may, therefore, experience end-of-day withdrawal symptoms and/or the re-emergence of craving.

It has been suggested that medications such as bupropion and the monoamine oxidase inhibitors (MAOIs) could be effective in the treatment of cocaine dependence because they exert their effects, at least in part, by enhancing catecholaminergic activity. The prescribing of MAOIs also carries certain risks. The use of MAOIs in combination with stimulant drugs, for example, may precipitate a hypertensive crisis (Hersh and Modesto-Lowe 1998). The MAOIs have the potential to cause a hypertensive crisis. Bupropion can lower the seizure threshold. The TCAs have well-known risks of fatality when used in overdose. It could be argued that the use of these agents with cocaine misusers carries unwarranted risks under any circumstances. Since the selective serotonin-reuptake inhibitors (SSRIs) are less dangerous if taken with cocaine or in overdose, these may be more suitable for the treatment of depression among cocaine abusers.

A number of potential difficulties may arise when using benzodiazepines and MAOIs with drug misusers. Because of this, and also because of the proven efficacy of both the TCAs and the SSRIs, it has been suggested these drugs may have more potential as treatments for anxiety disorders, and especially with cocaine misusers (Deas-Nesmith *et al.* 1998). However, caution is also required when prescribing antidepressants such as TCAs and SSRIs since these may cause an initial activation leading to a worsening of anxiety, and this may increase the risk of relapse to drug use. The TCAs and SSRIs also have a latency of onset with maximal effectiveness taking as long as 2–6 weeks, and this delay may also put the drug-misusing patient at increased risk of relapse.

Some studies have found that TCAs can reduce depression in cocaine misusers. In a study of outpatient cocaine users, Carroll *et al.* (1995) randomly assigned patients to receive desipramine or a placebo, combined with either cognitive–behavioural relapse prevention therapy or case management, to evaluate the treatment response of depressed and non-depressed groups. Desipramine was found to reduce depressive symptoms compared with placebo, but it had no effect upon cocaine use in either depressed or non-depressed patients. Cognitive–behavioural therapy resulted in less cocaine use and enhanced treatment retention, but did not reduce depressive symptoms.

There are few rigorous studies of the efficacy of antidepressant medications in opiate-dependent patients, though several trials of pharmacotherapies for the treatment of depression in opiate addicts have been conducted with patients in methadone programmes. In a study of methadone-maintained patients with dysthymia and/or major depression, Nunes *et al.* (1991) found that imipramine produced improvements in mood and reduced drug use among more than half (53 per cent) of the treated sample. Petrakis *et al.* (1994) evaluated the effects of fluoxetine in the treatment of depression in methadone-maintained patients and found significant improvements in mood, but no reduction in substance use.

In a review of the efficacy of TCAs in the treatment of depressed methadone maintained patients, Nunes *et al.* (1991) concluded that, although depressive symptoms appeared to improve with medication, there were many methodological problems that complicated the interpretation of these findings and that, despite improvements in mood, there was little evidence of reductions in use of illicit drugs among patients treated with these medications. None of these pharmacotherapies has been shown to have clearly demonstrated indications or efficacy in the treatment of cocaine dependence.

Despite the lack of controlled studies of their efficacy in the treatment of depression among drug dependent patients, Hersh and Modesto-Lowe (1998) suggested that the SSRIs may be useful because of their relative safety and ease of use. The use of cognitive–behavioural interventions should also be considered in this context since these may be equally effective with fewer potential adverse effects. The balance of risks versus benefits for pharmacotherapies requires careful consideration.

Because of the lack of consistent findings regarding the effectiveness of desipramine and because of the absence of demonstrated efficacy for other antidepressants in the treatment of cocaine dependence without comorbid depression, it has been suggested that the use of antidepressants should be restricted to cocaine abusers with clearly diagnosed depressive disorders (Hersh and Modesto-Lowe 1998).

Most anxiety disorders are responsive to non-pharmacological treatment. Cognitive–behavioural techniques, such as exposure and systematic desensitization, have been found to be effective in the treatment of anxiety disorders (Barlow and Lehman 1996). Non-pharmacological treatments can be especially useful with patients who also have drug use disorders. In their review of the literature on the treatment of dual anxiety and drug use disorders, Deas-Nesmith et al. (1998) suggested that forms of pharmacotherapy and psychotherapy may be used to complement each other in maximizing patient outcomes.

Finally, it should be borne in mind that some of the psychological problems experienced by drug misusers may be directly related to their drug use problems. Strain et al. (1991b) found that the depressive symptoms reported by opiate addicts decreased significantly during the first 4 weeks after admission to a methadone treatment programme, with depression scores remaining stable over subsequent weeks. Similarly, Kosten et al. (1990) found that depressed opiate abusers experienced a rapid improvement in their mood when maintained on buprenorphine. A more accurate assessment of the nature and severity of psychiatric symptoms may be obtained by waiting 1 or 2 weeks after starting the addiction treatment programme.

Combined treatments

One obstacle to the use of medications in the treatment of substance use disorders is what has been called the 'pharmacophobia' of many substance misuse treatment professionals and paraprofessionals (Rawson et al. 2000). In its more generalized form, this resistance to drug treatments can apply to all forms of medication for the treatment of addiction, and sometimes even to the use of medications for the treatment of other psychological and psychiatric disorders.

Carroll *et al.* (1995) suggested that there may be a number of potential advantages to using a combined therapy package of psychotherapy and pharmacotherapy in the treatment of drug dependence. Psychotherapy and pharmacotherapy may be assumed to work through different mechanisms. The prescription of an opiate agonist such as methadone may reduce the need to use illicit heroin. Cognitive behavioural therapy such as relapse prevention may provide skills training to improve the individual's ability to cope with or avoid high-risk situations and relapse. As such the different types of treatment may affect different problem areas, and psychotherapy-plus-pharmacotherapy combinations may improve outcome for more symptom areas than either treatment alone. Combined treatments may be particularly useful with drug-addicted patients who present with complex mixtures of symptoms and problems. The offer of pharmacotherapy may also help to support treatment participation during the early stages of a programme where a developing therapeutic alliance may not be established, or until coping skills are mastered and integrated (Carroll 1993).

Chapter 12

Duration, intensity, and setting

Patient outcomes are extremely variable after drug misuse treatment. Some patients become drug-free and remain abstinent after treatment. Some become abstinent but relapse to drug use. Others achieve varying degrees of improvement in terms of reduced frequency of use, reduced quantity, or reductions in drug-related problems. Many move through complex cycles of improvement and deterioration in terms of the multiple domains of drug use, alcohol use, crime, social functioning, and mental and physical health problems. In recent years, researchers have made increasing efforts to identify and study specific factors that may account for this variability in posttreatment outcomes. McLellan *et al.* (1997*b*) asked, if treatment is effective, what makes it effective? And what are the 'active ingredients' of treatment?

If treatment is to produce improved outcomes, patients should stay for long enough to be exposed to and to participate in treatment components of sufficient quality and intensity to facilitate change. The issues of treatment engagement, retention, and compliance are problems for virtually all medical and psychological disorders. They can be especially problematic for drug addiction treatment. As Onken *et al.* (1997, p. 1) succinctly comment: 'Treatment won't work if it is not administered. Penicillin will not effectively treat streptococcal pneumonia if patients don't take it, and take it as prescribed. Insulin won't help a diabetic if it is not used. Cognitive therapy for panic disorder won't work if all the therapy sessions are missed. And treatment for drug addiction will not work if the addict is not engaged and retained in treatment.'

Many studies have shown that a greater 'therapeutic dose' of treatment is related to greater improvements in outcomes (McLellan *et al.* 1997*a*). However, the notion of a treatment dose should not obscure the fact that, for all types of addiction treatment, exposure is not in itself sufficient for change. The impact of treatment is more closely related to the patient's engagement with treatment, and it is engagement that is associated with positive outcomes (Joe *et al.* 1999). Patient engagement has been related to both the intensity and duration of treatment participation. Also, the strength of the relationship between most treatment treatment process factors and subsequent outcomes has generally been found to be rather weak (McLellan *et al.* 1994). The ways in which individual patients benefit from treatment are often idiosyncratic.

Treatment duration (and treatment retention)

Length of time in treatment is one of the factors that is predictive of favourable posttreatment outcomes among drug users (Simpson 1997). Time in treatment is linked to improved outcomes both when compared to the patients' own pretreatment baseline behaviours and with comparison groups (Simpson 1981; DeLeon 1989a; Hubbard *et al.* 1989; Simpson *et al.* 1997). Patients who stay in treatment longer and who complete a course of therapy have been found to be more likely to achieve the best outcomes, regardless of the outcome measure (Simpson and Savage 1980; Hubbard *et al.* 1989). In a study of 21 000 patients with substance use disorders, Moos *et al.* (2000) found that patients who received longer periods of care improved more than those who had shorter episodes.

Similar findings have been reported from studies of residential and out-patient drug-free programmes (Joe *et al.* 1999), methadone maintenance programmes (Ball and Ross 1991), methadone plus day-care therapeutic community programmes (De Leon *et al.* 1995b), and residential alcohol-treatment programmes (Moos *et al.* 1990). Etheridge *et al.* (1999) found that duration of treatment was related to improved outcomes in a study of treatment for cocaine problems. In studies of alcoholics, longer stays in treatment and treatment completion have also been shown to be associated with greater reductions in posttreatment alcohol use, even after controlling for pretreatment severity of alcoholism (McKay *et al.* 1994; Moos *et al.* 1990). Patients from the NTORS (National Treatment Outcome Research Study) residential programmes who remained in treatment for longer periods of time achieved better 1-year outcomes than those who left earlier in terms of abstinence from opiates and stimulants, reduced injecting, and reduced criminal behaviour (Gossop *et al.* 1999b). The effect of time in treatment was confirmed after controlling for the influence of other potential predictive factors.

It has also been suggested that continuity of care may play an important role in determining treatment effectiveness. This has been shown in the psychosocial treatment of other chronic problems (Bachrach 1992). The requirement for continuity of care may imply that the termination of contact with treatment services may result in the loss of rehabilitative gains for the individual. McLellan (2002).

In a randomized trial of residential drug abuse treatment, two programmes differing in planned duration were compared (McCusker *et al.* 1995). The 3- and 6-month programmes comprised 21 and 42 sessions, respectively. The 3-month programme was more concentrated, with group meetings three times a week, compared to twice a week for the 6-month programme. Improved outcomes were found for patients in both the 3- and the 6-month relapse prevention programmes and, for these patients, continued treatment beyond 3 months appeared to be beneficial, at least in terms of delaying time to first drug use. There were also some trends towards lower severity of drug, alcohol, legal, and employment problems in the 6- versus the 3-month programme. A further study showed little additional benefit for a 12- versus a 6-month therapeutic community programme (McCusker *et al.* 1997). The authors suggested that their results provided support for continuing treatment for up to 6 months.

Better retention tends to be associated with better outcomes in terms of reductions in substance abuse (Simpson and Sells 1983), and it has been suggested that the critical treatment retention period for long-term residential and out-patient drug-free programmes may be 3 months or longer, and 12 months in out-patient methadone programmes (Simpson 1981).

It is unclear whether treatments can be too long, either in terms of providing diminishing returns, or even in terms of undoing the benefits gained during earlier stages of treatment. There is undoubtedly a real danger that, within very long treatment programmes, both staff and patients may lose direction and focus. If long-term treatments are used with patients who are lacking in motivation or commitment, those who drop out of treatment early may derive little benefit from the programme. It is interesting that in the trial of McCusker *et al.* (1997) the outcomes were often worse among short-stay patients who had been assigned to the longer treatment duration. Where patients dropped out of treatment prematurely, those from the long-stay (12-month) programmes tended to have worse outcomes than those assigned to the 6-month programme.

As well as longer durations of treatment, treatment completion has also been linked to better outcomes after treatment (Moos *et al.* 1990; McLellan *et al.* 1997*b*). Such findings have been confirmed in various clinical subsamples. In a study of treatment outcomes of men and women randomly assigned to two therapeutic communities of different treatment durations, Messina *et al.* (2000) found that treatment completers achieved better outcomes in terms of reduced drug use and arrests, and increased employment. Longer treatment durations appeared to be particularly beneficial for women. Treatment completion has been found to be related to improved outcomes in studies with adolescent drug abusers (Williams and Chang 2000), and Grella *et al.* (1999) also found that, whereas treatment retention was related to increased abstinence in patients treated in long-term residential and out-patient drug-free programmes, treatment retention was more strongly predictive of abstinence in younger adults.

In certain respects, treatments for drug addiction are considered effective to the extent they are able to retain patients. Methadone maintenance, for example, is successful partly because it is able to retain patients in treatment. In contrast, despite the fact that it is (technically) an effective, safe, and long-acting treatment, naltrexone is infrequently used because of its poor ability to retain patients in treatment.

Research into methadone maintenance clearly shows an association between longer stays in treatment and positive posttreatment outcomes. One of the first large-scale studies to investigate this issue examined the long-term outcomes of more than 1500 patients admitted to methadone maintenance programmes in New York in the late 1960s (Dole and Joseph 1978). Among the patients who had been discharged or had left the methadone programmes, reductions in drug misuse and criminal behaviour outcomes were associated with having spent a longer time in methadone maintenance. In their comprehensive review of the literature, Ward *et al.* (1998) concluded that patients who remained in treatment for at least 2–3 years of continuous maintenance were more likely to benefit than patients who received briefer periods of maintenance, and that this was unlikely to be due merely to processes of selective attrition. However, although the evidence indicates that longer stays are better than shorter stays, and that being in methadone maintenance is better than not being in methadone maintenance, the literature does not indicate any optimum duration for methadone maintenance that would be applicable to all individuals.

Some methadone maintenance programmes are more successful than others at retaining their patients (Ball and Ross 1991). Rapid and ready access to treatment, higher methadone doses, a flexible policy regarding dosage, a non-punitive approach to illicit drug use, and an explicit orientation toward maintenance rather than abstinence have been found to lead to increased retention rates (Ward *et al.* 1998).

Time in treatment is not, in itself, sufficient for clinical improvement (Joe and Simpson 1975). Time in treatment is a complex measure, and one that should, in many respects, be regarded as a proxy indicator of other factors. Many of the factors that predict treatment retention may also be predictive of improved outcomes. The findings regarding a treatment threshold for improved outcomes may reflect the tendency of the more motivated patients to stay longer and engage better with treatment. Patients who actively participate in the programmes and make cognitive and behavioural changes during treatment achieve superior outcomes to others who stay for comparable periods but who do not make such changes (Simpson *et al.* 1995; McLellan *et al.* 1993).

Although patients who remained in treatment for longer periods of time showed better outcomes, some of those who left treatment at an earlier stage also showed improvements at follow-up (Gossop *et al.* 1999*b*). More than

Fiorentine and Hillhouse (2000) found an additive effect of treatment and twelve-step involvement in the process of recovery. Those drug users who spent longer periods in treatment, who successfully completed treatment, and who attended twelve-step meetings on a weekly or more frequent basis were more likely to maintain abstinence than those who participated only in treatment, or only in the twelve-step programmes. From the evidence of these and other similar studies, and with respect to frequent participation in group counselling, treatment completion, and regular attendance at twelve-step meetings, Fiorentine (2001) suggested that 'more is better', or even that 'much more is much better' (Fiorentine and Hillhouse 2000).

Several studies have looked at whether patients who receive additional treatment services do better than those who receive 'standard' treatment only. Abbott *et al.* (1998) found that methadone maintenance patients who also received community reinforcement treatment did significantly better than the standard treatment group in terms of reduced illicit drug use, and the authors suggest that community reinforcement interventions may confer additional benefit for patients on methadone maintenance.

In a comparison of a standard methadone maintenance programme with a combined methadone maintenance plus day-care therapeutic community programme, De Leon *et al.* (1995*b*) found that the enhanced programme led to greater reductions in heroin use, cocaine use, needle use, criminal activity, and psychological dysfunction. The patients who remained in the enhanced treatment condition for at least 6 months showed the most marked overall improvement. De Leon *et al.* (1995*b*) suggested that the degree of exposure to treatment was a key factor in leading to the improved functioning.

Such findings have also been found in other areas. In a study of community-based psychosocial support programmes for people with chronic mental illnesses, Brekke *et al.* (1997) found that patients in programmes of greater intensity showed higher rates of improvement on a range of outcome measures than those in a low-intensity programme. The authors suggested that, in the treatment of patients with schizophrenia, psychosocial programmes that provided more services were more effective than those that provided fewer services.

Saxon *et al.* (1996) found only modest effects of enhanced psychosocial services upon illicit drug use outcomes among methadone maintenance patients. The authors suggest that treatment outcome may depend upon some threshold level of services, and that surpassing that threshold may not lead further treatment gains. McLellan *et al.* (1998) have emphasized that treatment enhancements should not be seen merely as increases in the number of sessions, and that outcomes should not be measured simply in terms of illicit drug use but should encompass other outcome domains (e.g. social functioning, criminal behaviour, physical and mental health). Other studies have also failed to show any benefit from increased numbers of sessions when outcomes are measured only in terms of illicit drug use (Alterman *et al.* 1994).

As with time in treatment, these findings about treatment dose may also reflect a tendency for the more motivated patients to remain in treatment for longer periods and to involve themselves more actively in treatment. Patient characteristics and treatment factors can both be associated with engagement. Patients who engage with treatment may be more receptive to treatment or see treatment as being more helpful. The issue of engagement may be important during the earlier phases of the treatment process, especially in helping to retain patients within treatment (Simpson *et al.* 1997b). It is at this time that the patient establishes a therapeutic alliance and learns how to become an active participant in the treatment programme.

It is possible to reinterpret intensity of treatment and treatment participation simply as behavioural indicators of high levels of motivation for recovery, and to see better outcomes as a consequence of motivation rather than treatment involvement. This view is not open to empirical refutation if treatment involvement and participation are themselves seen as indicators of motivation. However, although motivation is often regarded as an important determinant of outcomes, the observed associations between measures of motivation and posttreatment outcomes have generally been found to be rather low (DeLeon and Jainchill 1986; Simpson and Joe 1993). The pretreatment motivation of the patient may be less important than what happens during treatment (Fiorentine *et al.* 1999).

The outcomes of treatment delivered in standard clinical settings have been compared in controlled clinical trials where the 'dose' of treatment services has been systematically varied. In a study of individual psychotherapy and counselling services during methadone maintenance treatment, Woody *et al.* (1984) randomly assigned patients to receive standard drug counselling alone, or drug counselling plus one of two forms of professional psychotherapy. These were supportive–expressive psychotherapy or cognitive–behavioural psychotherapy over a 6-month period. Patients who received psychotherapy showed greater reductions in drug use, more improvements in health and personal functioning, and greater reductions in crime than those receiving counselling alone. These differences were found throughout treatment and at follow-up (Woody *et al.* 1987).

The quantity and range of treatment services within a programme (e.g. counselling, medical care, assistance with employment, housing, and family therapy) are important factors contributing to the effectiveness of treatment programmes (McLellan *et al.* 1997b). The nature and quality of treatment services may also facilitate patient engagement. Increasing the opportunity for counselling, providing useful treatment and ancillary services, and strengthening the patient–counsellor relationship are likely to improve the effectiveness of drug treatment (Fiorentine *et al.* 1999).

Patients with drug misuse problems who received specialist out-patient mental health care have been found to achieve better outcomes than patients who did not receive such care, and intensity of care was found to be particularly related to improved outcomes among patients with both substance use and mental health problems. In a comparison of a standard treatment consisting of twice-weekly out-patient group counselling versus an enhanced programme (standard treatment plus individualized case management with access to extra services), the patients receiving enhanced care were found to show improved outcomes in terms of reduced substance use, fewer physical and mental health problems, and better social functioning (McLellan *et al.* 1998). Such findings have been replicated in various different groups. In a study of women with children, for example, Marsh *et al.* (2000) found that enhanced access to and use of drug abuse treatment services (number of services used) was related to reductions in the use of drugs and alcohol.

Studies of patients being treated for cocaine dependence have also found that greater amounts of treatment services can improve treatment outcomes. Higgins *et al.* (1991) randomly assigned cocaine-dependent patients seeking out-patient treatment to either standard drug counselling and referral to AA, or to a multicomponent behavioural treatment integrating contingency-managed counselling, community-based incentives, and family therapy. The enhanced treatment condition retained more patients in treatment, produced more abstinent patients and longer periods of abstinence, and produced greater improvements in personal functioning than the standard treatment. Further studies of the components of treatment found that family therapy (Higgins *et al.* 1994), incentives (Higgins *et al.* 1993), and the contingency-based counselling (Higgins *et al.* 1991) each contributed to the improved outcomes.

Etheridge *et al.* (1999) found that duration of treatment for cocaine abusers was related to improved outcomes, but failed to find any relationship between either frequency of counselling or frequency of attendance at NA/AA and improved outcomes. This failure to find a treatment intensity effect may suggest that the effectiveness of treatment may be less influenced by the amount of counselling *per se* than by the provision of targeted interventions that are specifically directed towards the problems of the individual patient. Treatment interventions and services should be appropriate to the needs and problems of the patients.

McLellan *et al.* (1997*a*) randomly assigned patients either to a standard treatment or to 'matched' treatment services that were directed towards their important psychiatric, family, or employment problems. The matched patients stayed longer in treatment, were more likely to complete treatment, and had better posttreatment outcomes than the patients who received a standard package of care. In the study of Woody *et al.* (1984), the main effect of psychotherapy was seen in those with more severe psychiatric problems. These patients showed few gains with counselling alone. In contrast, patients with less severe psychiatric problems often improved after counselling alone and, among the less psychiatrically disordered drug users, there were no differences between the treatment types.

Another controlled study showed that the treatment programmes that provided the most services in particular problem areas (alcohol, social, psychiatric problems) achieved the best outcomes in those areas (McLellan *et al.* 1993). Opiate-dependent patients were allocated to three levels of psychosocial services while in methadone maintenance. They either received methadone only with no counselling or other services, methadone plus regular addiction counselling, or methadone plus addiction counselling plus other (psychiatric, employment, and family therapy) services. After 6 months of treatment, the methadone alone group showed some reductions in opiate use but few other improvements. The methadone plus addiction counselling group showed improvements in drug and alcohol use, improved employment, and reduced crime. The patients who received the most treatment services showed the greatest improvement, particularly in the areas of personal adjustment and public health and safety risk.

Brief interventions

In apparent contrast to the use of longer and/or more intense treatment interventions, there has been considerable interest in recent years in the potential uses of brief interventions to tackle substance abuse problems. One rationale for such interventions is that, although their success rate may not be high, neither will it be negligible. Although only a relatively small proportion of drug users who receive the intervention may change their behaviour, the ready accessibility and potentially high recruitment rates may provide important public health benefits (Heather 1998).

Brief interventions may have a potentially useful role with drug addicts by providing an acceptable option for individuals who would otherwise receive no assistance at all for their problems, either because they refuse referral to treatment, or who accept referral but subsequently fail to attend the service.

Under these circumstances, the provision of a brief intervention is preferable to no therapeutic intervention.

Heather (1998) discussed the possible uses of brief interventions provided in medical settings as a means of initiating change in addictive behaviours. Interventions may consist of no more than basic advice and support for behaviour change, or even just providing information. The intervention should be delivered in a sympathetic and non-judgemental fashion, and need last no longer than 5–10 minutes. Brief interventions may be used to provide information about ways of avoiding dangerous practices or reducing levels of risk associated with drug taking. Many brief interventions, including printed information and instructional materials or self-help manuals, can be delivered by personnel who have received relatively modest amounts of training.

These sorts of short and inexpensive interventions have been used almost entirely with cigarette smokers, heavy drinkers, and long-term benzodiazepine users. Heather (2002) suggested that brief interventions can work but whether they actually work in day-to-day clinical practice depends upon the manner in which they are provided and upon the particular characteristics of the health-care system. The effectiveness of such interventions is still somewhat uncertain. For example, although Wutzke *et al.* (2002) reported short-term changes among problem drinkers after brief interventions when compared to a no-treatment control group, there were no differences in long-term outcomes for the brief intervention and untreated groups. Also, these approaches have not yet been used systematically with people with illicit drug problems. It is not known to what extent such interventions are applicable or effective with people who are long-term, dependent users of illicit drugs, often with co-dependence upon other substances, and possibly with serious medical and mental health problems.

Many drug addicts seek treatment only after they have first attempted to come off drugs on their own, and there may be much to learn from investigating the ways in which people stop taking drugs without formal treatment (Biernacki 1986). With some addictive behaviours, self-managed cessation plays an important role. Most cigarette smokers, for example, give up smoking entirely on their own without any formal treatment intervention (US Surgeon General's Report 1988). Many people with alcohol problems also give up without treatment (Saunders and Kershaw 1979). Some 'natural recoveries' are related to life events such as changes in family milieu, vocation, or health. However, some may also be associated with less prominent events, described by Knupfer (1972) as 'strangely trivial' factors.

In a study of self-detoxification attempts, Gossop *et al.* (1991*b*) found that almost all (94 per cent) of the opiate addicts attending a treatment centre had made previous self-detoxification attempts. These appeared to be more common during the earlier stages of their drug-taking career. Nearly two-thirds had succeeded on at least one occasion in becoming drug-free without any medical assistance, though many of these attempts failed at a relatively early stage.

Various approaches were used. The single most widely reported method was 'cold turkey' involving the abrupt cessation of opiate use with no drug cover. Benzodiazepines were also frequently used to self-medicate the withdrawal syndrome, and these drugs were described as being helpful, particularly in dealing with sleep problems. Non-pharmacological means were also used to cope with withdrawal. Among the more common strategies were distraction through exercise or physical activity, taking hot baths, or having a massage. The majority of the coping strategies tended to be very practical in nature. Because self-detoxification attempts are common among drug addicts and because these attempts have a relatively low probability of success, self-help detoxification materials for opiate addicts could play a useful role in supporting these efforts at self-change.

Another category of brief interventions is sometimes referred to as 'brief therapies' (Institute of Medicine 1990b). These differ in several respects from brief interventions. Brief therapy may involve instruction in specific behavioural procedures (such as goal-setting, self-monitoring, identification of high-risk situations). Brief therapy is usually preceded by a comprehensive assessment and may involve up to six out-patient sessions. One form of brief therapy (guided self-change treatment) consisted of an assessment interview followed by two 90-minute sessions (Sobell and Sobell 1998). This was developed for use with non-dependent problem drinkers, and it is unclear (as the authors note) whether this form of treatment would be applicable with other, or more severely dependent users.

Brief therapy can be seen as an approach that stands between brief interventions and specialized treatments. It requires much more in the way of training than does brief intervention, and probably requires therapists with relatively high levels of professional training. Because of its greater intensity, it is not as easily incorporated into the standard operations of non-addiction services.

Single-session interventions represent another type of brief therapy. In one respect, single-session interventions are something that all drug and alcohol workers are involved with whether they like it or not since this is what is being provided to all of those drug users who do not return for a second session. For this reason, the development of a planned and effective single-session intervention may be seen both as an opportunity to strengthen a particular way of working, and also as a way of responding to an existing but frequently unacknowledged problem.

Current practice often fails to make best use of the first session, which for many patients may also be the only session. Out-patient programmes for drug problems usually assume that the patient will attend on more than one occasion, and the first session is used for problem identification and history-taking procedures. The actual delivery of 'therapy' tends to be left to subsequent sessions. For some of the people who attend drug treatment services, this way of working may be inappropriate because they may attend only the first session and not return for any further sessions. One study of a London out-patient drug clinic found that, of the patients who attended the first appointment, about one-third did not return for a further session (Love and Gossop 1985). This is a high (but not untypical) attrition rate and, for the patients who only attended the first session, it raises questions about how productively the time was used during that session. Time spent gathering information to guide subsequent interventions is wasted if the patient does not return. Where it can be delivered immediately following identification of the problem, an appropriate form of brief intervention may be valuable and worthwhile.

Setting

Treatment consists of more than just clinical procedures and interventions. Treatment may also be influenced by other factors, including the programme's location, facilities, policies, services, and the aggregate characteristics of the patients and staff (Moos 1997). These factors combine to influence the objective and psychological quality of the programme and they may have an important impact on responses to treatment and posttreatment outcomes. Treatment is provided both by specialists in dedicated drug treatment services, and by generalists. It is provided in medical, psychiatric, and a variety of non-medical settings. It is also delivered in both residential and in community settings.

General practitioners (GPs) are increasingly being urged to play a major role in the care and treatment of drug misusers (Department of Health 1986) and British GPs currently have a substantial and increasing involvement with drug users (Hutchinson et al. 2000; Gruer et al. 1997). In a recent UK survey, more than 40 per cent of the methadone prescriptions given to addicts and filled by retail pharmacists were issued by GPs (Strang et al. 1996a). Current national policy in the UK is to encourage and expand the role of GPs.

One of the most frequently used and recommended forms of GP response is that of 'shared care'. This involves primary care and secondary care clinicians having joint and contemporaneous responsibility for care of the patient (Edwards et al. 1996), and it differs from the usual relationship between primary care and secondary care clinicians in which responsibility for the care of the patient may be referred from one clinician to the other. There are many examples of shared care, and it is used with patients who have a variety of medical problems including thyroid disease, rheumatoid arthritis, diabetes, and hypertension (Hickman *et al.* 1994).

Among the potential advantages of shared care schemes for the treatment of addiction is that they permit patients to be seen close to where they live, and allow ongoing medical care to be incorporated with methadone treatment programmes (Hutchinson *et al.* 2000). Shared care also gives drug clinics a greater opportunity to concentrate on the assessment of new patients, and the treatment of more severe and complex cases. The GPs take responsibility for the patient's medical management including the prescribing of methadone. Cooper (1995), for example, has suggested that the provision of 'methadone medical maintenance' (methadone prescribing with minimal or no additional therapy services) may be ideally conducted in a primary health care setting rather than in a specialist clinic.

The provision of methadone medical maintenance (MMM) may sometimes be appropriate for selected groups of patients. In a study of highly stable methadone maintenance patients (all were fully employed and none had tested positive for any form of illicit drug use during the previous year), King *et al.* (2002) randomly assigned them to one of three groups. These were methadone medical maintenance in either a general practice or a drug clinic setting, or standard methadone maintenance in a clinic setting. The results showed that patients who received MMM in both the GP and in the clinic settings continued to do extremely well despite the substantial reduction in the intensity of their care. Indeed, in terms of increased time spent in employment, family, and other social activities, the GP sample did better. It should be noted that this result was obtained with a highly selected subgroup of high-functioning patients. It is not clear what treatment outcomes would have been obtained with other samples.

In a study of clinically stable patients (no illicit drug use for the past year, and no psychiatric comorbidity), Fiellin *et al.* (2001) randomly assigned patients to continuing methadone maintenance in a clinic or in a GP setting. The results showed the feasibility of transferring stable methadone patients to treatment in a primary care setting with similar outcomes for the two groups. It has been suggested that standard clinic procedures may be 'inordinately restrictive' for clinically stable, high functioning patients and that treatment in primary care settings may be more appropriate for this subgroup (King *et al.* 2002).

Within a stepped care approach, it is appropriate to provide the least intensive treatment necessary to produce the required level of clinical improvement. Stepped care approaches are frequently used in other areas of medical and mental health care and these fit well within the structure of a comprehensive treatment delivery system (McLellan *et al.* 2000).

As part of NTORS, data were collected on the treatment outcomes of patients receiving standard community-based methadone treatments in specialist drug clinics or in general practice settings (Gossop *et al.* 1999*a*). The patients who received methadone substitution treatment from GPs or from clinics were very similar in their demographics, and in the type and severity of substance use behaviours and other presenting problems at intake. Patients treated in both settings showed similar improvements, with substantial reductions in their frequency of use of illicit drugs, alcohol consumption, in criminal activity, and improvements in mental and physical health.

The important potential role of GPs in the detection and treatment of problem drug use has been repeatedly emphasized in the UK, and policy makers and planners have placed great reliance upon the presumed willingness of GPs to become actively involved in these issues. This policy trend has not been matched by the willingness of the majority of British GPs to become actively involved. Although drug misusers often have contact with their GPs, many GPs have shown great reluctance to becoming involved with the treatment of drug problems. Policy makers may have underestimated the reluctance of GPs to take on the treatment of opiate addicts, especially when this requires long-term care. The extent to which GPs are actively involved in the treatment of drug addicts tends to be very uneven. In a study of GPs in south London, Groves *et al.* (1996) found that a small number of GPs were seeing many opiate misusers, with the rest seeing few or none. Other studies have found a GP workforce that was only minimally involved with problem drug users, and that did not wish to become involved in this work.

Many GPs continue to have negative attitudes towards drug-misusing patients (Roche *et al.* 1991) and see them as exhibiting 'difficult' behaviour (McKeganey 1988). Many GPs feel that they are already overstretched and have insufficient time to treat drug misusers. Commonly they feel they lack appropriate training (Bell *et al.* 1990; Roche *et al.* 1991). GPs may be more willing to become involved with opiate misusers where there is a lack of specialist services (Martin 1987; Scott *et al.* 1995), inadequate specialist services, or long waiting lists (Cohen and Schamroth 1990), or due to a public health need because of a high prevalence of blood-borne infections (Greenwood 1992).

The mirror image of this is that many drug misusers are dissatisfied with the attitudes and responses of their GPs. In a survey of London drug misusers, Fountain *et al.* (2000*b*) found that only 15 per cent of their sample were satisfied with the GP services that they received. This compared unfavourably with their satisfaction with specialist addiction services. Whereas 91 per cent of the respondents said they would go to a specialist clinic for treatment of a drug problem, only 23 per cent said they would go to their GP.

Various attempts have been made to facilitate greater GP involvement. An addiction liaison service was set up in London to provide support and training for primary care staff to help to tackle some of the barriers that limit primary care involvement (Groves *et al.* 2002). Generally the service was well received. More than half of the GP practices made use of the service. However, other than a subjective appreciation and a general welcome, the study failed to show changes in either the clinical practices or even the attitudes of primary care staff towards substance-abusing patients. In Scotland Gruer *et al.* (1997) described a different approach, in which GPs received additional payment as an inducement to provide maintenance treatment to opiate addicts.

There remain considerable doubts about the extent to which the national treatment response to problem drug use can make proper use of the network of GP services. The development of 'GP specialists' in the UK who provide treatment for substantial numbers of problem drug users constitutes a form of service that is very different from traditional GP responses where treatment for problem drug users is likely to be offered to numbers of patients that are deliberately kept very low. The growth of 'GP specialists' in addiction treatment also raises questions about the extent to which this development either attempts to, or ought to re-create conventional drug clinic services in a limited number of GP practice settings.

One of the obvious issues raised by providing addiction treatment in a GP setting is that of limited resources. This is most evident in terms of the time available for treatment contact. If an average GP consultation takes 5–7 minutes (Balint and Norell 1973), there are obvious and powerful constraints upon what might realistically be attempted or achieved.

Treatment in a residential setting provides the potential for an intensive and comprehensive treatment programme. The residential setting can provide a place of safety, and a psychological and social respite for patients by removing them from their drug-taking environments, and by supporting their drug-free functioning. De Leon (2000) identified this as an important role of the therapeutic community—to remove the addict from the physical, social, and psychological surroundings previously associated with a dysfunctional, negative lifestyle. The recovery process may involve withdrawal, not just from the psychopharmacological effects of drugs but also from the people, places, and things associated with drug use.

Detoxification can be conducted in either in-patient/residential or in out-patient/community settings. There has been considerable enthusiasm for out-patient detoxification and, in a major review of the literature, the US Institute of Medicine (1990a) noted that 'detoxification of most illicit drugs in most cases can occur as safely and effectively on an ambulatory [i.e. out-patient] basis as in a bedded setting'. In the UK, as in many other countries, the detoxification of opiate addicts on an out-patient basis is widely used as part of the national treatment response. In practice, however, the success rate for out-patient detoxification programmes is often poor. Many opiate addicts who receive out-patient detoxification treatments fail to complete their treatment programme. Only 17 per cent of the patients who received out-patient detoxification treatment at a London drug clinic achieved even short-term abstinence, compared to 81 per cent of a comparable in-patient sample (Gossop *et al.* 1986).

Attempts have been made to improve this poor outcome rate for out-patient detoxification. For example, the use of a 'flexible' reduction schedule was introduced whereby the patients could negotiate with the prescribing doctor to increase or decrease the rate at which dose reductions occurred (Dawe *et al.* 1991). This failed to produce any improvement in outcome when compared to the use of a 'fixed' withdrawal schedule; both groups continued to do badly with very few subjects successfully completing the out-patient detoxification programme.

There are several distinct advantages to inpatient treatment settings. This allows more intensive medical observation, supervision and control. Importantly, it also is much more likely to ensure that abstinence is actually initiated (Maddux *et al.* 1980; Gossop *et al.* 1986). Complicated detoxification treatment regimens may be required for patients who are co-dependent upon two or more drugs. Co-dependence upon more than one type of drug is an increasingly common clinical problem (Gossop 2001), though it has seldom been explicitly studied. In such cases it is often advisable that dual (or multiple) detoxification treatments should be administered in a hospital setting because of the risks of complex drug and withdrawal interactions, and the possible need for re-evaluation and adjustment of detoxification regimens (Weiss 1999).

Paradoxically, the protectiveness of treatment in a residential setting also represents a potential disadvantage. The availability of drugs and other drug-related cues in the normal environment can be powerful determinants of craving (Meyer and Mirin 1979). Patients in drug-free residential settings may not experience urges to take drugs because they are removed from such cues. This may not prepare them for the drug cravings they may experience after discharge when they are confronted by the availability (or potential availability) of drugs.

In this respect, there are, at least in principle, advantages to leaving the patient in, rather than removing them from their environment. Out-patient treatment may allow a better assessment of the environmental and other antecedents of drug-taking behaviours, allow new coping strategies to be practised in the real world, and permit greater generalization of learning (Annis 1986). The choice between in- and out-patient settings should not be seen as a choice between better and worse alternatives. The issue is choosing a treatment setting appropriate to the circumstances, needs, and problems of individual patients at specific times.

Among the rationales that have been put forward for residential treatment, Finney *et al.* (1996) suggest that residential settings, in general, provide a context in which treatment interventions can be delivered more intensively and represent an opportunity to provide practical and emotional support to patients who otherwise would not have access to such care or support. In-patient settings provide a place where patients can receive appropriate medical and psychiatric care.

In-patient treatments are an intensive form of treatment provided in a hospital, or similar medical setting. In the UK, such services are mostly provided in psychiatric teaching hospitals. In-patient treatment usually consists of a combination of detoxification and psychosocial rehabilitation (either simultaneously, or one followed by the other). In-patient treatments have several potential advantages over less intensive programmes. A hospital setting permits a high level of medical supervision and safety for patients needing intensive psychiatric care. In this respect, such services may be appropriate for the treatment of patients with complex dual diagnosis disorders. Residential treatment may also useful for patients who do not respond to less intense interventions (Weiss 1999).

In a study of a opiates addicts treated in a specialist in-patient unit, more than half were found to be drug-free at 6-month follow-up (Gossop *et al.* 1989*a*). In a subsequent study, heroin addicts were randomly allocated to either a specialist in-patient drug dependence unit or a general (i.e. not addiction-specialist) psychiatric in-patient ward in the same hospital (Strang *et al.* 1997*d*). Patients in the specialist setting were more likely to accept the treatment to which they were allocated, to enter hospital treatment, to complete detoxification, and to be opiate-free at both 2- and 7-month follow-up points.

The effects of treatment setting upon outcome may be largely due to such other treatment factors as modality type, treatment intensity, and treatment duration (Finney *et al.* 1996). In their literature review, Finney *et al.* found treatment setting effects in 7 of 14 studies. However, in all but one of these studies, the treatment setting that produced the better outcomes was also the one that provided the more intensive treatment.

Most treatment responses take place within a clinical setting, but some interventions may occur in other settings. Community pharmacists both in the UK (Roberts *et al.* 1997) and in other countries (Myers *et al.* 1998) have considerable involvement with drug-dependent patients through their dispensing of prescribed drugs and through their provision of needle exchange services. In a study in Glasgow, Roberts *et al.* (1997) reported the widespread use of pharmacist supervision of methadone consumption. Community pharmacies have the potential to offer interventions to 'hard-to-reach' and 'recreational' injectors who do not attend treatment agencies and for whom pharmacy-based needle exchanges may be the first or the only point of contact with a primary health-care professional. This setting could also be used for the provision of brief interventions.

Drug misusers frequently come into contact with the law. By definition, the use of illegal substances makes them liable to arrest. There are also other links between drug misuse and crime (Hall *et al.* 1993*a*). Drug dependence imposes a huge financial expenditure on the user, or requires them to commit illegal acts to obtain drugs. Addictive use of drugs is often associated with high levels of acquisitive crime (Ball *et al.* 1983; Speckart and Anglin 1985; Stewart *et al.* 2000*a*). When addicts are taken into police custody, some treatment interventions may be required (e.g. to prevent the onset of acute withdrawal syndromes). There is often uncertainty and disagreement among police surgeons about how to respond to drug withdrawal syndromes. A survey of police doctors (Stark 1994) found a range of (often conflicting) views about methadone prescribing, coupled with negative attitudes towards drug addicts and a lack of knowledge of current drug misuse treatment practice.

Although the treatment of opiate withdrawal symptoms presents few clinical problems when conducted in a medical setting, there are, unquestionably, practical problems involved in providing treatment to drug addicts in police custody. The accuracy of self-reported drug use may be compromised by the factors that operate in the police situation. Typically, police doctors stay with the suspect for only a few minutes and the next doctor to attend may be a different one. In most cases it is unlikely that adequate resources or facilities will be available to permit trained staff to observe the medical and physical state of the addict. Nonetheless, not providing drug cover to a physically dependent opiate addict will necessarily lead to the onset of the withdrawal syndrome. The management of drug addicts in police custody is also important for practical reasons. There are concerns to prevent the complications of drug use and, in particular, deaths in custody. This includes suicide. Many addicts are troubled by depressed mood and specifically by thoughts of killing themselves (Gossop *et al.* 1998*b*).

One of the most restrictive of 'residential' treatment settings is prison. Treatment provided within prisons has also been found to reduce post-release drug use and reoffending (Wexler *et al.* 1990; Knight *et al.* 1997). However, the issues involved in providing effective treatment in prison are similar to those for treating addicts in a more normal clinical setting. In studies of therapeutic community programmes provided within prisons, programme participation, time spent in treatment, programme completion, and the provision of aftercare were all found to lead to much greater effectiveness than simple exposure to treatment (Martin *et al.* 1999; Wexler *et al.* 1999; Knight *et al.* 1999).

Chapter 13

Causes for concern: issues for attention

Several issues have been identified as requiring further attention within addiction treatment services. Some have been defined in structural terms (e.g. gender or ethnicity). Some have been defined in functional or behavioural terms (homelessness, drug addicts with drinking problems, patients who are non-responsive to treatment). Some are organizational issues (liaison between different health-care services, coordination of treatment interventions, or problems of treatment planning and implementation).

One such issue is that of so-called 'special groups', though it is more useful to think of patients with special needs rather than of special groups. In certain respects, every patient is 'special'. If the definition of special populations is based on demographic, social, or biological factors, everyone belongs to one or more special groups. Nor is it known whether the notion of special groups has heuristic value for treatment. In a study of treatment for cocaine users, Sterling *et al.* (2001), for example, investigated the effects of patient–therapist matching on the basis on both race and sex. The study provided no results to support matching. However, the concept has helped to develop services and programmes that are more attractive, culturally specific, and relevant to the needs of users within different groups.

The problems of different groups are multidimensional, and members of those groups vary in many ways related to treatment outcome. It is simplistic to assume that they would benefit from a homogeneous treatment based upon their special population membership. Where attempts are made to identify special populations, programme planners and clinicians should avoid categorizing individuals only in terms of their age, gender, or racial or ethnic group. Systems of segregated treatment programmes, each serving a particular special subgroup, are neither cost-effective nor realistic: there is a limit to the number of separate programmes that can be funded. At worst, a segregated treatment system may be anti-therapeutic (Institute of Medicine 1990*b*).

Ethnicity

Ethnicity is an important factor in relation to addiction problems in many countries (e.g. the USA). Although various recommendations have been made regarding the need for separate, culturally specific programmes for ethnic groups, there is little agreement about what constitutes a culturally sensitive programme, given the heterogeneity within this apparent category. Africans, Asians, and other 'ethnic' groups may come from vastly different national and socio-cultural backgrounds, each of which has developed different attitudes towards types of drugs, and about appropriate treatment.

There is, for example, great ethnic diversity across Asian (and other) populations, not least in terms of geographical and cultural origins. Discussion of ethnic issues has often not distinguished between Asian ethnic groups and has treated Asians as a single homogeneous group. More detailed studies have found differences in drug use behaviours among Chinese, Filipino, and Vietnamese drug takers, with patterns of drug use that are specific to their ethnicity, gender, immigrant status, and age groups (Nemoto *et al.* 1999). Generational factors are also important. Third-generation descendants of immigrants typically differ from current immigrants in their beliefs and behaviours.

Correctly interpreting ethnic distinctions is fraught with difficulty. Moise *et al.* (1982) investigated differences between African-American and white addicts. They found that African-American women had fewer family problems than white women and were more likely to have partners who were not drug takers, but they suffered more economic hardships, more social isolation, and had more child-care responsibilities than white women. It was suggested that African-American women addicts could benefit from pragmatic, problem-centred approaches focusing upon issues such as housing, childcare, and employment. When broader social, environmental, and economic factors are taken into account, what appear to be ethnic distinctions may be found to mask more pervasive socio-economic disadvantages that differentially affect ethnic groups (Iguchi *et al.* 1988).

One theme that recurs regularly in the discussion of special groups is that of poverty. Poverty is commonly linked to drug dependence. It is a problem for many women who are dependent upon drugs. It is found among almost all of those who are homeless. Poverty is essentially about social exclusion. It is about being denied the expectation of decent housing, good health, education, and a satisfying social life. The poverty of many people who are dependent upon drugs represents a major obstacle to their opportunities to improve their situation.

Women

Men have been found to outnumber women in both in-treatment and out-of-treatment samples of drug misusers (Powis *et al.* 1996; Chatham *et al.* 1999). The number of women seeking treatment for drug problems has increased over the past 15 years, though the ratio of men to women has remained similar, with men outnumbering women by between 2 : 1 and 3 : 1. This ratio varies according to the types of drugs, the intake criteria of treatment services, and the specific types of interventions being offered. About a quarter of drug-dependent patients in the UK are women (Gossop *et al.* 1998*b*). In the USA Chatham *et al.* (1999) found that 31 per cent of the patients in their methadone programmes were women. The observation that drug addiction predominantly affects men could be seen as a reason for giving emphasis to the problem as a 'men's issue'. If 2–3 times as many women as men were dependent upon heroin and crack cocaine, it would readily be seen as a 'women's issue' (Browne 2000).

Various reasons have been suggested for the lower numbers of women in treatment. These include the greater stigma of addiction among women, and the lack of specialized facilities, particularly child-care facilities (Swift *et al.* 1996). It has been suggested that fewer women enter treatment services, or that they leave treatment prematurely because services do not adequately meet their needs (Reed 1987), and that services fail to meet the needs of women because they have been developed for men (Hagan *et al.* 1994). A survey of addiction treatment services for women in the UK, found low levels of provision specifically orientated to the needs of women (DAWN 1994), with nearly a quarter of agencies providing no services for pregnant women or women with children.

Among the treatments sometimes proposed for women are family therapy, group therapy, separate women-only services, and female rather than male therapists. Few scientific studies have investigated or supported the superiority of such interventions, and there is little evidence supporting the superior efficacy of any particular treatment modality for women (Institute of Medicine 1990*b*).

Where men and women with comparable sociodemographic characteristics and similar problems have been treated, they appear to do equally well in the same treatment settings. There is little to support the widely held view that women are harder to treat than men, or are less likely to recover. Treatment outcome studies have found similar outcomes for women and men despite the fact that some of the women's pretreatment problems may be more severe than those of their male counterparts (Fiorentine *et al.* 1997; Stewart *et al.* 2003).

The lack of association between pretreatment gender differences in problems and treatment outcome has been described as 'the gender paradox'.

Many drug-dependent women have psychological problems. Nearly half of the women in NTORS had received previous treatment for a psychiatric problem, about-one third had been prescribed drugs for depression, and one-fifth had suicidal thoughts (Gossop *et al.* 1998*b*; Marsden *et al.* 2000). Other studies have found high levels of depression among women drug misusers (Degen *et al.* 1993; Griffin *et al.* 1989).

Many women drug misusers have a relationship with partners who are drug-dependent, and not infrequently with men who are physically violent towards them (Powis *et al.* 2000). Drug-dependent women are more likely to have been severely beaten as an adult (often by their partner) than non-drug-misusing women (Regan 1987). Taylor (1993) also found that many women drug misusers were in violent, abusive (and sometimes life-threatening) relationships but felt unable to leave such relationships. Drug-dependent women with physically violent partners are less likely to respond well to treatment (Ravndal and Vaglum 1994).

Female drug misusers, like other drug takers, are a heterogeneous group. They differ from one another on important dimensions, including age, social and educational background, occupational status, patterns of drug use, severity of drug problems, and psychological and physical health. There are many sub-groups within the population of women that may have needs for differential treatment services in addition to those required by all women.

It is uncertain both how much of what we know about treatment and recovery applies equally to men and women, and the extent to which special interventions and services are needed for women. Nonetheless, treatment programmes that specifically address issues of particular relevance to women may be more effective for some women, or at least, more attractive to many women. Examples of this could include treatment services that offer child care facilities, assessment (and treatment where required) for psychiatric disorder, and work with partners and family.

Pregnancy

Pregnancy among drug addicts presents difficult clinical and other problems. Drug misuse can adversely affect the mother, the foetus, and eventually the baby. An important concern is the reduction of adverse consequences to the foetus. The treatment goals listed in the US Institute of Medicine (1990*a*) report include reducing the number of infants born with drug dependence symptoms and other impairments due to intrauterine exposure to drugs.

Obstetrical and medical complications and lack of antenatal care contribute to the health problems of infants born to drug-dependent women. Medical complications are seen in about 40–50 per cent of American pregnant women abusing drugs (Finnegan 1982), and infants born to drug-dependent women have generally poorer outcomes than those born to non-dependent women (Finnegan et al. 1977; Ryan et al. 1987). Babies born to opiate-dependent mothers have been found to have increased rates of intrauterine growth retardation, prematurity, meconium staining, jaundice, infection, seizures, and idiopathic respiratory distress syndrome (Oleske 1977). Morbidity in infants born to drug-dependent women is related to the amount of prenatal care as well as to types of drugs used (Connaughton et al. 1977). Increased prenatal care can reduce some maternal and neonatal adverse effects of illicit drug use (Jansson et al. 1996).

The difficulties of intervening with pregnant drug addicts are compounded by the limited time available (9 months). The clinical management of pregnancy in opiate addicts can be further complicated by the fact that drug addicts may not follow medical advice. Also, most addicts who become pregnant seek treatment relatively late in their pregnancies. Green and Gossop (1988) found that contact with addiction services often occurred in the middle trimester of pregnancy. Use of antenatal facilities was generally poor: some women never attended an antenatal clinic. Several babies required medical treatment immediately after birth, including treatment for opiate withdrawal symptoms.

Maternal opiate withdrawal can lead to serious complications (Rementeria and Nunag 1973). Episodes of overdose and/or withdrawal make the intrauterine environment unstable and cause hypoxia to the foetus (Finnegan 1982). Hypoxia may predispose the infant to meconium staining and subsequent aspiration pneumonia, which increases the risk of injury or death. Many medical complications among neonates born to drug misusers are linked to premature delivery. From the standpoint of the foetus it would be best if the woman were to abstain from drugs during the pregnancy. Unfortunately, many drug-dependent women continue to use a variety of illicit drugs, often in variable doses.

Neonatal withdrawal is influenced by many factors, including the type of drug(s) used, dosage and timing of dose before delivery, type of analgesia given in labour, and presence of intrinsic disease in the infant. Neonatal withdrawal symptoms usually occur shortly after birth or within 72 hours (Finnegan 1982). Infants born with a heroin withdrawal syndrome tend to be irritable; they often have feeding disturbances, sleeplessness, attention deficits, and can be difficult to parent (Finnegan 1976; Kandall et al. 1976). Disturbed neonatal behaviour may reduce the care-giver's responsiveness to the infant and exacerbate other problems for drug-using parents.

The issue of whether the pregnant heroin addict should be maintained upon prescribed opiates or withdrawn from drugs remains a matter of contention.

What is clear is that someone should take responsibility for the monitoring and supervision of the woman's drug status throughout pregnancy. Whether the woman is maintained on opiates or withdrawn from drugs, care should be taken to avoid sporadic drug use, especially if it involves street drugs, or uncontrolled withdrawal episodes.

Communication and liaison between addiction services, antenatal clinics, and obstetric hospitals is often unsatisfactory (Green and Gossop 1988). Services concerned with the care of pregnant addicts should maintain good channels of communication to optimize care during the antenatal period. Involvement of a key worker, especially within the first 6 months of pregnancy, can help to improve antenatal attendance and allow assessment of psychological and social problems prior to the birth of the infant. Providing interventions to develop parenting skills may reduce the possibility of child neglect. The mother should be offered support, and her ability to care for her infant should be assessed during her stay in hospital, and after discharge. Jannson *et al.* (1996) described a single, multidisciplinary service that incorporated treatment specialists for addiction, mental health, obstetric/gynaecological, family planning, and paediatrics, within a 'one-stop shopping' programme.

Women with children

The responsibility for looking after children falls disproportionately upon women. Women drug users who are bringing up children are likely to face many special difficulties, especially when they are physically dependent upon drugs, and the mothers' problems may have an impact upon their children that carries forward for decades into the future.

In a study of opiate-dependent women with parental responsibility for at least one child, Powis *et al.* (2000) found that these women faced many serious problems. Almost all were living in poverty, and many in conditions of extreme poverty. More than half of them reported having to pawn their possessions to support themselves and their children, and others reported prostitution and begging as means of financial support. Many women drug users lack access to the economic and social resources required to remove themselves from abuse and chaotic or oppressive situations (Hagan *et al.* 1994).

Such difficulties represent profound barriers to change. Women drug users with children have less time for their own needs because of their child-care responsibilities (Taylor 1993). Many have the constant fear of their children being taken into care (Powis *et al.* 2000), and they often believe that social services regard them all as unfit mothers purely on the basis of their drug use, and regardless of their parenting capabilities (Taylor 1993). For many women, concern over their children's welfare is a major motivating force for entering treatment (Swift *et al.* 1996). Rosenbaum and Murphy (1981) found that the major motivating force to enter treatment was concern over their children's welfare, but the most important obstacle to them actually entering treatment was the lack of child-care facilities.

Powis *et al.* (2000) found that the women who were most severely dependent upon heroin felt that if they sought treatment this might help them to avoid having their children taken into care. At the same time, they were afraid that, by approaching treatment, they might expose their problems and possible failings and increase the risk of their children being taken from them. This is an uncomfortable dilemma and one to which there are no easy solutions. Whereas no firm assurances can be given to women about the consequences of seeking treatment, the probability of children being taken into care is much lower than many women think, and services should seek to reduce the barrier to treatment presented by the anxieties of women with children.

The children of drug-abusing mothers often have higher levels of psychological disturbance than other children, greater behavioural problems, and learning difficulties (Kolar *et al.* 1994; Davis 1990). Children of drug abusers may show symptoms of neglect, and often report being left without adult supervision, even at very young ages (Davis 1990). Children are often present when their parents are using drugs and are able to describe their parents' drug-taking activities in detail (Nictern 1973).

Although Powis *et al.* (2000) found that most women reported never injecting in front of their children, it is disturbing that even a small minority did so. It was also worrying that less than half of the women had received advice about the importance of storing their drugs safely. Although prescribed drugs were usually provided in a child-proof container, several mothers said that drugs had been left within the reach of their children during the previous year. More than a quarter of the women reported that they sometimes bought drugs when their children were present. In more than half of the cases, the children were said to be aware of their mother's drug taking. Such findings are clearly disturbing.

Drug use by children and adolescents

There is a lack of precision and agreement regarding the definition of drug problems and drug dependence in children and adolescents, and few studies have investigated different treatment approaches for younger drug users. As with other treatment populations, diversity and heterogeneity are key issues. No special treatment intervention or approach is applicable to all cases of drug problems among young people.

Great care is required in the assessment of drug problems among young people. When children or adolescents are caught in possession of or using drugs, this usually creates serious concern. However, overresponse leading to a diagnosis of drug abuse or dependence may be an unnecessarily stigmatizing and traumatizing experience. It may also be incorrect. It is not known, for example, which of the youths who misuse drugs will continue to do so as adults and which of them will 'mature out' without formal treatment or other interventions. The provision of drug treatment for young people is based largely upon intuitive clinical judgements and moral values, rather than on the findings of empirical research.

One of the first tasks in the assessment of adolescent drug misuse involves the determination of whether the adolescent has a drug problem and whether there is need for further assessment (Meyers *et al.* 1999). Among the questions that require attention during assessment are the following.

- Does the youth have (or is there a high probability of them developing) a specific drug problem?
- What precisely is the nature and severity of the problem?
- Are they in need of protection (e.g. domestic violence issues)?
- Are they in need of crisis intervention (e.g. suicidal intent)?
- What are the safety, flight, and recidivism risks?
- Is there a need for further assessment by other specialist services?

Adolescents and their families often contact treatment services because of a crisis (e.g. arrest for a drug-related offence). In such circumstances, it can be useful to conduct the initial assessment as soon as possible after the precipitating event. In those circumstances in which it is appropriate, immediate referral or admission to treatment can make good use of this window of treatment opportunity (Meyers *et al.* 1999).

One type of drug problem that is especially likely to be found among children and adolescents is volatile substance abuse (sniffing glues, aerosol sprays, lighter fuel, petrochemicals, or other solvents). This problem may come to notice as the result of an accidental injury, or even the death of a young person. Volatile substance abuse is also sometimes identified as occurring in clusters among groups of children (e.g. in playgrounds of schools).

For adolescents assessment should include measures of school (or job) performance, as well as measures of the adolescent's living situation. This will require closer attention to details of family circumstances and functioning than is often necessary for many adults. Young people who have drug problems of sufficient severity to require treatment are likely to be struggling with the developmental tasks of adolescence, and their drug use is usually part of a network of interconnected issues and problems. Indeed, for most adolescents, drug taking tends to be the most visible symptom of a range of other difficulties. These may include problems in the areas of physical and mental health, family relationships, educational performance, social and peer relationships, sexual behaviour, and criminal activity (Hawkins *et al.* 1992; Newcomb 1995).

As for adults with a drug problem, treatment interventions may include behavioural, cognitive behavioural, operant conditioning, social learning, psychosocial, and other psychotherapies. There is a lack of agreement about the need for a drug-focused versus a broader developmental approach to treatment, and about the need for age-segregated facilities. However, young people may often be more appropriately treated in separate programmes to those of the standard addiction services. Very few addiction treatment programmes offer services specifically geared to the needs of adolescents. Indeed, many drug treatment services are reluctant to admit adolescents to programmes in which they may come into contact with older, more experienced drug users who may be seen by them as role models and who may teach them new (and more risky) drug-taking behaviours. Consequently, adolescent drug users tend to be distributed across diverse health and social service systems, including mental health services, child welfare, education, and juvenile justice. There is insufficient research evidence to evaluate the effectiveness of programmes that either segregate or integrate younger patients.

The elderly

Drug addiction is most often regarded as a problem affecting young people and, where drug misuse occurs among children and adolescents, this creates special concerns and may require special responses. What is less often recognized is that drug problems also occur among older people.

Ageing and its losses can affect psychological well-being. Many elderly people outlive their spouses, friends, and even children. They also have to cope with loss of employment, economic problems, failing health, loneliness, and social isolation. Many elderly people also have visual and hearing problems, and lose vital communication skills, which serves to aggravate problems of depression, isolation, and loneliness. Drugs, alcohol, or both may be used as ways of dealing with or forgetting the problem. Many elderly people with drug use disorders have concurrent depression (Holroyd and Duryee 1997).

The elderly are more likely to suffer from multiple health problems, and physical ailments leading to disability and pain. Osteoporosis affects millions of elderly women and predisposes to fractures. Arthritis is one of the most common problems of the elderly. Neuropathies, recurrent gout attacks, and cancer may also predispose older people to substance use. Chronic pain is a daily problem for many elderly people.

Assessment of the elderly should consider the possibilities of substance misuse since substance misuse and illnesses may cause the same problems. Also, illnesses may present atypically or non-specifically during later life. Changes in cognition, behaviour, or physical functioning may be wrongly blamed on underlying medical conditions, with substance misuse being overlooked. Elderly patients who present with symptoms of self-neglect, cognitive and affective impairment, and social withdrawal should be properly screened for substance abuse.

Between 1 and 3 per cent of hospital in-patients aged 65 and older have been found to have substance abuse disorders (Moos *et al.* 1993; Brennan *et al.* 2000). Studies of geriatric psychiatry services have reported high rates of substance abuse disorders, and benzodiazepine misuse is one of the most common disorders (Holroyd and Duryee 1997). Prescribed drugs, especially when taken in high doses or in inappropriate ways, may affect functional capacity and cognition. Such difficulties may put the older person at greater risk of falling, with fractures and subsequent institutionalization. Benzodiazepine misuse by elderly people, for instance, may lead to impaired cognitive function and an increased risk of falling (Tinetti *et al.* 1988).

Elderly people often take over-the-counter medications, or unused medications belonging to family and/or friends. Sedative–hypnotics, anxiolytics, and analgesics are among the more commonly misused prescribed or diverted drugs in this group. Many elderly people who take such drugs have been found to do so for more than 5 years (Gambert 1997), and they may only recognize their dependence when they stop taking their medication. As a group, the elderly are amongst heaviest consumers of both prescription and over-the-counter medications (Miller *et al.* 1991). 'Classical' patterns of drug misuse such as the use of street heroin or crack cocaine or the use of drugs by injection are believed to be rare among the elderly. However, some survivors from earlier generations of drug addicts are growing old, and some elderly addicts are now being treated in methadone treatment programmes.

Drug dependence can also be more problematic among the elderly because tolerance to drugs decreases with age. The use of multiple prescriptions and combined use of prescription drugs with heavy drinking may also put elderly people at increased risk of accidents and adverse reactions (Brennan *et al.* 2000). Where drug taking is excessive, or where drug interactions, including drug–alcohol interactions, lead to drug-related delirium or dementia, this can be wrongly seen as indicative of Alzheimer's disease.

It is useful to distinguish between early- and late-onset drug use among the elderly. Early-onset users typically have a history of long-term and often problematic drug use, and many have chronic physical and psychological health problems. Late-onset drug users have no history of drug problems prior to their identification, and typically begin misusing drugs in response to lifestyle problems associated with ageing.

Elderly drug misusers often try to hide their drug taking. This increases the difficulties of identifying such behaviours, and such problems are very often not recognized by clinical staff (McInnes and Powell 1994). When appropriately treated, elderly people with substance misuse problems have been found to be as likely as other patients with the same problems to remain in treatment and to recover (Fitzgerald and Mulford 1992). Where older drinkers are treated in programmes specially tailored to their needs, they may have an even higher rate of success (Kashner *et al.* 1992).

In studies of alcohol problems among the elderly, characteristics that have been found to be associated with poorer outcomes include chronic physical problems, psychiatric comorbidity, family drinking practices, and isolation (Schuckit 1983*b*; Hurt *et al.* 1988). As an example of how 'special problems' may cluster together, Brennan *et al.* (2000) found that, among the elderly patients in their study, substance use disorders affected a disproportionately high number of Black people and a significant number of women.

The homeless

In the USA, on any given night, 200 000–700 000 persons may be homeless (Institute of Medicine 1990*a*). People find themselves homeless for many reasons, including lack of adequate, affordable housing for people on low incomes, chronic unemployment, personal and family crises, and the deinstitutionalization of the mentally ill without adequate follow-up services. Many homeless women and young people run away from home because of verbal, physical, and sexual abuse.

Individuals have been defined as homeless if they live at night in emergency shelters, on the streets, in parks, subways, railway stations, abandoned buildings without utilities, or as squatters in property belonging to others (Joseph and Paone 1997). It can be useful to distinguish between the temporarily, episodically, and the chronically homeless. This last group tends to have the highest rate of people with serious mental illnesses.

Drug problems are commonly found among the homeless, and they frequently exacerbate the adverse consequences of homelessness and act as a barrier to social rehabilitation (Galaif *et al.* 1999). Prevalence estimates among homeless women, for example, range between 25 and 50 per cent for drug abuse (Galaif *et al.* 1999). Many of the homeless are also suffering from mentally illnesses. A study in eight different countries of prevalence rates for schizophrenia found an average prevalence of 11 per cent with higher rates in younger persons, women, and the chronically homeless (Folsom and Jeste 2002).

In a survey of homeless people currently or recently sleeping rough (on the streets) in London, almost two-thirds of them had been homeless for 6 years or more, and more than half had first become homeless when aged 18 or younger (Fountain *et al.* 2002). Almost half had slept rough for more than 6 months in the year before the interview. Drug use was prevalent with 83 per cent of the sample having used drugs in the month prior to interview (Fountain *et al.* 2003). Polydrug use was common. The longer they had been homeless, the more severe their drug problems (daily use, injecting, and drug dependence). Among those who were dependent or regular users of heroin, less than one-third had been in contact with addiction treatment services, though more of them had been in contact with needle exchange schemes. The main reason given for not contacting treatment services was that they did not want to stop using drugs.

Being homeless (as well as some of the factors leading to homelessness) creates additional problems in avoiding further complications and adverse effects of drug misuse and drug addiction, and creates a barrier to accessing treatment services. Homeless persons are a medically underserved group without access to primary care. Their medical conditions tend to be undiagnosed and untreated, leading to further complications and increased rates of mortality (Redliner 1994). Where homeless people are admitted to addiction treatment programmes, their medical conditions put additional strain on the resources of the services.

Homeless addicts face practical difficulties that make it hard for them to use safe injecting or safe sex practices to protect themselves from becoming infected with and transmitting infections such as HIV, hepatitis, sexually transmitted diseases, and tuberculosis. The link between homelessness and HIV infection has led to the reappearance of tuberculosis as a serious public health concern. The rate of tuberculosis (often involving drug-resistant mycobacterium tuberculosis) among homeless persons in the USA has been estimated at 20 times that of the general adult population (Brewer *et al.* 2001). The incidence of hepatitis C and HIV/AIDS among the homeless has also been found to be much higher than in the general population (Cheung *et al.* 2002). Many homeless people have concealed their health problems when applying for services because of fears that, if they revealed their HIV serostatus, or other infectious diseases, they could be denied access to sheltered accommodation, or suffer physical harm in the shelters.

Outreach services provided outside of institutional settings are important in reaching and responding to the needs of the homeless. Outreach services can provide a bridge to mainstream services and institutions for these who otherwise may lack the skills or motivation to approach such services. The homeless often tend to congregate in railway or bus stations, and outreach programmes can contact many of them at such sites.

Alcohol, the 'hidden drug'

Within the polydrug-using repertoire of many drug addicts, some drugs assume greater prominence than others. Heroin and crack cocaine are often identified as 'main' drugs. Other drugs are more easily overlooked, especially when their use is more widespread and less socially stigmatized. Such drugs may represent problems in their own right, they may aggravate other problems, or they may be latent problems that, if not dealt with, emerge when the main drug problems are removed.

Alcohol problems are often underrated and neglected in the treatment of drug addiction (De Leon 1989*b*; Lehman and Simpson 1990; Gossop *et al.* 2000*b*). Alcohol is among the most frequently reported 'secondary' substance problems among drug addicts, and alcohol abuse is often found among addicts after treatment for drug addiction problems.

There is wide variation in drinking patterns among drug misusers. A surprisingly large number of drug addicts do not drink. Within the NTORS cohort, about one-third had been abstinent from alcohol throughout the 3-month period prior to treatment (Gossop *et al.* 2000*b*). This abstinence rate is much higher than for age-matched samples from the normal population. However, many of those who were drinkers reported problematic patterns of drinking. Nearly one-fifth were co-dependent on alcohol and were regularly drinking excessively: on average, they were drinking daily amounts equivalent to a bottle of spirits. Many others were drinking heavily and regularly, or extremely heavily but infrequently.

Excessive drinking among drug addicts may aggravate other problems and adversely affect outcomes after treatment. Dually (drug and alcohol) dependent patients have worse treatment outcomes than those who are not heavy drinkers (Rawson *et al.* 1981), and co-dependence upon alcohol among opiate misusers in methadone treatment programmes has been found to affect treatment response and treatment outcome (Chatham *et al.* 1997). Chronic alcohol abuse is an important cause of medical complications during methadone treatment and is frequently linked to the premature discharge of patients from methadone programmes (Kreek 1981; McLellan 1983; Joe *et al.* 1991). Alcohol use among methadone patients has been linked to increased criminal activity (Roszell *et al.* 1986). Cocaine misusers who also have drinking problems have been found to be more likely to relapse to cocaine use after treatment, and drinking is often closely linked to relapse episodes (McKay *et al.* 1999).

Drug users who are also dependent on alcohol have worse physical and psychological health than other drug addicts. Drug addicts who were severely dependent on alcohol were found to be more likely to have had drug-related problems such as abscesses, vein scarring, and overdoses (Gossop *et al.* 2002c). Fatal and non-fatal overdoses that are commonly attributed to the use of opiates are seldom due simply to the use of opiates, and are more likely to involve the combined use of opiates and alcohol or other sedatives (Darke and Zador 1996; Gossop *et al.* 1996). The interrelationship of drinking and illicit drug use is not well understood, though it has been suggested that some drug misusers may substitute alcohol for drugs (Simpson and Lloyd 1977; De Leon 1987), and that in some circumstances, there may be an inverse relationship between the frequency of use of alcohol and drugs (Anglin *et al.* 1989a).

Drinking outcomes after treatment for drug addiction are often poor with many drinkers making little or no change from their pretreatment drinking (Gossop *et al.* 2000b). Even where reductions in alcohol use occurred, this was often unsatisfactory in that it consisted mainly of reductions from very heavy drinking to heavy, rather than to moderate levels of drinking. For example, the average amount of alcohol consumed at follow-up on a typical drinking day was between 10 and 19 units (equivalent to about half a bottle of spirits). This level of drinking represents a serious threat to the health of this group, especially since so many of them have liver disease and impaired liver function.

The continued heavy drinking of so many patients after treatment stands in contrast to the widespread changes and substantial improvements that were found within the same group in terms of reduced use of illicit drugs (Gossop *et al.* 1998a). The results of these and other studies suggest that changes in illicit drug misuse and drinking outcomes may be independent, with drinking behaviour after treatment being more reflective of pretreatment drinking patterns (Simpson and Lloyd 1981; Hubbard *et al.* 1989; Gossop *et al.* 2000b).

Drinking problems often receive insufficient attention in the treatment of illicit drug misusers (Simpson 1997). Drug misusers and clinical staff may either deliberately or unintentionally focus upon what is perceived to be a main illicit problem drug (notably heroin or cocaine) and neglect or minimize the use of other substances. The extent and severity of heavy drinking among drug misusers both before and after treatment point to the need to develop programmes and interventions that are specifically designed to tackle alcohol-related problems in this patient group.

Drug problems among people with severe mental illness

Regier *et al.* (1990) reported that the prevalence of substance abuse disorders was almost twice as high among people with mental illness as among the general population. People with a severe mental illness were most at risk. Those with schizophrenia were more than four times as likely to have a lifetime substance use disorder than people in the general population, and those with bipolar disorder were more than five times more likely to have a substance use disorder. More than half of the people diagnosed with a bipolar disorder (56 per cent) and almost half of those with schizophrenia (47 per cent) had a lifetime diagnosis of substance abuse or dependence.

Despite these high rates of substance abuse, many general psychiatrists and mental health clinicians fail to obtain a thorough history of drug use, and drug problems are often overlooked and underdiagnosed in mental health treatment settings (Ananth *et al.* 1989; Shaner *et al.* 1993). Several factors contribute to this. Drug misuse often occurs within the broader context of other psychosocial problems associated with mental illnesses, and the negative psychological and social consequences of drug misuse may be less evident than in others without comorbid mental illness. The cognitive, emotional, and behavioural effects of drugs can also mimic those of mental illnesses, and interactions between drugs and underlying psychiatric problems can create difficulties in identifying the primary causes of presenting symptoms. Anxiety, depression, confusion, delusions, and even hallucinations can occur with drug use and, in people with mental illnesses, such adverse effects may be misattributed to psychiatric conditions (Schuckit 1983*a*). For example, cocaine withdrawal can produce depressive episodes, and excessive stimulant use can lead to psychotic states. These difficulties are made worse since mental health staff often lack the training, the expertise, and the confidence to respond appropriately to drug misuse among their patients.

Mentally ill drug misusers are frequently in a pre-motivational state regarding their drug taking even if they are otherwise participating well in mental health treatment programmes. People with mental illnesses may also underreport their substance use problems when they present for treatment (Carey and Correia 1998). Current or past psychiatric disorders may be less reliably reported by current drug users than by non-drug-users (Bryant *et al.* 1992; Corty *et al.* 1993). Patients with schizophrenia have shown substantial underreporting of cocaine use, which was detected only when the results of urine screening were compared with their self-reported drug use (Shaner *et al.* 1993; Stone *et al.* 1993). Urine screening can help to identify some patients who have not reported substance use and serve to alert mental health staff to the possibility of problematic drug use.

Mentally ill drug misusers often have financial and housing problems, destabilization of their illness, and difficulties in participating in rehabilitation (Mueser *et al.* 1997). Treatments that are effective in reducing or eliminating drug use may confer positive benefits in other areas such as psychiatric symptomatology, social functioning, treatment adherence and service utilization. Delays in problem identification and in the effective treatment of underlying psychiatric disorders may contribute to increased problems of disrupted personal and social functioning and therefore lead to an increased risk of addiction relapse.

Where treatment is provided in in-patient or residential units, it may be possible to withdraw the patient from drugs for a period of observation to see if their psychological disturbances moderate or disappear during a period of abstinence. Clinical features may sometimes help to differentiate between primary psychiatric and drug-induced disorders. Clinical features that are suggestive of a primary rather than a drug-induced mental disorder may include having symptoms not typically associated with the drug or the doses used, and a family history of the mental disorder. Atypical presentations of a primary psychiatric disorder when associated with drug use, such as a first psychotic episode or manic episode late in life, may be suggestive of a drug-induced disorder.

The usual dimensions of drug use (quantity and frequency of use, consequences, signs of dependence, etc.) may be qualitatively different among drug misusers with mental illness compared to those who are not mentally ill. Mentally ill drug misusers often use lower amounts, with less frequent and less regular patterns of drug taking. In particular, they are less likely to develop and present with a drug *dependence* disorder (Lehman *et al.* 1994; Mueser *et al.* 1997).

Treating dually diagnosed patients in separate mental health and addiction treatment services is often unsatisfactory, especially for those with severe psychiatric disorders. In a study of dually diagnosed patients with severe mental illness, Bartels *et al.* (1995) found little improvement in drug use or alcohol use disorders. Poor outcomes for such patients may often be, at least partly, due to barriers within the treatment service system (Ridgely *et al.* 1990). The reliance upon separate services systems can lead to a lack of liaison and agreement over treatment practices and treatment goals between mental health and addiction treatment services. Where professionals are unclear about how best to combine psychiatric and addiction treatments, the burden of accessing the different services tends to fall upon the patients, who are often poorly equipped for this demanding task.

Drake *et al.* (1993) found improved outcomes among substance abusers with severe mental illnesses who were treated in integrated programmes compared to a comparison group who received a traditional service intervention. Recent developments in integrating mental health and addiction treatment within comprehensive programmes, with both types of treatment being provided simultaneously (and not sequentially), by the same person, team, or organization have been described by Mueser *et al.* (1997).

Non-responsive patients

Even in studies that have demonstrated the efficacy of various treatment interventions, some patients typically fail to respond to the effective intervention (Morral *et al.* 1997; Belding *et al.* 1998). Such patients may continue to behave in seriously problematic ways (using street heroin, sharing needles). They may turn up at the clinic when drunk, fail to meet routine programme requirements by missing appointments, failing to give urine specimens when requested, or using abusive language.

In a study of methadone patients, Gossop *et al.* (2000*a*) identified several subgroups with different clinical response profiles corresponding to the amount of improvement in drug use between admission to treatment and follow-up. More than half of the sample, showed clear improvements. For example, their illicit opiate use at follow-up had fallen to about one-quarter of pre-intake levels. However, about one-fifth of the sample (18 per cent) failed to show improvement on virtually all outcome measures. These treatment non-responders showed poor outcomes in terms of continued use of illicit drugs; they had the highest rate of injecting at intake (72 per cent), and this increased to 76 per cent at 1 year; they showed no improvement in either their physical or psychological health; and they also fared badly in terms of their continued involvement in crime. The patients in the poor response group were also more likely than other patients to have dropped out of treatment.

Belding *et al.* (1998) found that 22 per cent of their sample of methadone maintenance patients continued to use illicit opiates despite having been in treatment for at least 6 months, and Gerstein and Harwood (Institute of Medicine 1990*a*) also suggested that about one in four patients tended to show a poor response to treatment. In some respects it is encouraging that only a minority of patients showed such poor outcomes. On the other hand, the failure of these patients to improve on a range of different outcome measures despite their access to, and often extensive input from treatment services, is a matter for concern.

A common dilemma within clinic services involves the large amount of staff time and effort taken up by the most severely problematic and/or disruptive drug users. Patients with less severe problems, or who are responding well to treatment may be ignored. Conversely, if more attention is paid to those with less severe problems, the needs of the most problematic cases may be neglected. This issue creates organizational problems, as well as tensions among both staff and other patients. Some services require abstinence from illicit drugs (or other behaviours) from programme participants, and discharge patients from treatment if they fail to achieve these goals. This can aggravate problems among the discharged patients. Zanis *et al.* (1996) found that, among a sample of patients who had been discharged from methadone treatment for such reasons, the majority had very poor outcomes, and 12 per cent had died.

Limitations in treatment resources may tempt staff to select patients who are believed to be more likely to respond well to treatment. It is extremely difficult to predict who will respond well or fail to respond to treatment. 'Clinical judgement' provides a poor basis for such predictions (Gossop and Connell 1983). It has also proved difficult to identify treatment non-responders on the basis of pre-treatment patient characteristics, behaviours, and problems (Belding *et al.* 1998).

One approach to non-responsive patients is to provide different types of treatment. Contingency management, for example, has been used specifically to tackle the problem behaviours of non-responders (see Chapter 8). This has been described as one of the most effective and generally useful interventions in this context (Robles *et al.* 1999).

Another approach has been to provide treatments of increased intensity. A trial that involved the prescribing of increased doses of maintenance drugs (including injectable heroin) for 'problematic' and 'treatment-resistant' addicts was conducted by Gossop *et al.* (1982*b*). The clinical goals for patients included reduced illicit drug taking, reduced dangerous injecting practices, reduced alcohol consumption, and various changes in social behaviour. The results were equivocal, with some patients showing improved responses and others showing continuing problem behaviours. Strain *et al.* (1999) also found that high doses of methadone may not be sufficient to solve the problems of illicit drug taking during treatment. More than half of the patients in their high-dose condition continued to use illicit heroin even though most were receiving doses of more than 80 mg.

One of the purposes of the Swiss and the Dutch heroin-prescribing trials was to address the problems of drug addicts for whom previous treatment attempts had already failed (Uchtenhagen *et al.* 1999; van den Brink *et al.* 2002).

Treatment delivery: treatment integrity

Despite the substantial literature demonstrating the effectiveness of many types of interventions for addiction problems, treatments are often delivered in ways that could politely be described as 'suboptimal'. Treatment services that apparently provide similar interventions vary greatly both in their treatment practices and in their patients' treatment outcomes (Gossop *et al.* 1998*a*). Patients in some treatment programmes have been found to achieve three times as great a reduction in heroin use as patients in other, apparently very similar programmes (see Fig. 13.1). Such variation in patient outcome is obviously of great interest. The reasons for this variation are not properly understood.

Specifying the rationale and goals of therapy, the mutual agreement of these between therapist and patient, delineating treatment procedures, and providing feedback about progress are core features of cognitive–behavioural therapies.

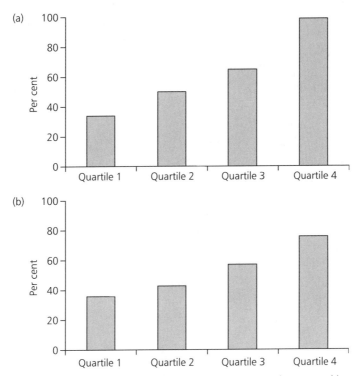

Fig. 13.1 There is marked variation in patient outcomes even when treated in similar sorts of treatment programmes. (a) The variation in outcomes for patients treated in residential programmes. (b) The variation in outcomes for patients treated in out-patient methadone programmes. The data are from NTORS (National Treatment Outcome Research Study; Gossop *et al.* 1998*a*).

Indeed, they are probably common features of most effective treatments. The marked and often unacceptable variation in programme delivery can lead to key elements of treatment being neglected or even omitted. The use of treatment manuals can help to improve treatment integrity.

A weakness concerning the provision of many treatments is the limited availability of properly trained staff with the skills to provide such treatments effectively. One way of improving the standard of treatments delivered in existing services (under conditions of, typically, restricted resources) involves the use of treatment manuals. Treatment manuals have been called a 'small revolution' in psychotherapy research and the potential uses of manual-based therapies within clinical practice have been widely discussed in clinical psychology (Wilson 1996). Manuals can provide direction about treatment methods and procedures by specifying what the therapist should do within sessions, and how the sessions should proceed. Manuals are particularly useful where interventions are delivered by therapists with limited training and expertise. An important distinction to be made here is that between the ideals of 'best practice' and the reality of treatment interventions delivered under day-to-day conditions in existing services.

On the other hand, treatment manuals are no panacea. They tend to be more suited to the treatment of clearly defined focal problems rather than the diverse and diffuse problems presented by many drug-addicted patients. The advantage of manuals is their concrete and specific descriptions of procedures. This can also be a weakness in that they find it difficult to allow flexibility for differing patient needs. Strict adherence to treatment 'according to the manual' does not guarantee good outcomes. Barber *et al.* (1996) showed that therapeutic competence is more likely to produce improved outcomes than simple adherence to procedures taken from a manual.

A final word is necessary on the threat of cost-cutting. In recent years, there have been increasing demands that addiction treatments should demonstrate value for money. The calculation of the types and extent of treatment benefit may be made separately, and in different ways by the treatment purchaser, by public health agencies, by clinicians, and by the individual patient. In some instances, these calculations may lead to quite different conclusions.

The job of the clinician is to deliver the most effective treatment for the individual patient. The job of the health purchaser is to maximize the health gains of the population being served within the available financial resources. The job of the manager is to deliver the agreed volume of product (e.g. occupied bed days, treatment slots). The patient seeks to obtain the most personally suitable and most clinically effective treatment, regardless of the considerations of organization and finance that may impinge upon the decisions of others.

Sometimes, these four perspectives are in accord. But sometimes they are in conflict (Gossop and Strang 2000). This mismatch between different perspectives on treatment requires further exploration and, ultimately, resolution.

Many changes have been forced upon the drug treatment systems of Britain, the USA, and other countries during the past 2 decades. Changes in treatment financing and other policy changes have often contributed to the erosion of the ability of treatment programmes to exercise control over the types of patients being treated, length of stay, types of treatment and services provided, and other clinically relevant dimensions of treatment.

Etheridge *et al.* (1997) reported significant decreases in the amount and in the range of treatment services provided to patients in the USA in the early 1990s compared to the level of services provided a decade earlier. This was linked to a corresponding decrease in the proportion of patients who reported that services were able to meet their treatment needs. There are undoubted dangers associated with a naive adherence to cost and cost-containment considerations, and the priority given to cost containment by treatment purchasers has led to treatment programmes becoming substantially shorter. As part of the drive to cost-containment, out-patient treatment has increasingly become the modality of choice for the treatment of drug abuse. In its worst form, the changes within addiction services have led to a 'ledger clerk culture' in which treatment provision is determined by price rather than effectiveness.

Where drug-dependent patients have special needs, this creates further difficulties within 'stripped-down' services. Patients with multiple drug problems, and those who have psychological and physical health problems are particularly likely to be found within the residential treatment programmes (Simpson *et al.* 1997*a*; Gossop *et al.* 1998*b*). Such patients frequently require intensive treatment and multiple services. These interventions may be costly to provide, and are not available in many services, especially within typical community-based programmes operating with limited resources. Other studies have also shown a decline in the provision of out-patient treatment services (D'Aunno and Vaughn 1995).

Time spent in treatment has been repeatedly found to relate to improved treatment outcomes (Hubbard *et al.* 1989; Simpson and Sells 1983). Paradoxically, the time permitted to patients within treatment programmes is one of the features of treatment that has been most eroded by managed care initiatives (Etheridge *et al.* 1997). This drive towards reduced treatment durations can adversely affect the clinical goals and procedures of treatment programmes. In some instances, it has been necessary to make radical alterations to existing treatments to meet the requirement for shorter treatment durations.

The planned durations of some in-patient programmes in the UK have now been reduced to the point at which they are too brief to provide the most effective potential outcomes for their patients (Gossop *et al.* 1999*a*). This is largely due to decisions about treatment duration being made not on clinical grounds, but by outside treatment purchasers (Leshner 1997; Swift and Miller 1997).

Chapter 14

Treatment effectiveness and social policy

Treatment effectiveness: the evidence base

Large-scale, prospective, multi-site treatment outcome studies have played an important role in improving our understanding of treatment effectiveness (Simpson 1997). They provide valuable information about drug misusers, the separate stages of their addiction careers, their various and complicated involvements with treatment services, and, of course, the changes that occur in their drug use and other problem behaviours across extended periods of time after treatment. Such studies are rare, however, because of the high costs in money, effort, and organizational commitment necessary to implement, coordinate, and sustain such data collection systems over many years.

Among the earliest follow-up studies were the investigations of 100 New York City male addicts admitted to Lexington Hospital in 1952 and 1953 (Vaillant 1966, 1973), and another study, also of a sample of Lexington patients, but this time with a very different group of 266 addicts from rural Kentucky (O'Donnell 1969). Although the samples studied by Vaillant and O'Donnell were different in a number of important respects, they shared some similar characteristics and outcomes. The majority of both samples relapsed after leaving Lexington, but drug use trends over time were toward reduced opiate use. Vaillant found 22 per cent were abstinent after 5 years, and 37 per cent after 10 years. In O'Donnell's sample, the corresponding figures were 15 and 25 per cent, respectively.

More recently, four major studies have been conducted—DARP (the Drug Abuse Reporting Programme), TOPS (Treatment Outcome Prospective Study), NTORS (National Treatment Outcome Research Study), and DATOS (Drug Abuse Treatment Outcome Study). These all showed that drug-addicted patients were able to make a broad range of improvements in their problem behaviours after receiving treatment (Simpson and Sells 1983; Hubbard *et al.* 1989; Gossop *et al.* 1998*a*; Etheridge *et al.* 1997).

The Drug Abuse Reporting Programme (DARP)

The origins of DARP lie in the unsolicited proposal submitted in 1968 by Saul B. Sells to the National Institute of Mental Health to monitor and evaluate the emerging US federal addiction treatment system. DARP collected admission records for 44 000 patients at the time of entry into 52 treatment agencies, and recorded their status every 2 months until treatment termination. The programmes were located throughout the USA and in Puerto Rico. Data were collected through intake interviews, during-treatment progress reports, and a series of follow-up interviews from 3 to 12 years after treatment. Over 6000 patients were selected to participate in the first wave of posttreatment follow-up interviews, which were conducted, on average, 6 years after admission to DARP, and 4657 (77 per cent) were located and successfully interviewed. Follow-up data were available at 1, 2, and 3 years after treatment, and provided information for the year before the follow-up interview. In 1982, a second wave of follow-ups was conducted with a sample of 697 addicts, approximately 12 years after admission, with a follow-up rate of 70 per cent (Simpson and Sells 1990).

DARP investigated four treatment types as well as a comparison group that enrolled but never started treatment. The four treatments were methadone maintenance, therapeutic communities, out-patient drug-free (services that rely on counselling with an emphasis on abstinence), and out-patient detoxification.

Reductions were found in the use of opiates and other drugs after treatment. Among those patients who had been daily users of opioids before treatment, more than half (53 per cent) reported no daily opioid use at one year. Opioid use continued to decline over time until year 6, when it stabilized at 40 per cent for 'any' use and 25 per cent for 'daily' use. At some point during the 12 years following treatment, three-quarters of the sample had relapsed to daily opioid use, but at the year 12 interview, nearly two-thirds (63 per cent) had not used opioids on a daily basis for a period of at least 3 years.

DARP found that time in treatment was an important determinant of outcome, and that a minimum of 3 months in treatment was necessary to effect positive changes in drug use behaviour. Posttreatment outcomes became more favourable as the length of time spent in treatment increased. No long-term effect was found for 21-day detoxification. For methadone maintenance, drug-free out-patient treatment, and the therapeutic communities, significantly higher percentages of patients who stayed in treatment for longer than 90 days had favourable outcomes. For methadone, a significant linear relationship was found, with those staying longer having better outcomes (Simpson 1981).

One of DARP's contributions was its demonstration that methodologically rigorous longitudinal, field-based research could be successfully carried out with this difficult population to evaluate drug abuse treatment.

The Treatment Outcome Prospective Study (TOPS)

TOPS also provided longitudinal data on patients entering US federally funded drug abuse treatment programmes, and assessed short- and long-term treatment outcomes. Its design and core data elements were closely modelled upon those of DARP, and it built upon the earlier research by obtaining more data on patient characteristics, programme environments, and treatment services. Fieldwork to refine the TOPS methodology was carried out in 1978, and the first intake data were collected in 1979 (Hubbard *et al.* 1989).

TOPS enrolled a total of 11 750 patients entering treatment in 41 addiction treatment programmes in 10 US cities. The sample was recruited in three cohorts in 1979, 1980, and 1981. The four treatment modalities originally selected for investigation were methadone maintenance, detoxification, and residential and out-patient drug-free programmes. The programmes were purposely selected to represent the optimal types of these programmes. This rationale differed somewhat from DARP and yielded a sample of stable, established programmes that were more likely to be affiliated to hospitals and somewhat larger than average. The detoxification modality was subsequently excluded from the study as there were only four participating programmes.

Patients were interviewed on admission into treatment, and at 1 month, 3 months, 6 months, 9 months and 1 year after admission. For the follow-up interviews over 4000 patients were selected for participation and, after leaving treatment, a sample was followed up at 3 months, 1 year, 2 years, and then 3–5 years after treatment had terminated. Between 70 and 80 per cent of the patients from the treatment modalities were successfully followed up.

TOPS showed that treatment was effective in reducing use of heroin and other illicit drugs during and after treatment. Levels of predatory crime were reduced during treatment, and these remained lower than baseline levels after treatment. TOPS also reflected some of the changes in illicit drug use that were taking place in the USA at the time. Patterns of drug use among TOPS patients had changed substantially from DARP, though more than three-quarters (77 per cent) of TOPS admissions still reported opiates as their primary drug of abuse (Hubbard *et al.* 1989).

TOPS examined profiles of those patients entering the different treatment modalities and identified a number of differences between those starting on methadone maintenance programmes and those entering residential treatment. Patients entering residential treatment were more likely to be younger than those in the methadone maintenance group, and had more serious medical, mental health, family, and legal problems. There were also differences between the patients in these two modalities in their drug use prior to treatment. Approximately two-thirds of the methadone patients reported weekly or more frequent heroin use in the year before treatment compared to only about one-third of the residential patients. The residential patients were more likely to be users of drugs other than opioids and to be multiple drug users.

Length of time in treatment was found to be one of the most important predictors of positive outcomes, with relatively long periods in treatment necessary to effect changes. Significant reductions in regular heroin use were only evident for methadone and residential patients following one year of treatment.

The National Treatment Outcome Research Study (NTORS)

Because of cross-national differences in patterns of drug use, in the types of treatment services provided, and in socio-environmental factors, it was unclear to what extent the US findings could be generalized to different patient groups, with different treatment systems, and in different countries. It was for these reasons, that the National Treatment Outcome Research Study (NTORS) was established in the UK. NTORS was commissioned by a Department of Health Task Force in 1994, and is the largest prospective longitudinal cohort study of treatment outcome for drug abusers to be conducted in the UK.

NTORS investigated a cohort of problem drug users treated in four treatment modalities provided in either residential or community treatment settings throughout England. The modalities were selected to be representative of the main treatment modalities within the UK. Residential modalities were specialist in-patient treatment and rehabilitation programmes. The community treatments were methadone maintenance and methadone reduction programmes.

NTORS provided detailed information about the pretreatment behaviours and problems of the cohort, the operational characteristics of treatment programmes, and, particularly, the patient outcomes across a range of measures. As in the American studies, a central feature of NTORS was its concern with the impact of existing national treatment programmes delivered under day-to-day operating conditions.

Between March and July 1995, 1075 patients were recruited by 54 treatment programmes. Patients presented with a range of extensive, chronic, and serious drug-related problems. The most common drug problem was long-term opiate dependence, often in conjunction with polydrug and/or alcohol problems. Many patients had psychological and physical health problems, and high rates of criminal behaviour were reported.

One year after intake to treatment, outcome data were obtained for 769 patients (72 per cent). Of these, 753 successfully completed a research interview conducted by field interviewers from the Office for National Statistics; a further 16 patients (1.5 per cent) died during the year. Subsequent follow-ups at 2 and 4–5 years were conducted with a random stratified sample of 650 patients based upon a sampling frame of 894 patients for whom definite locator information was confirmed by contact during the first year after intake.

Clinical improvements were found in a wide range of problem behaviours, including reductions in use of heroin and other illicit drugs, reduced injecting and sharing of injecting equipment, improvements in psychological health, and reductions in crime. Frequency of heroin use after 1 year, for example, was reduced to about half of the intake levels, and heroin use remained at this lower level throughout the full 4–5 year follow-up period. The sharing of injecting equipment was more than halved among patients who had been treated in both residential and community settings.

Rates of abstinence from illicit drug use increased among the patients from both the residential and the methadone programmes. Among the residential patients, for instance, almost half (49 per cent) were abstinent from heroin after 4–5 years, and the percentage of residential patients who were abstinent from all six illicit target drugs had increased from 1 per cent at intake to 38 per cent after 4–5 years. As in the American outcome studies, time in residential treatment was related to improved posttreatment outcomes.

Although many patients showed improvements, these were not found for all patients, and they were not found for all outcome measures. Many patients were drinking excessively at intake to treatment. Although there were some improvements in alcohol use at follow-up, the changes in alcohol consumption were disappointing and many patients were still drinking heavily at follow-up. Greater improvements in drinking behaviour were found among the patients who had been treated in residential settings. There was no overall improvement in drinking among those treated in the methadone programmes. NTORS recommended that drug treatment services should introduce or strengthen interventions specifically targeted at drinking problems among drug misusers.

The Drug Abuse Treatment Outcome Study (DATOS)

DATOS was initiated in 1989 as a continuation of the US National Institute on Drug Abuse's long-term investment in national treatment outcome studies, and built on the foundations provided by DARP and TOPS. DATOS is a longitudinal prospective study of adults who entered drug treatment programmes between 1991 and 1993, and investigated the links between patient outcome, treatment process, and programme structure. Treatment programmes were purposely chosen to represent treatment delivered in typical programmes. Intake data were collected on 10 010 adults, from 99 treatment programmes in 11 cities across the USA. Data were collected at 1 and 3 months during treatment and 12 months after treatment. The four types of treatment programmes were: methadone maintenance, short-term residential (hospital in-patient and chemical dependency), long-term residential (therapeutic community), and out-patient drug-free treatment. The 12-month follow-up sample of 4500 was drawn from 85 programmes, with the follow-up stratified by treatment modality, drug pattern, impairment level, and length of time in treatment (Hubbard *et al.* 1997).

DATOS provided further data on the changes in the drug use patterns and problems of patients that occurred between the 1960s and the 1990s. The patient populations in TOPS and DATOS had some common features but also differed in certain sociodemographic and background characteristics (Craddock *et al.* 1997). Compared to TOPS patients, DATOS patients were older, and the proportion of women in treatment had also increased. One of the most obvious changes during these decades, was in the trend away from opiates to use of crack cocaine. TOPS patients were more likely to use multiple drugs than were those in DARP, and they were more likely to be frequent users of drugs other than, or in addition to opioids. In DATOS, cocaine was the predominant drug.

The patients treated in long-term residential, short-term in-patient, and out-patient drug-free programmes reported 50 per cent less weekly or daily cocaine use in the follow-up year than in the pre-admission year. Reductions were greater for patients treated for 3 months or more. Among the long-term residential patients, reductions in illegal activity and increases in full-time employment were related to treatment stays of 6 months or longer. The patients who remained in methadone maintenance programmes reported less heroin use than patients who left treatment.

DATOS was designed not only to enable replication of previous outcome studies but to investigate research and policy issues about treatment effectiveness and treatment processes. DATOS drew further attention to the potential importance of differences in programme size, treatment setting, programme organization, philosophy, structure, and therapeutic approach, which had been identified in the earlier projects. The DATOS treatment programmes also varied in the nature and intensity of core therapies and comprehensive services provided, types of therapists and therapies offered, average length of stay, and inclusion of aftercare (Etheridge *et al.* 1997). In particular, the study showed a marked decrease in the number and variety of services received by patients in 1991–93 compared to those received by TOPS patients in 1979–81 (Etheridge *et al.* 1995).

The assessment of treatment effectiveness

An important feature of these treatment outcome studies is that they investigated the outcomes for patients after treatment provided in existing services under day-to-day clinical circumstances. The complex and complicated environment in which treatment policy is made and implemented requires this sort of information, and there is increased acknowledgment of the need for evidence of effectiveness to guide decisions about treatment policy and provision. The investigation of treatment outcome in field settings has been valuable in helping to identify what works in practice, even though the possibilities for control over treatment assignment and other aspects of evaluation design are more limited than in clinical trials or other experimental studies (Simpson 1997).

The study of treatment in normal clinical settings creates complex problems for research design, measurement, and analysis, which have no perfect solution. The limitations of non-experimental prospective longitudinal studies revolve around the sampling frame, the absence of random assignment and of a non-treated control sample, and the wide variability between patients in terms of services received and length of time spent in treatment. In addition, the index treatment episode may represent only one of multiple treatment exposures over time.

This is not the appropriate place to enter into a detailed exposition of different research methods, and of their attendant advantages and disadvantages. However, a few words are perhaps in order regarding two of the most commonly voiced criticisms of treatment outcomes studies: that they are seriously handicapped by the absence of random allocation procedures and a non-treated control group.

Random assignment is widely regarded as one of the most powerful research procedures and sometimes as a *sine qua non* for a properly designed clinical trial. There are circumstances in which randomized experiments are both appropriate and necessary. One area of clinical research in which they undoubtedly have a useful place is in the evaluation of pharmacological treatments for clearly delineated medical conditions. When used correctly, the randomized trial offers one way of dealing with the massive uncertainty inherent in the evaluation of addiction treatments. Like all techniques, the randomized trial has its strengths. But it also has weaknesses. It is not the only way of doing research. The questions to which it provides answers are limited in scope, and the answers that it gives are not the only answers worth having. There are, however, circumstances in which randomization may be neither appropriate nor necessary. Randomization is a means to an end, and not an end in itself.

There are certain general principles that apply to the evaluation of treatment effectiveness. One of the most important is that the research designs should be matched to research question(s). D.L. McLellan, a specialist in rehabilitation medicine noted that 'Sometimes it is claimed that some methodologies are better or 'more scientific' than others. The proposition that randomized double-blind prospective quantitative group trials are better than . . . observational studies is of course absurd' (McLellan 1997). Conducting useful and informative research into treatment effectiveness does not necessarily depend upon using the most advanced methods, but rather depends upon using the most appropriate methods. The key issue is how to choose the best and most appropriate methodology to answer the specific research question. Using the wrong method is unhelpful, no matter how powerful the design, nor how systematically the method is applied.

The distinction between efficacy and effectiveness has long been established. Efficacy refers to evidence from carefully controlled trials where threats to internal validity have been minimized. In effectiveness research, the design is weighted towards high generalizability. Internal validity refers to the extent to which the study design was sufficiently rigorous that conclusions can confidently be drawn about main treatment effects within this specific experiment. External validity, on the other hand, refers to the degree to which the results can be generalized beyond the confines of the specific study, for example, to other populations or settings. Clinicians or policymakers are generally more interested in the extent to which a study's findings can be generalized to other populations and settings, or about its replicability, and less about issues of internal validity.

The randomized trial focuses upon internal validity to the detriment of external validity and, whilst efficacy studies are essential in establishing if an intervention can work under ideal conditions, they often tell us little about how the results relate to real-world clinical practice (Gilbody *et al.* 2002). Orford (1999) also commented that overconcern with internal validity at the expense of external validity, can result in close attention being paid to the minutiae of the experiment while the wider context of the study is ignored. There is a growing recognition that treatment evaluation is more than just a technical enterprise (Moos *et al.* 1990).

The process of randomly allocating patients to a treatment condition, for example, is quite different from what happens in normal clinical practice (Sperry *et al.* 1996). Drug users in treatment generally enter a type of treatment and a type of agency that they have actively sought. Treatment consumers can shop around for a treatment or self-help group of their own choosing (Seligman 1995). Even where services are few in number and restricted in choice, most patients are still able to exercise some choice about which treatment programme they attend. This is likely to affect factors such as treatment satisfaction and programme participation that are known to influence subsequent outcomes (Joe and Friend 1989; Joe *et al.* 1999). The reliance upon randomization, in which patients are passively assigned to treatment, can lead evaluation research to neglect the role played by self-selection.

Treatment samples that are created by random assignment may behave differently from those selected through clinical need and motivation for treatment (De Leon *et al.* 1995*a*). The process of randomization may reduce the effectiveness of the intervention when this depends upon the patient's cognitions and behaviours, leading to an artificial experiment with little relevance to circumstances in the real world.

Many biases and problems of covert selection can also occur prior to randomization. Under such circumstances, the inclusion/exclusion criteria of a study, and the processes of selection that lie hidden behind them make it difficult or impossible for a therapist to know the extent to which any particular patient is of the same type, or is likely to respond in the same way as those who entered a particular study (Finney *et al.* 1996).

The starting point for many substance abuse treatment evaluations is a comparison of treatment and control conditions, or of alternative treatment programmes: unfortunately, that is often all that the evaluation seeks to achieve (Finney 1995). The randomized trial offers a sort of race between two treatments and asks which one gets to the finishing post first. It is a serious drawback of the randomized clinical trial that it usually provides only a very small amount of useful or relevant information about treatment effectiveness or about how treatment can be improved, especially since results often show very small main effects of treatment.

The requirement that treatment outcome studies should be designed with a no-treatment control condition is usually made without an understanding of the inherent problems. From a practical point of view it is extremely difficult to see how drug misusers seeking treatment could not only be randomly allocated to receive no treatment from the programme that they approached, but could also be prevented from seeking the same or a similar treatment from another treatment service. In addition, there are many who would argue that the withholding of treatment from such individuals would not be ethically acceptable.

Drug users not seeking treatment do not provide a properly comparable control group. However, there are several 'natural experiments' that provide information that has relevance to the issue of non-treated controls. Many addiction treatment services are overburdened, and sometimes have relatively lengthy waiting lists for treatment. This provides an opportunity to study drug use and other problem behaviours of patients who were seeking, but not yet receiving treatment. In a study of heroin addicts who were waiting to be admitted to an out-patient treatment programme, there were no changes in the levels or severity of drug use problem behaviours during the waiting period (of approximately 2 months), and no evidence of 'spontaneous' improvement in drug use (Best *et al.* 2002). After treatment entry, there were rapid and substantial reductions in the quantity and frequency of drug use that were maintained during the 6 months after starting treatment.

Studies of untreated, dependent drug users provide information about the natural course of addiction. Metzger *et al.* (1993) investigated the drug-using patterns, needle-sharing practices, and HIV infection rates of two samples of opiate-dependent injectors. One group consisted of drug users receiving methadone maintenance. None of the out-of-treatment heroin users had previously received treatment, but were matched to the treatment group in terms of age, race, sex, neighbourhood, and other relevant background factors. Both groups were followed up for 7 years. At the initial assessment, 13 per cent of the treatment sample and 21 per cent of the out-of-treatment group were HIV positive. After 7 years, 21 per cent of the treatment group tested HIV positive compared to more than half (51 per cent) of the out-of-treatment group. It is not possible to attribute this difference to treatment since the out-of-treatment users may have differed from those in treatment in important ways, for example, in terms of lower motivation for change.

One way of separating the effects of drug dependence treatment from the effects of motivation is to compare treated and untreated substance-dependent individuals who were explicitly not interested in treatment. In a study of about 3000 drug injectors who sought HIV testing, Booth *et al.* (1996) randomly assigned them either to standard HIV testing alone, or to testing plus three sessions of motivational counselling. Those who received additional counselling were less likely to be injecting drugs at 6-month follow-up (20 versus 45 per cent), and four times more likely to be abstinent than those who received HIV testing only.

Similarly, in a study of women who had applied for prenatal care and were found to be positive for cocaine use as a result of routine drug screening, Svikis *et al.* (1997) offered a drug treatment package of 1 week of residential care followed by twice-weekly addiction counselling during scheduled prenatal visits. They were compared with another group of pregnant women, matched by demographic characteristics, who also tested positive for cocaine and received standard prenatal care, but who received no addiction treatment. At delivery, rates of cocaine use were twice as high among the untreated women (63 per cent) as among those who received treatment (37 per cent).

The babies of the treated women averaged higher birth weights and longer gestational periods than those of the comparison group, and 10 per cent of the babies of the treated women required intensive neonatal care for an average of 7 days, compared to 26 per cent of the babies of the untreated women who required intensive care for an average of 39 days. The average costs of care were $14 500 for the treated women and $46 700 for the comparison group.

Costs and cost-effectiveness of treatment

As in other areas of medicine, there are increasing demands for evidence about value for money. This legitimate interest in cost-effectiveness, however, has limitations and unintended side-effects. Calculations of the types and extent of treatment benefit may be made in different ways by the treatment purchaser, by public health agencies, by clinicians, and by the individual patient. Different calculations lead to different conclusions.

Hodgson and Meiners (1982) identified three types of costs that can be included in cost-of-illness studies. *Direct costs* included medical care costs for the diagnosis and treatment of addiction and its related medical conditions, and non-medical costs such as prison and law enforcement costs. *Indirect costs* included loss of earnings due to premature mortality or imprisonment, and *psychosocial costs* included those due to reduced quality of life for the heroin addict and their family. These last costs are important but extremely difficult to quantify.

Drummond *et al.* (1997) suggested that the societal costs of drug treatment can be considered in four main areas.

- Costs to the agency providing the intervention.
- Costs to other agencies directly related to the intervention (e.g. referrals to other agencies, and costs associated with treatment but not borne by the agency).
- Costs borne by the patients (e.g. travel costs, treatment fees, costs of patient's time while in treatment or travelling to treatment).
- Productivity costs. For those in residential treatment there is a loss of potential time in employment. Out-patient programmes may also affect availability for work. Whether to include these effects and the valuation of such lost productivity remains controversial.

Consequences of treatment can also be divided into four main categories.

- Consequences for the individual in terms of their quality and quantity of life.
- Resources saved as a result of treatment (e.g. health care and criminal justice expenditures).

- Other value created (including the wider impacts on other members of society, such as potential victims of crime, and improvements in local communities resulting from reductions in drug use).
- Increased productivity of the individual as they may re-enter the legitimate labour market.

Although only about 5 per cent of illicit drugs users take heroin, approximately 20 per cent of the total economic costs of illicit drug use has been found to be linked to heroin use (Harwood *et al.* 1988). Based on 1996 figures, Mark *et al.* (2001) estimated the total economic costs of heroin addiction in the USA as US$21.9 billion. Of this, the largest portion (53 per cent) was due to the indirect costs of lost productivity. Crime costs were the next largest component of total costs (24 per cent). Medical care costs associated with heroin addiction accounted for 23 per cent of the total, of which the largest amount (16 per cent) was spent on treating associated medical complications, including HIV/AIDS, tuberculosis, hepatitis B and C, and pregnancy complications. Direct addiction treatment costs accounted for only 6 per cent of costs.

Cost-effectiveness and cost-benefit studies were carried out on TOPS modalities. These studies showed that, when the crime-related costs of drug abuse were calculated, treatment was cost-effective and cost-beneficial. In most cases, the cost of treatment was recouped during treatment, and further cost-benefits accrued as a result of reduced posttreatment drug use (Harwood *et al.* 1988).

Similarly, the economic costs imposed upon society by the NTORS cohort were largely due to their criminality. High rates of criminal behaviour were found prior to treatment, and crime costs prior to treatment greatly outweighed all of the treatment costs. After treatment there was a marked reduction in criminal activity. The savings to society in terms of reduced criminal behaviour and reduced demands upon the criminal justice system were estimated to be worth many millions of pounds per year. The increased expenditure for treatment interventions yielded an immediate cost saving in terms of the reduced victim costs of crime, as well as cost savings within the criminal justice system. For every extra UK£1 spent on drug misuse treatment, there was a return of more than £3 in terms of costs savings associated with victim costs of crime, and reduced demands upon the criminal justice system (Gossop *et al.* 1998*a*).

In a study based upon the behaviour of DATOS participants, Flynn *et al.* (1999) also calculated that there was a range of economic benefits from treatment for cocaine dependence, based solely on costs of crime. These reduced costs of crime during and after treatment substantially outweighed the costs of treatment and demonstrated the value of investing in the treatment of cocaine addiction. Flynn *et al.* concluded that, even without the numerous other tangible and intangible benefits that may have occurred in addition to the reductions in costs of crime to society, the fiscal resources expended in treating cocaine-dependent patients provide a return that justified the cost of treatment.

The true cost savings to society are likely to be even greater than these crime-focused estimates. Using the NTORS data, the changes in crime and health-care consequences that were associated with specific costs of the index treatment were calculated. This suggested net savings of UK£27 million for an investment in index treatment of £2 million. The cohort could also been seen as having received a further investment of £2.4 million pounds in non-index treatment during the follow-up period. However, this cohort also received investment in treatment in the 2 years prior to treatment. The most useful ratio may be the consequences related to the net change in total treatment investment. This yields a net treatment investment in the 2 years after intake of about £1.5 million, and a ratio of consequences to net treatment investment of 18:1 (Godfrey *et al.* 2001).

Health- and social-care costs seem small in comparison to the crime costs. However, this highlights an important omission of the potential value of treatment—the estimate of the impact on the individual's quantity and quality of life. Estimates of the monetary value of life are significant. If as a result of index treatment some 26 patients of the NTORS sample had not died who would have been predicted to die without their index treatment, then the 'savings' from treatment would have been much greater and would match those from the drop in the social costs of crime (Godfrey *et al.* 2001).

However, quality of life as well as quantity is important. Most studies claiming to use cost–benefit methodology fail to include estimates for the individual outcome gains (Godfrey and Sutton 1996; Cartwright 2000). This is a major omission. It is equivalent to suggesting that drug-misusing individuals have a zero value, and that drug treatments are only offered to drug misusers because of the potential value to the rest of society whatever the consequences to the individual and their families. Ethically, this contrasts with other health service codes.

In a study of the costs and effectiveness of drug addiction treatments, Gossop and Strang (2000) focused upon the links, but also, and more importantly, upon the tension and sometimes the conflict that can exist between the priorities of cost effectiveness and those of clinical effectiveness.

One of the most conspicuous differences between a treatment delivered in an in-patient setting and that delivered in an out-patient setting is that of cost. Gossop and Strang (2000) calculated that the unadjusted weekly cost of an in-patient detoxification is 24 times greater than that of an out-patient detoxification. Even when adjustment is made for the possibility that withdrawal treatment may be implemented more rapidly in an in-patient setting, the crude costs are still much higher than for out-patient treatment. When adjustments are made for outcome, the differences in cost become less marked. The costs of a 10-day in-patient programme when adjusted for successful programme completion rates are almost identical to those of the out-patient programme. Discussion of treatment costs is misleading if not informed by, and adjusted for, evidence of effectiveness. This is especially important where there are marked differences in outcome between treatment options.

Where in-patient treatment was provided either in a dedicated drug dependence unit or on a general psychiatry ward, the difference in unadjusted costs per week was less marked than for the contrast between in- and out-patient settings (Gossop and Strang 2000). However, the duration of treatment in these two in-patient settings was such that, when adjustment was made for the actual length of stay, the cost of a treatment episode on the drug dependence unit was about three times greater than that on the general psychiatry ward. When adjusted for different clinical outcomes, the cost difference dropped considerably, though the dedicated drug dependence unit continued to be the more costly of the two options. For individual patients, however, the outcomes were consistently superior for treatment on the drug dependence unit.

Such analyses illustrate the dangers of naive adherence to cost and cost-containment considerations. Provision of in-patient detoxification in a non-specialist setting may be easier to establish, and probably cheaper to run than a specialist service. Provision of out-patient-only detoxification provides opportunities for substantial cost-cutting, but at a huge cost to the individual patient, his or her family, and society. The logic of purchasing a cheaper detoxification programme with significantly worse completion rates is difficult to understand.

For some time, and in many countries, treatment services have been exposed to pressures that have used the terminology of cost-effectiveness but that have often placed greater weight upon accountancy administration, or upon the simple issue of costs. It has been as if cost and cost minimization were considered to be synonymous with cost-effectiveness. In the USA, changes in the availability and funding of addiction treatment services have led to in-patient and residential treatments often being replaced by community-based treatment services, and with clinical decisions being directly influenced by cost considerations rather than clinical need (Swift and Miller 1997).

The patient's own interests (and those of family and other patient advocates) may be irreconcilable with the crude calculations of the accountant.

Ultimately, the patient will still rightfully pursue the treatment with the best outcome for themselves, regardless of the broader strategic considerations by others of health purchase across the wider population. For the individual patient, it is the probability of a successful outcome that is paramount. It is little consolation to be told of the more widespread provision of care if the price to be paid is treatment with a suboptimal outcome. The patient purchasing private health would consider this an unacceptable argument, and the patient receiving state-funded health care should be similarly dissatisfied. An ineffective service is inefficient and cannot be cost-effective no matter how cheaply it is provided.

An 'outcome funding' or 'outcome purchase' approach represents an interesting option for commissioning of health care in the addictions. If health purchasers were to purchase successful outcomes, this would provide incentives to the care providers to make best use of the available resources. If longer in-patient care or more expensive specialist care were associated with sufficiently better outcome, then the clinician, administrator, and purchaser would all be pursuing similar objectives to those that interest the patient.

Treatment and social policy

A report by the Royal Colleges of Psychiatrists and Physicians (2000) suggested that UK national expenditure on tackling drug problems was not being used to full effect. For example, 12 per cent of the UK's overall drug budget was spent on drugs education in 1997–98, almost as much as on treatment and rehabilitation. Despite the scale of the expenditure on educational programmes, drug education programmes have been evaluated less fully and rigorously than treatment, and there is little evidence of beneficial results. Where drugs education programmes have been evaluated, they have usually produced only short-lived improvements in knowledge and attitudes, with little evidence of changes in behaviour. The Royal Colleges' report questions whether current levels of expenditure on education and prevention are justified in the absence of evidence of their effectiveness.

Out of a total annual expenditure (in 1997–98) of about £1.4 billion devoted to tackling drug misuse in the UK, law enforcement and customs/interdiction accounted for 75 per cent of expenditure, with 12 per cent spent on education and prevention, and 13 per cent on treatment (Fig. 14.1; Department of Health 1998). In the USA, where total federal expenditure spent on law enforcement, interdiction, and crime intervention was 69 per cent of the budget, prevention received the same as in Britain, but treatment received half as much again with19 per cent.

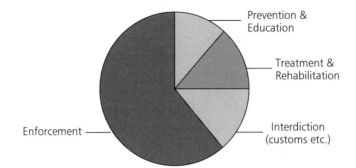

Estimated UK expenditure for 1997/98 was £1.4 billion

Fig. 14.1 National UK expenditure to tackle drug problems for the year 1997–98. About two-thirds of national expenditure was used for enforcement measures. When enforcement and interdiction activities are combined, this accounts for three-quarters of national expenditure. Expenditure on treatment remains proportionately very low. The data are from Department of Health (1999a) drug misuse statistics.

Very little is known about the effectiveness of law enforcement, and the Royal Colleges' report also argued that the balance of investment between supply and demand reduction approaches should be altered. In return for the huge sums spent on law enforcement and attempts to discourage or prevent the international trade in illicit drugs, the usual indicators of 'success' are the numbers of arrests or quantities and hypothetical 'street values' of drugs seized. Such indicators are used without evidence to show how (if at all) these are related to levels of drug use. In contrast, there is now good evidence of benefit resulting from the treatment of drug addicts. If sufficient funding were available, it is probable that twice as many drug addicts could be drawn into, and treated within treatment services.

One study of the impact of law enforcement measures reported the response of drug misusers to a major police operation that targeted drug dealers across ten London boroughs (Best *et al.* 2001*b*). Within the first 14 days of the operation, more than 241 people had been arrested and drugs seized with an estimated street value of £1.5 million. In spite of the scale of the operation, the majority of drug users living in target areas noticed no changes in the price or availability of heroin or crack cocaine. Indeed, most were unaware of increased police activity in the areas directly affected by the operation.

Those who were aware of the increased police activity (about one-third of the sample), reported no knowledge of market changes, and made no changes in their own drug use. Such findings suggest that the markets for heroin, crack, and cannabis are not sensitive, at least in the short term, to increased police activity, even when such activity is associated with a number of significant drug seizures, and with the removal of a large number of dealers from the street. Even the lesser ambition of supply reduction strategies, the harassment and disruption of local markets, cannot be guaranteed by concerted police activity. What the Metropolitan Police described as 'the biggest ever drug operation' in London and as a 'spectacular success' actually appeared to have little or no observable impact on drug markets or drug users.

The question of how addiction treatment interventions influence criminal behaviour is important both for the implementation and evaluation of treatment programmes and for the development of policies to tackle drug misuse problems. Drug-related crime imposes substantial economic and psychological costs upon society and upon the victims of crime, and it has high priority in public opinion, media, and political views of the problem. Although clinical services focus more upon tackling drug misuse and health problems, the reduction of crime is currently also seen as a goal of drug misuse treatment (Institute of Medicine 1990a).

The reductions in criminal activity found in DARP were less marked than those for illicit drug use. High levels of criminal activity were found in year 12, even amongst those who were drug-free. Studies since DARP have consistently found a positive impact of treatment on criminal activity. Hubbard et al. (1989) and Ball and Ross (1991) found major reductions in the most common forms of income-generating crime such as shoplifting and other forms of theft. Hubbard et al. (1989) found that the proportion of patients committing property crimes during treatment was reduced to 10 per cent of pretreatment levels, and to about one-third in the year after treatment. Ball and Ross (1991) reported that the number of offences fell to about 20 per cent of pretreatment levels during methadone maintenance. Less crime is committed by patients in methadone maintenance treatment than by comparable groups of addicts out of treatment (Hunt et al. 1984), and involvement in crime and the amount of crime committed during periods of addiction far exceed that committed during periods of non-addiction (Ball et al. 1983; Nurco et al. 1989). The meta-analytic study conducted by Marsch (1998) showed that methadone maintenance treatment appeared to have one of its strongest effects in terms of reducing drug-related criminal behaviours.

Among NTORS patients, substantial reductions in crime were found after treatment. This was shown both by the reduced numbers of crimes committed and in the reduced percentage of patients engaged in acquisitive crime. Overall, acquisitive crimes were reduced to one-third of intake levels, and the rate of involvement in crime was reduced to about half of intake levels (Gossop et al. 2000c). The number of shoplifting offences was reduced to about one-third of intake levels and, for the more serious offence of burglary, offending was reduced to less than one-quarter of intake levels. Much of this change was linked to reductions in drug use after treatment, and especially to reduced heroin use.

In any population of addicts, not all will be involved in crime. Half of the NTORS patients committed no acquisitive crimes during the 3 months prior to intake and, of those who were involved in crime, the majority were relatively low-rate offenders. The vast majority of acquisitive crimes were committed by a small minority of the patients, with 10 per cent of the patients committing 76 per cent of the crimes (Stewart *et al.* 2000*a*). At intake, the patients who were most heavily involved in crime were the most frequent users of heroin and cocaine. Stewart *et al.* also reported more severe dependence on drugs, poorer psychological health, and lower rates of employment. NTORS showed that many of the greatest reductions in criminal activity occurred within this highly active group of offenders (Gossop *et al.* 2000*c*). Among the high-rate offenders, crimes were reduced to 13 per cent of intake levels. By any standards, this represents a huge reduction in criminal behaviour.

Just as concerns about drugs and crime have had a strong influence upon drugs policy, other issues have also had a profound effect. Without doubt, one of the most powerful events of recent years was the appearance and identification of HIV infection among injecting drug users. The problem was identified in the early 1980s, and a systematic response to the threat was rapidly put together in the UK (and in many other countries). HIV forced all who were involved in treatment to rethink of the nature of the drug problem and to look again at the appropriateness and effectiveness of existing services.

Unlike some other countries, the UK was relatively open to the ideas and practices of harm reduction. There were no major political or community objections, and no major legal obstacles. The implementation of harm reduction in the UK was typified by having appropriate, attractive, and accessible treatment services, by the need to increase contact with drug misusers, and the use of innovative methods for doing so. Outreach services were used to contact hard-to-reach groups and to facilitate the passing of health promotion information through social networks (Stimson 1998).

In general, the period since the rapid changes of the 1980s has been characterized more in terms of the consolidation of addiction treatment responses. Recent developments have tended to involve a gradually improved understanding of problems and responses rather than the discovery or implementation of radical new interventions. There remains a need for further research to strengthen what is still a rather impoverished understanding of what are the active ingredi-ents of treatment, and how they produce an effect. More research is also required into the effectiveness of new treatment methods that are being developed.

It is surprisingly difficult to determine how much is spent on addiction research in the UK. Government reports provide the sums spent on deterrence, prevention, and treatment, but do not give any figures for research. The best recent estimate suggests that the total annual addiction research by government departments, research councils, and the major charitable foundations was £2.5–3 million in 1998. This represented only 0.02 per cent of the £1.4 billion annual expenditure (Royal Colleges of Psychiatrists and Physicians 2000).

To put these figures in perspective, in 1995, the US Government spent $542 million on addiction research. This represented 4 per cent of their annual drugs budget. Even this level of expenditure was criticized as inadequate by the US General Accounting Office. Current UK expenditure on addiction research is trivial compared with the scale and importance of the problem. Research is conspicuously the most underfunded component of the UK's response to drugs and, without doubt, there is an urgent need for increased research funding.

Undoubtedly we have made much progress since the 1960s, and have learned a good deal about the treatment of addiction. There is a sizeable body of evidence that gives grounds for confidence about the effectiveness of a number of the current treatments. However, there is also a great deal that we do not know and that continues to hamper our efforts to provide more effective treatments. In a field in which the problem itself is so mutable, evidence from studies conducted in previous decades may not be a secure foundation for current practice. Whereas addiction treatment research gradually accumulates, it also gradually ages. It is imperative that addiction research is properly funded and that our knowledge of addiction treatment interventions is kept up to date.

References

Abbott, P.J., Weller, S.B., Delaney, H.D., and Moore, B.A. (1998). Community reinforcement approach in the treatment of opiate addicts. *American Journal of Drug and Alcohol Abuse* **24**, 7–30.

ACMD (1982). *Treatment and rehabilitation. Report by the UK Advisory Council on the Misuse of Drugs.* HMSO, London.

ACMD (1988). *AIDS and drug misuse: Part 1. Report by the UK Advisory Council on the Misuse of Drugs.* HMSO, London.

ACMD (2000). *Reducing drug related deaths. Report of the UK Advisory Council on the Misuse of Drugs.* The Stationery Office, London.

Aghajanian, C. (1978). Tolerance of locus coeruleus neurons to morphine and suppression of withdrawal responses by clonidine. *Nature* **276**, 186–8.

Ahmed, A., Gruer, L., McGuigan, C., Penrice G., *et al*. (2000). *Clostridium novyi* and unexplained illness among injecting drug users—Scotland, Ireland and England, April–June 2000. *Morbidity and Mortality Weekly Report* **49**, 543–5.

Alter, M.J., Kruszon-Moran, D., Nainan, O.V., McQuillan, G.M., Gao, F., Moyer, L.A., Kaslow, R.A., and Margolis, H.S. (1999). The prevalence of hepatitis C virus infection in the United States 1988 through 1994. *New England Journal of Medicine* **341**, 556–62.

Alterman, A. and Cacciola, J. (1991). The antisocial personality disorder diagnosis in substance abusers: problems and issues. *Journal of Nervous and Mental Disease* **179**, 401–9.

Alterman, A., McLellan, A., and Shifman, R. (1993). Do substance abuse patients with more psychopathology receive more treatment? *Journal of Nervous and Mental Disease* **181**, 576–82.

Alterman, A., O'Brien, C., McLellan, A.T., August, D., Snider, E., Droba, M., Cornish, J., Hall, C., Raphaelson, A., and Schrade, F. (1994). Effectiveness and costs of inpatient versus day hospital cocaine rehabilitation. *Journal of Nervous and Mental Disease* **182**, 157–63.

Ananth, J., Vandewater, S., Kamal, M., Brodsky, A., Gamal, R., and Miller, M. (1989). Missed diagnosis of substance abuse in psychiatric patients. *Hospital and Community Psychiatry* **40**, 297–9.

Andree, R. (1980). Sudden death following naloxone administration. *Anesthesia and Analgesia* **59**, 782–4.

Anglin, M.D. (1988). A social policy analysis of compulsory treatment for opiate dependence. *Journal of Drug Issues* **18**, 527–45.

Anglin, M.D., Almog, I., Fisher, D., and Peters, K. (1989*a*). Alcohol use by heroin addicts: evidence for an inverse relationship: a study of methadone maintenance and drug-free treatment samples. *American Journal of Drug and Alcohol Abuse* **15**, 191–207.

Anglin, M.D., Brecht, M., and Maddahian, E. (1989*b*). Pretreatment characteristics and treatment performance of legally coerced versus voluntary methadone maintenance admissions. *Criminology* **27**, 537–57.

Annis, H. (1986). A relapse prevention model for the treatment of alcoholics. In *Treating addictive behaviors* (ed. W. Miller and N. Heather). Plenum, New York.

Annis, H. and Davis, C. (1988). Self-efficacy and the prevention of alcoholic relapse. In *Addictive disorders: psychological research on assessment and treatment* (ed. T. Baker and D. Cannon). Praeger, New York.

Aronson, T.A. and Craig, T.J. (1986). Cocaine precipitation of panic disorder. *American Journal of Psychiatry* **143**, 643–5.

ASAM (2001). *ASAM placement criteria for the treatment of substance-related disorders.* American Society of Addiction Medicine, Chevy Chase, Maryland.

Ashton, C.H. (1990). Solvent abuse. *British Medical Journal* **300**, 135–6.

Auriacombe, M. (2001). Deaths attributable to methadone vs buprenorphine in France. *Journal of the American Medical Association* **285**, 45.

Avants, S., Margolin, A., Kosten, T., and Cooney, N. (1995). Differences between responders and non-responders to cocaine cues in the laboratory. *Addictive Behaviors* **20**, 215–24.

Ayllon, T. and Azrin, N. (1968). *The token economy: a motivational system for therapy and rehabilitation.* Appleton Century Crofts, New York.

Babor, T.F., Brown, J., and DelBoca, F.K. (1990). Validity of self-reports in applied research on addictive behaviors: fact or fiction? *Behavioral Assessment* **12**, 5–31.

Babor, T.F., Steinberg, K., Anton, R., and Del Boca, F. (2000). Talk is cheap: measuring drinking outcomes in clinical trials. *Journal of Studies on Alcohol* **61**, 55–63.

Bachrach, L. (1992). Psychosocial rehabilitation and psychiatry in the care of long-term patients. *American Journal of Psychiatry* **149**, 1455–63.

Baker, A., Boggs, T., and Lewin, T. (2001). Randomized controlled trial of brief cognitive behavioural interventions among regular users of amphetamine. *Addiction* **96**, 1279–87.

Bale, R., van Stone, W., Kuldau, J., Engelsing, T., Elashoff, R., and Zarcone, V. (1980). Therapeutic communities vs methadone maintenance. *Archives of General Psychiatry* **37**, 179–93.

Balint, E. and Norell, J. (1973). *Six minutes for the patient: interactions in general practice.* Tavistock, London.

Ball, J. (1967). The reliability and validity of interview data obtained from narcotic drug addicts. *American Journal of Sociology* **72**, 650–4.

Ball, J. and Ross, A. (1991). *The effectiveness of methadone maintenance treatment.* Springer-Verlag, New York.

Ball, J., Shaffer, J., and Nurco, D. (1983). The day to day criminality of heroin addicts in Baltimore: a study in the continuity of offence rates. *Drug and Alcohol Dependence* **12**, 119–42.

Bandura, A. (1977). *Social learning theory.* Prentice Hall, Englewood Cliffs, New Jersey.

Bandura, A. (1997). *Self-efficacy.* Freeman, New York.

Bandura, A. and Simon, K. (1977). The role of proximal intentions in self-regulation of refractory behavior. *Cognitive Therapy and Research* **1**, 177–94.

Banks, A. and Waller, T. (1988). *Drug misuse: a practical handbook for GPs.* Blackwells, Oxford.

Barber, J., Crits-Chistoph, P., and Luborsky, L. (1996). Effects of therapist adherence and competence on patient outcome in brief dynamic therapy. *Journal of Consulting and Clinical Psychology* **64**, 619–22.

Barber, J., Luborsky, L., Gallop, R., Crits-Chistoph, P., Frank, A., Weiss, R., Thase, M., Connolly, M., Gladis, M., Folz, C., and Siqueland, L. (2000). Therapeutic alliance as a predictor of outcome and retention in the National Institute on Drug Abuse

Collaborative Cocaine Study. *Journal of Consulting and Clinical Psychology* **69**, 119–24.

Barlow, D.H. and Lehman, C.L. (1996). Advances in the psychosocial treatment of anxiety disorders: implications for national health care. *Archives of General Psychiatry* **53**, 727–35.

Barrau, K. Thirion, X., Micallef, J. Chuniaud-Louche, C., Bellemin, B., and San Marco, J. (2001). Comparison of methadone and high dosage buprenorphine users in French care centres. *Addiction* **96**, 1433–41.

Barrio, G., de la Fuente, L., Royuela, L., Diaz, A., and Rodriguez-Artalego, F. (1998). Cocaine use among heroin users in Spain: the diffusion of crack and cocaine smoking. *Journal of Epidemiology and Community Health* **52**, 172–80.

Bartels, S., Drake, R., and Wallach, M. (1995). Long-term course of substance disorders among persons with severe mental disorder. *Psychiatric Services* **46**, 248–51.

Battersby, M., Farrell, M., Gossop, M., Robson, P., and Strang, J. (1992). 'Horse trading': prescribing injectable opiates to opiate addicts. A descriptive study. *Drug and Alcohol Review* **11**, 35–42.

Bearn, J., Gossop, M., and Strang, J. (1998). Accelerated lofexidine treatment regimen compared with conventional lofexidine and methadone treatment for in-patient detoxification. *Drug and Alcohol Dependence* **50**, 227–32.

Bearn, J., Gossop, M., and Strang, J. (1999). Rapid opiate detoxification treatments. *Drug and Alcohol Review* **18**, 75–81.

Beck, A.T. (1976). *Cognitive therapy and emotional disorders*. International Universities Press, New York.

Belding, M., McLellan, A.T., Zanis, D., and Incmikoski, R. (1998). Characterising "nonresponsive" patients. *Journal of Substance Abuse Treatment* **15**, 485–92.

Belenko, S. (1979). Alcohol abuse by heroin addicts: review of research findings and issues. *International Journal of the Addictions* **14**, 965–75.

Belenko, S., Fagan, J., and Dumanovsky, T. (1994). The effects of legal sanctions on recidivism in special drugs courts. *Justice System Journal* **17**, 53–81.

Bell, G., Cohen, J., and Cremona, A. (1990). How willing are general practitioners to manage narcotic misuse? *Health Trends* **2**, 56–7.

Bennett, G. and Rigby, K. (1990). Psychological change during residence in a rehabilitation centre for female drug misusers. Part I. Drug misusers. *Drug and Alcohol Dependence* **27**, 149–57.

Benzer, D. and Cushman, P. (1980). Alcohol and benzodiazepines: withdrawal syndromes. *Alcoholism, Clinical and Experimental Research* **4**, 243–7.

Berglund, G., Bergmark, A., Bjorling, B., Gronbladh, L., Linberg, S., Oscarsson, L., Olsson, B., Segraeus, V., and Stensmo, C. (1991). The SWEDATE Project: interaction between treatment, client background, and outcome in a one-year follow-up. *Journal of Substance Abuse Treatment* **8**, 161–9.

Bergmark, A. (1998). Treatment in Sweden. In *Evaluation of treatment: an European overview* (ed. M. Coletti). ITACA, Rome.

Best, D., Gossop, M., Marsden, J., Farrell, M., and Strang, J. (1997). Time of day of methadone consumption and illicit heroin use. *Drug and Alcohol Dependence* **49**, 49–54.

Best, D., Lehmann, P., Gossop, M., Harris, J., Noble, A., and Strang, J. (1998). Eating too little, smoking and drinking too much: wider lifestyle problems among methadone maintenance patients. *Addiction Research* **6**, 489–98.

Best, D., Gossop, M., Greenwood, J., Marsden, J., Lehmann, P., and Strang, J. (1999a). Cannabis use in relation to illicit drug use and health problems among opiate misusers in treatment. *Drug and Alcohol Review* **18**, 31–8.

Best, D., Noble, A., Finch, E., Gossop, M., Sidwell, C., and Strang, J. (1999b). Accuracy of perceptions of hepatitis B and C status: cross-sectional investigation of opiate addicts in treatment. *British Medical Journal* **319**, 290–1.

Best, D., Gossop, M., Lehmann, P., Harris, J. Marsden, J., and Strang, J. (1999c). The relationship between overdose and alcohol consumption among methadone maintenance patients. *Journal of Substance Misuse* **4**, 41–4.

Best, D., Harris, J., Gossop, M., Manning, V., Man, L-H., Marshall, J., Bearn, J., and Strang, J. (2001a). Are the Twelve Steps more acceptable to drug users than to drinkers? A comparison of experiences of and attitudes to Alcoholics Anonymous (AA) and Narcotics Anonymous (NA) among 200 substance misusers attending inpatient detoxification. *European Addiction Research* **7**, 69–77.

Best, D., Strang, J., Beswick, T., and Gossop, M. (2001b). Assessment of a concentrated, high-profile police operation. No discernible impact on drug availability, price or purity. *British Journal of Criminology* **41**, 738–45.

Best, D., Noble, A., Ridge, G., Gossop, M., Farrell, M., and Strang, J. (2002). The relative impact of waiting time and treatment entry on drug and alcohol use. *Addiction Biology* **7**, 67–74.

Biernacki, P. (1986). *Pathways from heroin addiction: recovery without treatment.* Temple University Press, Philadelphia.

Biggam, A.G. (1929). Malignant maleria associated with the administration of heroin intravenously. *Transactions of the Royal Society of Tropical Medicine and Hygiene* **23**, 147–53.

Blachly, P. (1964). Procedure for withdrawal of barbiturates. *American Journal of Psychiatry* **120**, 894.

Blachly, P. (1973). Naloxone for diagnosis in methadone programs. *Journal of the American Medical Association* **224**, 334–5.

Blachly, P., Casey, D., Marcel, L., and Denney, D. (1975). Rapid detoxification from heroin and methadone using naloxone. A model for the study of the treatment of the opiate abstinence syndrome. In *Developments in the field of drug abuse* (ed. E. Senay, V. Shorty, and M. Alkesne). Schenkma Publishing, Cambridge, Massachusetts.

Black, S. and Casswell, S. (1993). Recreational drug use in New Zealand. *Drug and Alcohol Review* **12**, 37–48.

BMA (1998). *The misuse of alcohol and other drugs by doctors.* British Medical Association, London.

Booth, R., Koester, S., Brewster, J., Weibel W., and Fritz, R. (1991). Intravenous drug users and AIDS: risk behaviours. *American Journal of Drug and Alcohol Abuse* **17**, 337–53.

Booth, R., Crowley, T., and Zhang, Y. (1996). Substance use, treatment entry, retention and effectiveness. *Drug and Alcohol Dependence* **42**, 11–20.

Boyd, J. (1986). Use of mental health services for the treatment of panic disorder. *American Journal of Psychiatry* **143**, 1569–74.

Bradley, B., Phillips, G., Green, L., and Gossop, M. (1989). Circumstances surrounding the initial lapse to opiate use following detoxification. *British Journal of Psychiatry* **154**, 354–9.

Bradley, B., Gossop, M., Brewin, C., Phillips, G., and Green, L. (1992). Attributions and relapse in opiate addicts. *Journal of Consulting and Clinical Psychology* **60**, 470–2.

Brahams, D. (1992). Death of a remand prisoner. *Lancet* **340**, 1462.

Brekke, J., Long, J., Nesbitt, N., and Sobel, E. (1997). The impact of service characteristics on functional outcomes from community support programs for persons with schizophrenia: a growth curve analysis. *Journal of Consulting and Clinical Psychology* **65**, 464–75.

Brennan, P., Kagay, C., Geppert, J., and Moos, R. (2000). Elderly medicare inpatients with substance use disorders: characteristics and predictors of hospital readmissions over a four year interval. *Journal of Studies on Alcohol* **61**, 891–5.

Brewer, C. (1993). Naltrexone in the prevention of relapse and opiate detoxification. In *Treatment options in addiction* (ed. C. Brewer). Gaskell, London.

Brewer C. (1995). Recent developments in maintenance prescribing and monitoring in the United Kingdom. *Bulletin of the New York Academy of Sciences* **72**, 359–70.

Brewer, C. (1997). Ultra-rapid, antagonist-precipitated opiate detoxification under general anaesthesia or sedation. *Addiction Biology* **2**, 291–302.

Brewer, C., Rezae, H., and Bailey, C. (1988). Opioid withdrawal and naltrexone induction in 48–72 hours with minimal dropout, using a modification of the naltrexone–clonidine technique. *British Journal of Psychiatry* **153**, 340–3.

Brewer, T.F., Heymann, S.J., Krumplitsch, S.M., Wilson, M.E., Colditz, G.A., and Fineberg, H.V. (2001). Strategies to decrease tuberculosis in US homeless populations: a computer simulation model. *Journal of the American Medical Association* **286**, 834–42.

Brook, R.C. and Whitehead, I.C. (1980). *Drug-free therapeutic community*. Human Sciences Press, New York.

Brooner, R.K., King, V.L., Kidorf, M., and Schmidt, C.W. (1997). Psychiatric and substance use comorbidity among treatment seeking opioid abusers. *Archives of General Psychiatry* **54**, 71–80.

Brown, B., Kinlock, T., and Nurco, D. (2001). Self-help initiatives to reduce the risk of relapse. In *Relapse and recovery in addictions* (ed. F. Tims, C. Leukefeld, and J. Platt). Yale University Press, New Haven, Connecticut.

Brown, J., Kranzler, H.R., and DelBoca, F.K. (1992). Self-reports by alcohol and drug abuse inpatients: factors affecting reliability and validity. *British Journal of Addiction* **87**, 1013–24.

Brown, S. (1985). *Treating the alcoholic: a development model of recovery*. John Wiley and Sons, New York.

Brown, T., Seraganian, P., Tremblay, J., and Annis, H. (2002). Process and outcome changes with relapse prevention versus 12-Step aftercare programs for substance abusers. *Addiction* **97**, 677–89.

Browne, A. (2000). Why aren't men interesting? *The Psychologist* **13**, 546–7.

Bryant, K.J., Rounsaville, B., Spitzer, R., and Williams, J. (1992). Reliability of dual diagnosis: substance dependence and psychiatric disorders. *Journal of Nervous and Mental Disease* **180**, 251–7.

Buckalew, L. and Sallis, R. (1986). Patient compliance and medication perception. *Journal of Clinical Psychology* **42**, 49–53.

Buntwal, N., Bearn, J., Gossop, M., and Strang, J. (2000). Naltrexone and lofexidine combination treatment compared with conventional lofexidine for in-patient opiate detoxification. *Drug and Alcohol Dependence* **59**, 183–8.

Burroughs, W. (1953). *Junkie*. Ace Books, New York.

Callahan, E. (1980). Alternative strategies in the treatment of narcotic addiction: a review. In *The addictive behaviors* (ed. W. Miller). Pergamon, Oxford.

Camacho, M., Bartholomew, N., Joe, G., Cloud, M., and Simpson D.D. (1996). Gender, cocaine and during treatment HIV risk reduction among injecting opioid users in methadone maintenance. *Drug and Alcohol Dependence* 41, 1–7.

Capelhorn, J., Dalton, M., Cluff, M., and Petrenas, A. (1994). Retention in methadone maintenance and heroin addicts' risk of death. *Addiction* 82, 203–9.

Carey, K. and Correia, C. (1998). Severe mental illness and addictions: assessment considerations. *Addictive Behaviors* 23, 735–48.

Carnwath, T. and Hardman, J. (1998). Randomised double blind comparison of lofexidine and clonidine in the outpatient treatment of opiate withdrawal. *Drug and Alcohol Dependence* 50, 251–4.

Carroll, J.F. and Sobel, B.S. (1986). Integrating mental health personnel and practices into a therapeutic community. In *Therapeutic communities for addictions: readings in theory, research and practice* (ed. G. De Leon and J.T. Ziegenfuss), pp. 209–26. Charles C. Thomas, Springfield, Illinois.

Carroll, K.M. (1993). Psychotherapeutic treatment of cocaine abuse: models for its evaluation alone and in combination with pharmacotherapy. In *Cocaine treatment: research and clinical perspectives* (ed. F. Tims and C. Leukefeld), NIDA Research Monograph no. 135. NIDA, Rockville, Maryland.

Carroll, K.M. (1997). Enhancing retention in clinical trials of psychosocial treatments: practical strategies. In *Beyond the therapeutic alliance: keeping the drug-dependent individual in treatment*, NIDA Research Monograph no. 165. NIDA, Rockville, Maryland.

Carroll, K.M., Rounsaville, B.J., Nich, C., Gordon, L., and Gawin, F. (1995). Integrating psychotherapy and pharmacotherapy for cocaine dependence: results from a randomized clinical trial. In *Integrating behavioral therapies with medications in the treatment of drug dependence* (ed. L. Onken, J. Blaine, and J. Boren), NIDA Monograph no.150. NIDA, Rockville, Maryland.

Carroll, K.M., Libby, B., Sheehan, J., and Hyland, N. (2001). Motivational interviewing to enhance treatment initiation in substance abusers: an effectiveness study. *American Journal on Addictions* 10, 335–9.

Cartwright, W. (2000). Cost–benefit analysis of drug treatment services: review of the literature, *Journal of Mental Health Policy and Economics* 3, 11–26.

Cassani, M. and Spiehler, W. (1993). Analytical requirements, perspectives and limits of immunological methods for drugs in hair. *Forensic Science International* 63, 175–84.

Caulkins, J., Johnson, B., Taylor, A., and Taylor, L. (1999). What drug dealers tell us about their costs of doing business. *Journal of Drug Issues* 29, 323–40.

Central Drugs Coordinating Unit (1998). *Tackling drugs to build a better Britain: the government's 10-year strategy for tackling drug misuse*. HMSO, London.

Cerkoney, A. and Hart, K. (1980). The relationship betwen the health belief model and compliance of persons with diabetes mellitus. *Diabetes Care* 3, 594–8.

Chambers, R. and Belcher, J. (1992). Self-reported health care over the past 10 years: a survey of general practitioners. *British Journal of General Practice* 42, 153–6.

Chan, M., Sorensen, J., Guydish, J., Tajima, B., and Acampora, A. (1997). Client satisfaction with drug abuse day treatment versus residential care. *Journal of Drug Issues* 27, 367–77.

Chaney, E., Roszell, D., and Cummings, C. (1982). Relapse in opiate addicts: a behavioral analysis. *Addictive Behaviors* 7, 291–7.

Chatham, L.R., Rowan-Szal, G.A., Joe, G.W., and Simpson, D.D. (1997). Heavy drinking, alcohol dependent vs. nondependent methadone maintenance clients: a follow-up study. *Addictive Behaviours* 22, 69–80.

Chatham, L., Hiller, M., Rowan-Szal, G., Joe, G., and Simpson D.D. (1999). Gender differences at admission and follow up in a sample of methadone maintenance clients. *Substance Use and Misuse* 34, 1137–65.

Cheung, R., Hanson, A., Maganti, K., Keeffe, E., and Matsui, S. (2002). Viral hepatitis and other infectious diseases in a homeless population. *Journal of Clinical Gastroenterology* 34, 476–80.

Childress, A.R., McLellan, A., and O'Brien, C. (1984). Measurement and extinction of conditioned withdrawal-like responses in opiate dependent patients. In *Problems of drug dependence* (ed. L. Harris), NIDA Monograph no. 49, pp. 212–19. NIDA, Washington, DC.

Childress, A., McLellan, A., and O'Brien, C. (1986). Abstinent opiate abusers exhibit conditioned craving, conditioned withdrawal and reductions in both through extinction. *British Journal of Addiction* 81, 655–660.

Childress, A.R., McLellan, A., Ehrman, R., and O'Brien, C. (1988). Classically conditioned responses in opioid and cocaine dependence: a role in relapse? In *Learning factors in substance abuse* (ed. B. Ray), NIDA Monograph no. 84, pp. 25–43. NIDA, Washington, DC.

Chitwood, D., Clyde, B., McCoy, J., Inciardi, D., McBride, M., Trapido, E., McCoy, V., Page, B., Griffin, J., Fletcher, M., and Ashman, M. (1990). HIV-seropositivity of needles from shooting galleries in south Florida. *American Journal of Public Health* 80, 150–2.

Cho, A. (1990). Ice: a new dosage form of an old drug. *Science* 249, 631–4.

Christo, G. and Franey, C. (1995). Drug users' spiritual beliefs, locus of control and the disease concepts in relation to NA attendance and six-month outcomes. *Alcohol Dependence* 38, 51–6.

Christo, G. and Sutton, S. (1994). Anxiety and self-esteem as a function of abstinence time among recovering addicts attending Narcotics Anonymous. *British Journal of Clinical Psychology* 33, 198–200.

Chutuape, M., Silverman, K., and Stitzer, M. (1998). Survey assessment of methadone treatment services as reinforcers. *American Journal of Drug and Alcohol Abuse* 24 (1), 1–16.

Chutuape, M., Silverman, K., and Stitzer, M. (1999). Contingent reinforcement sustains post-detoxification abstinence from multiple drugs: a preliminary study with methadone patients. *Drug and Alcohol Dependence* 54, 69–81.

Clark, D.M. (2000). Anxiety states: panic and generalised anxiety. In *Cognitive behaviour therapy for psychiatric problems* (ed. K. Hawton, P. Salkovskis, J. Kirk, and D. Clark). Oxford Medical Publications, Oxford.

Clark, L. (1991). Improving compliance and increasing control of hypertension: needs of special hypertensive populations. *American Heart Journal* 121, 664–9.

Clayton, R. and Voss, H. (1981). *Young men and drugs in Manhattan: a causal analysis*, NIDA Research Monograph no. 39. US Government Printing Office, Washington, DC.

Cohen, J. (1991). Why women partners of drug users will continue to be at high risk for HIV infection. In *Cocaine, AIDS and intravenous drug use* (ed. S. Friedman and D. Lipton). Harrington Park Press, New York.

Cohen, J. and Schamroth, A. (1990). The challenge of illicit drug addiction for general practice. *Drug and Alcohol Dependence* **25**, 315–18.

Cohen, S. (1977). *Inhalant abuse: an overview of the problem*, NIDA Research Monograph no. 15, pp. 2–11. National Institute on Drug Abuse, Rockville, Maryland.

Cole, S.G. and James, L.R. (1975). A revised treatment typology based on the DARP. *American Journal of Drug and Alcohol Abuse* **2**, 37–49.

Collins, J. and Allison, M. (1983). Legal coercion and retention in drug abuse treatment. *Hospital and Community Psychiatry* **34**, 1145–9.

Conklin, C. and Tiffany, S. (2002). Applying extinction research and theory to cue-exposure addiction treatments. *Addiction* **97**, 155–67.

Connaughton, J., Reeser, D., Schut, J., and Finnegan, L. (1977). Management of the pregnant opiate addict: success with a comprehensive approach. *American Journal of Obstetrics and Gynecology* **129**, 679.

Connell, P.H. (1958). *Amphetamine psychosis*. Oxford University Press, London.

Connell, P.H. (1969). Drug dependence in Great Britain: a challenge to the practice of medicine. In *Scientific basis of drug dependence* (ed. H. Steinberg). Churchill Livingstone, London.

Connell, P.H. and Strang, J. (1994). The creation of the clinics: clinical demand and the formation of policy. In *Heroin addiction and drug policy: the British system* (ed. J. Strang and M. Gossop). Oxford University Press, Oxford.

Contoreggi, C., Rexroad, V.E., and Lange, W.R. (1998). Current management of infectious complications in the injecting drug user. *Journal of Substance Abuse Treatment* **15**, 95–106.

Cook, C. (1988). The Minnesota Model in the management of drug and alcohol dependency: miracle, method or myth? Part II. Evidence and conclusions. *British Journal of Addiction* **83**, 735–48.

Cooper, J.R. (1995). Including narcotic addiction treatment in an office-based practice. *Journal of the American Medical Association* **273**, 1619–20.

Cooper, J.R., Altman, F., Brown, B., and Czechowicz, D. (1983). *Research on the treatment of narcotic addiction: state of the art*, NIDA Treatment Research Monograph Series. US Department of Health and Human Services, Rockville, Maryland.

Corty, E., Lehman, A.F., and Myers, C.F. (1993). Influence of psychoactive substance use on the reliability of psychiatric diagnosis. *Journal of Consulting and Clinical Psychology* **61**, 165–70.

Courtwright, D., Joseph, H., and Des Jarlais, D. (1989). *Addicts who survived: an oral history of narcotics use in America, 1923–1965*. University of Tennessee Press, Knoxville.

Craddock, S., Rounds-Bryant, J., Flynn, P., and Hubbard, R. (1997). Characteristics and pretreatment behaviors of clients entering drug abuse treatment: 1969–1993. *American Journal of Drug and Alcohol Abuse* **23**, 43–59.

Crofts, N., Nigro, L., Oman, K., Stevenson, E., and Sherman, J. (1997). Methadone maintenance and hepatitis C virus infection among injecting drug users. *Addiction* **92**, 999–1005.

Croop, R., Faulkner, E., and Labriola, D. (1997). The safety profile of naltrexone in the treatment of alcoholism: results from a multicenter usage study. *Archives of General Psychiatry* **54**, 1130–5.

Crowley, T., Wagner, J., Zerbe, G., and MacDonald, M. (1985). Naltrexone-induced dysphoria in former opioid addicts. *American Journal of Psychiatry* **142**, 1081–4.

Cummings, N., Gordon, J., and Marlatt, G. (1980). Relapse: strategies of prevention and prediction. In *The addictive behaviors* (ed. W.R. Miller). Pergamon, Oxford.

Cunningham, D. and Persky, L. (1989). Penile ecthyma gangrenosum. Complications of drug addiction. *Urology* **34**, 109–10.

Curran, H. (2000). Is MDMA ('Ecstasy') neurotoxic in humans? An overview of evidence and methodological problems in research. *Neuropsychobiology* **42**, 34–41.

Daley, D., Salloum, I., Zuckoff, A., Kirisci, L., and Thase, M. (1998). Increasing treatment adherence among outpatients with cocaine dependence: results of a pilot study. *American Journal of Psychiatry* **155**, 1611–13.

Darke, S. and Hall, W. (1995). Levels and correlates of polydrug use among heroin users and regular amphetamine users. *Drug and Alcohol Dependence* **39**, 231–5.

Darke, S. and Ross, J. (1999). Heroin-related deaths in South Western Sydney, Australia, 1992–96. *Drug and Alcohol Review* **18**, 39–45.

Darke, S. and Zador, D. (1996). Fatal heroin 'overdose': a review. *Addiction* **91**, 1765–72.

Darke, S., Hall, W., Wodak, A., Heather, N., and Ward, J. (1992). Development and validation of a multi-dimensional instrument for assessing outcome of treatment among opiate users: the Opiate Treatment Index. *British Journal of Addiction* **87**, 733–42.

Darke, S., Swift, W., and Hall, W. (1994). Prevalence, severity, and correlates of psychological morbidity among methadone maintenance clients. *Addiction* **89**, 211–17.

Darke, S., Kelaher, M., Hall, W., and Flahert, B. (1996a). Characteristics of admissions to residential drug treatment agencies in New South Wales, 1988–1992: illicit drug problems. *Drug and Alcohol Review* **15**, 127–132.

Darke, S., Ross, J., and Hall, W. (1996b). Overdose among heroin users in Sydney, Australia: I. Prevalence and correlates of non-fatal overdose. *Addiction* **91**, 405–11.

Darke, S., Sunjic, S., Zador, D., and Prolov, T. (1997). A comparison of blood toxicology of heroin-related deaths and current heroin users in Sydney, Australia. *Drug and Alcohol Dependence* **47**, 45–53.

D'Aunno, T. and Vaughn, T. (1995). An organizational analysis of service patterns in outpatient drug abuse treatment units. *Journal of Substance Abuse* **7**, 27–42.

Davis, S. (1990). Chemical dependency in women: a description of its effects and outcome on adequate parenting. *Journal of Substance Abuse Treatment* **7**, 225–32.

Davison, S. and Gossop, M. (1996). The problem of interviewing drug addicts in custody: a study of interrogative suggestibility and compliance. *Psychology, Crime and Law* **2**, 185–95.

Dawe, S., Griffiths, P., Gossop, M., and Strang, J. (1991). Should opiate addicts be involved in controlling their own detoxification? A comparison of fixed versus negotiable schedules. *British Journal of Addictions* **86**, 977–82.

Dawe, S., Powell, J., Richards, D., Gossop, M., Marks, I., Strang, J., and Gray, J. (1993). Does post-withdrawal cue exposure improve outcome in opiate addiction? A controlled trial. *Addiction* **88**, 1233–45.

DAWN (1994). *A survey of drug and alcohol services for women*. Drug and Alcohol Women's Network, GLASS, London.

Deas-Nesmith, D., Brady, K., and Myrick, H. (1998). Drug abuse and anxiety disorders. In *Dual diagnosis and treatment* (ed. H. Kranzler and B. Rousaville). Marcel Dekker, New York.

Degen, H., Myers, B., Williams-Peterson, M., Knisely, J., and Schnoll, S. (1993). Social support and anxiety in pregnant drug abusers and nonusers: unexpected findings of a few differences. *Drug and Alcohol Dependence* **32**, 37–44.

Dekker, F., Dieleman, F., Kaptein, A., and Mulder, J. (1993). Compliance with pulmonary medication in general practice. *European Respiratory Journal* **6**, 886–90.

DelBoca, F. and Noll, J. (2000). Truth or consequences: the validity of self-report data in health services research on addictions. *Addiction* **95**, 347–60.

De Leon, G. (1985). The therapeutic community: status and evolution. *International Journal of the Addictions* **20**, 823–44.

De Leon, G. (1987). Alcohol use among drug abusers: treatment outcome in a therapeutic community. *Alcoholism* **11**, 430–6.

De Leon, G. (1988). Legal pressure in therapeutic communities. *Journal of Drug Issues* **18**, 625–40.

De Leon, G. (1989*a*). Therapeutic communities for substance abuse: overview of approach and effectiveness. *Psychology of Addictive Behaviors* **3**, 140–7.

De Leon, G. (1989*b*). Alcohol: the hidden drug among substance abusers. *British Journal of Addiction* **84**, 837–40.

De Leon, G. (1995). Therapeutic communities for addictions: a theoretical framework. *International Journal of the Addictions* **30**, 1603–45.

De Leon, G. (1996). Integrative recovery: a stage paradigm. *Substance Abuse* **17**, 51–63.

De Leon, G. (2000). *The therapeutic community: theory, model, and method.* Springer, New York.

De Leon, G. and Jainchill, N. (1982). Male and female drug abusers: social and psychological status two years after treatment in a therapeutic community. *American Journal of Drug and Alcohol Abuse* **8**, 465–97.

De Leon, G. and Jainchill, N. (1986). Circumstance, motivation, readiness and suitability as correlates of treatment tenure. *Journal of Psychoactive Drugs* **18**, 203–8.

De Leon, G. and Rosenthal, M. S. (1979). Therapeutic communities. In *Handbook on drug abuse* (ed. R. DuPont, A. Goldstein, and J. O'Donnell), pp. 39–48. National Institute on Drug Abuse, Rockville, Maryland.

De Leon, G., Jainchill, N., and Wexler, H. (1982). Success and improvement rates 5 years after treatment in a therapeutic community. *International Journal of Addictions* **17** (4), 703–47.

De Leon, G., Inciardi, J., and Martin, S. (1995*a*). Residential drug abuse treatment research: are conventional control group designs appropriate for assessing treatment effectiveness? *Journal of Psychoactive Drugs* **27**, 85–91.

De Leon, G., Staines, G., Perlis, T., Sacks, S., McKendrick, K., Hilton, R., and Brady, R. (1995*b*). Therapeutic community methods in methadone maintenance (Passages): an open clinical trial. *Drug and Alcohol Dependence* **37**, 45–57.

Department of Health (1986). *Health service development. Services for drug misusers*, Health Circular HC(86)3. Department of Health, London.

Department of Health. (1991). *Drug misuse and dependence—guidelines on clinical management.* Department of Health, London.

Department of Health. (1998). *Tackling drugs to build a better Britain: the government's ten-year strategy for tackling drugs misuse.* Department of Health, London.

Department of Health (1999*a*). *Drug misuse statistics.* Department of Health, London.

Department of Health. (1999*b*). *Drug misuse and dependence—guidelines on clinical management.* Department of Health, London.

DesJarlais, D., Wish, E., Friedman, S., Stoneburner, R., Yancovitz, S., Mildvan, D., El-Sadr, W., and Cuadrado, M. (1987). Intravenous drug use and heterosexual transmission of immunodeficiency virus. *New York State Journal of Medicine* **87**, 283–6.

DesJarlais, D., Casriel, C., Friedman, S., and Rosenblum, A. (1992). AIDS and the transition to illicit drug injection—results of a randomized trial prevention program. *British Journal of Addiction* **87**, 493–8.

DiClemente, C.C. (1993). Alcoholics Anonymous and the structure of change. In *Research on Alcoholics Anonymous* (ed. B.S. McCrady and W.R. Miller), pp. 113–35. Rutgers Center of Alcohol Studies, New Brunswick, New Jersey.

Dole, V. (1989). Methadone treatment and the acquired immunodeficiency syndrome epidemic. *Journal of the American Medical Association* **262**, 1681.

Dole, V. and Joseph, H. (1978). Long-term outcome of patients treated with methadone maintenance. *Annals of the New York Academy of Sciences* **311**, 181–9.

Dole, V.P. and Nyswander, M. (1965). A medical treatment for diacetylmorphine (heroin) addiction. *Journal of the American Medical Association* **193**, 80–4.

Dole, V.P. and Nyswander, M. (1967). Heroin addiction—a metabolic disease. *Archives of Internal Medicine* **120**, 19–24.

Dole, V.P., Nyswander, M.E., and Kreek, M.J. (1966). Narcotic blockade. *Archives of Internal Medicine* **118**, 304–9.

Dole, V.P., Nyswander, M., and Warner, A. (1968). Successful treatment of 750 criminal addicts. *Journal of the American Medical Association* **206**, 2708–11.

Donoghoe, M., Stimson, G., and Dolan, K. (1989). Sexual behaviour of injecting drug users and associated risks of HIV infection for non-injecting sexual partners. *AIDS Care* **1**, 51–8.

Dowling, G., McDonough, E., and Bost, R. (1987). Eve and Ecstasy: a report of five deaths associated with the use of MDEA and MDMA. *Journal of the American Medical Association* **257**, 1615–17.

Drake, J. and Ballard, R. (1988). Misuse of temazepam: manufacturer's response. *British Medical Journal* **297**, 1402.

Drake, R., McHugo, G., and Noordsy, D. (1993). Treatment of alcoholism among schizophrenic outpatients: four year outcomes. *American Journal of Psychiatry* **150**, 328–9.

Drummond, D.C. (1992). Problems and dependence: chalk and cheese or bread and butter? In *The nature of alcohol and drug related problems* (ed. M. Lader, G. Edwards, and D.C.Drummond). Oxford Medical Publications, Oxford.

Drummond, D.C. (1999). Treatment research in the wake of Project MATCH. *Addiction* **94**, 39–42.

Drummond, D.C. and Glautier, S. (1994). A controlled trial of cue exposure treatment in alcohol dependence. *Journal of Clinical and Consulting Psychology* **41**, 809–17.

Drummond, D.C., Turkington, D., Rahman, M.Z., Mullin, P.J., and Jackson, P. (1989). Chlordiazepoxide vs. methadone in opiate withdrawal: a preliminary double blind trial. *Drug and Alcohol Dependence* **23**, 63–71.

Drummond, D.C., Tiffany, S., Glautier, S., and Remington, B. (1995). Cue exposure in understanding and treating addictive behaviour. In *Addictive behaviours: cue exposure theory and practice* (ed. D.C. Drummond, S. Tiffany, S. Glautier, and B. Remington). Wiley, London.

Drummond, M., O'Brien, B., Stoddart, G., and Torrance, G. (1997). *Methods for the economic evaluation of health care programmes.* Oxford University Press, Oxford.

DSM-III-R (1987). *Diagnostic and statistical manual of mental disorders,* revised 3rd edn. American Psychiatric Association, Washington, DC.

DSM-IV (1994). *Diagnostic and statistical manual of mental disorders,* 4th edn. American Psychiatric Association, Washington, DC.

Duchene, H. (1955). The need to drink. *Quarterly Journal of Studies on Alcohol* 16, 47–51.

Dumont, M. (1974). Self-help treatment programs. *American Journal of Psychiatry* 131, 631–5.

Dunbar, J. and Stunkard, A. (1979). Adherence to diet and drug regimen. In *Nutrition, lipids, coronary heart disease* (ed. R. Levy, B. Rifkind, B. Dennis, and N. Ernst). Raven Press, New York.

Dunn, C., DeRoo, L., and Rivara, F. (2001). The use of brief interventions adapted from motivational interviewing across behavioural domains: a systematic review. *Addiction* 96, 1725–42.

DuPont, R. and McGovern, J. (1994). *A bridge to recovery: an introduction to 12-step programs.* American Psychiatric Association, Washington, DC.

Durante, A.J., Hart, G.J., Brady, A.R. Madden, P.B., and Noone, A. (1995). The Health of the Nation target on syringe sharing: a role for routine surveillance in assessing progress and targeting interventions. *Addiction* 90, 1389–96.

Dyll, L. (1990). Neurologic perspective on cocaine. *Trauma* 32, 85–8.

Edwards, G. (1969). The British approach to the treatment of heroin addiction. *Lancet* i, 768–72.

Edwards, G. (1987). *The treatment of drinking problems.* Blackwells, Oxford.

Edwards, G. and Gross, M.M. (1976). Alcohol dependence: provisional description of a clinical syndrome. *British Medical Journal* 1 (6017), 1058–61.

Edwards, G., Arif, A., and Hodgson, R. (1981). Nomenclature and classification of drug- and alcohol-related problems: a WHO Memorandum. *Bulletin of the World Health Organization* 59 (2), 225–42.

Edwards, G., Marshall, E.J., and Cook, C.C.H. (1997). *The treatment of drinking problems.* Cambridge University Press, Cambridge.

Edwards, P., Jones, S., Shale, D., and Thursz, M. (1996). *Shared care: a model for clinical management.* Radcliffe, Oxford.

Egelko, S., Galanter, M., Dermatis, H., Jurewicz, E., Jamison, A., Dingle, S., and De Leon, G. (2002). Improved psychological status in a modified therapeutic community for homeless MICA men. *Journal of Addictive Diseases* 21, 75–92.

Eikelboom, R. and Stewart, J. (1982). Conditioning of drug-induced physiological responses. *Psychological Review* 89, 507–28.

Einstein, S. (1966). The narcotics dilemma: who is listening to what? *International Journal of the Addictions* 1, 1–6.

Eissenberg, T., Bigelow, G., Strain, E., Walsh, S., Brooner, R., Stitzer, M., and Johnson, R. (1997). Dose-related efficacy of levomethadyl acetate for treatment of opioid dependence. A randomized clinical trial. *Journal of the American Medical Association* 277, 1945–51.

Eldred, C. and Washington, M. (1976). Interpersonal relationships in heroin use by men and women and their role in treatment outcome. *International Journal of the Addictions* 11, 117–30.

Ellinwood, E.H. (1967). Amphetamine psychosis. I. Description of the individuals and process. *Journal of Nervous and Mental Disease* **144**, 273.

Ellis, A. (1962). *Reason and emotion in psychotherapy.* Lyle Stuart, New York.

Emrick, C.D. (1987). Alcoholics Anonymous: affiliation processes and effectiveness as treatment. *Alcoholism Clinical and Experimental Research* **11**, 416–23.

Emrick, C.D. (1999). Alcoholics Anonymous and other 12-step groups. In *The American Psychiatric Press textbook of substance abuse treatment,* 2nd edn (ed. M. Galanter and H.D. Kleber), pp. 403–12. American Psychiatric Press Inc, Washington, DC.

Eraker, S., Kirscht, J., and Becker, M. (1984). Understanding and improving patient compliance. *Annals of Internal Medicine* **100**, 258–68.

Etheridge, R., Craddock, G., Dunteman, G., and Hubbard, R. (1995). Treatment services in two national studies of community-based drug abuse treatment programs. *Journal of Substance Abuse* **7**, 9–26.

Etheridge, R., Hubbard, R., Anderson, J., Craddock, G., and Flynn, P. (1997). Treatment structure and program services in the Drug Abuse Treatment Outcome Study (DATOS). *Psychology of Addictive Behaviors* **11**, 244–60.

Etheridge, R., Craddock, S., Hubbard, R., and Rounds-Bryant, J. (1999). The relationship of counseling and self-help participation to patient outcomes in DATOS. *Drug and Alcohol Dependence* **57**, 99–112.

Farrell, M., Ward, J., Mattick, R., Hall, W., Stimson, G., DesJarlais, D., Gossop, M., and Strang, J. (1994). Methadone maintenance treatment in opiate dependence: a review. *British Medical Journal* **309**, 997–1001.

Farrell, M., Neeleman, J., Griffiths, P., and Strang, J. (1996). Suicide and overdose among opiate addicts. *Addiction* **91** (3), 321–3.

Farrell, M., Howed, S., Taylor, C., Lewis, G., Jenkins, R., Bebbington, P., Jarvis, M., Brugha, T., Gill, B., and Meltzer, H. (1998). Substance misuse and psychiatric comorbidity: an overview of the OPCS National Psychiatric Morbidity Survey. *Addictive Behaviors* **23**, 909–18.

Feinberg, M. (1999). Pharmacotherapy of depression. In *Handbook of comparative interventions for adult disorders* (ed. M. Hersen and A. Bellack). Wiley, New York.

Ferri, C. and Gossop, M. (1999). Route of cocaine administration: patterns of use and problems among a Brazilian sample. *Addictive Behaviors* **24**, 815–21.

Fhima, A., Henrion, R., Lowenstein, W., and Charpak, Y. (2001). Two-year follow-up of an opioid user cohort treated with high-dose buprenorphine (Subutex). *Annales de Médecine Interne* **152**, 26–36.

Fiellin, D., O'Connor, P., Chawarski, M., Pakes, J., Pantalon, M., and Schottenfeld, R. (2001). Methadone maintenance in primary care. *Journal of the American Medical Association* **286**, 1724–31.

Finn, P. and Alcorn, J. (1986). Noncompliance to hemodialysis dietary regimens. *Rehabilitation Psychology* **31**, 67–79.

Finn, P. and Wilcock, K. (1997). Levo-alpha acetyl methadol (LAAM): its advantages and drawbacks. *Journal of Substance Abuse Treatment* **14**, 559–64.

Finnegan, L. (1976). Management of the drug dependent pregnancy and effects on neonatal outcome. In *NIDA symposium on comprehensive healthcare for addicted families and their children* (ed. G. Beschner and R. Brotman). US Government Printing Office, Washington, DC.

Finnegan, L. (1982). Outcome of children born to women dependent upon narcotics. In *The effects of maternal alcohol and drug abuse on the newborn* (ed. B. Stimmel). Haworth, New York.

Finnegan, L., Reeser, D., and Connaughton, J. (1977). The effects of maternal drug dependence on neonatal mortality. *Drug and Alcohol Dependence* **2**, 131–40.

Finney, J.W. (1995). Enhancing substance abuse treatment evaluations: examining mediators and moderators of treatment effects. *Journal of Substance Abuse* **7**, 135–50.

Finney, J.W., Hahn, A.C., and Moos, R.H. (1996). The effectiveness of inpatient and outpatient treatment for alcohol abuse: the need to focus on mediators and moderators of setting effects. *Addiction* **91**, 1773–96.

Finney, J.W., Ouimette, P.C., Humphreys, K., and Moos, R.H. (2001). A comparative, process-effectiveness evaluation of VA substance abuse treatment. *Recent Developments in Alcoholism* **15**, 373–91.

Fiorentine R. (1999). After drug treatment: are 12-step programs effective in maintaining abstinence? *American Journal of Alcohol Abuse* **25**, 93–116.

Fiorentine, R. (2001). Counselling frequency and the effectiveness of outpatient drug treatment: revisiting the conclusion that 'more is better'. *American Journal of Drug and Alcohol Abuse* **27**, 617–31.

Fiorentine, R. and Anglin, D. (1996). More is better: counseling participation and the effectiveness of outpatient drug treatment. *Journal of Substance Abuse Treatment* **13**, 341–8.

Fiorentine, R. and Anglin, D. (1997). Does increasing the opportunity for counseling increase the effectiveness of outpatient drug treatment? *American Journal of Drug and Alcohol Abuse* **23**, 369–82.

Fiorentine, R. and Hillhouse, M. (2000). Drug treatment and 12-step program participation: the additive effects of integrated recovery activities. *Journal of Substance Abuse Treatment* **18**, 65–74.

Fiorentine, R., Anglin, M.D., Gil-Rivas, V., and Taylor, E. (1997). Drug treatment: explaining the gender paradox. *Substance Use and Misuse* **32**, 653–78.

Fiorentine.R., Nakashima, J., and Anglin, D. (1999). Client engagement in drug treatment. *Journal of Substance Abuse Treatment* **17**, 199–206.

Fitzgerald, J. and Mulford, H. (1992). Elderly vs younger problem drinkers 'treatment' and recovery experiences. *British Journal of Addiction* **87**, 1281–91.

Flemming, P. (1998). Prescribing amphetamine to amphetamine users as a harm-reduction measure. *International Journal of Drug Policy* **9**, 339–44.

Flemming, P. and Roberts, D. (1994). Is the prescription of amphetamine justified as a harm reduction measure? *Journal of the Royal Society of Health* 127–31.

Flynn, P., Kristiansen, P., Porto, J., and Hubbard, R. (1999). Costs and benefits of treatment for cocaine addiction in DATOS. *Drug and Alcohol Dependence* **57**, 167–74.

Folsom, D. and Jeste, D.V. (2002). Schizophrenia in homeless persons: a systematic review of the literature. *Acta Psychiatrica Scandinavica* **105**, 404–13.

Fountain, J., Griffiths, P., Farrell, M., Gossop, M., and Strang, J. (1999). Benzodiazepines in polydrug using repertoires: the impact of the decreased availability of temazepam capsules. *Drugs: Education, Prevention and Policy* **6**, 61–9.

Fountain, J., Strang, J., Gossop, M., Farrell, M., and Griffiths, P. (2000*a*). Diversion of drugs prescribed to drug users in treatment: analysis of the UK market and new data from London. *Addiction* **95**, 393–406.

Fountain, J., Strang, J., Griffiths, P., Powis, B., and Gossop, M. (2000*b*). Measuring met and unmet need of drug misusers: integration of quantitative and qualitative data. *European Addiction Research* **6**, 97–103.

Fountain, J., Howes, S., Marsden, J., and Strang, J. (2002). Who uses services for homeless people? An investigation amongst people sleeping rough in London. *Journal of Community and Applied Social Psychology* **12**, 71–5.

Fountain, J., Howes, S., and Strang, J. (2003). Unmet drug and alcohol service needs of homeless people in London. *Substance Use and Misuse* **38**, 377–93.

Frank, J. (1961). *Persuasion and healing*. Johns Hopkins University Press, Baltimore.

Franks, C. and Barbrack, C. (1991). Behavior therapy with adults: an integrative perspective for the nineties. In *Clinical psychology handbook* (ed. M. Hersen, A. Kazdin, and A. Bellack). Pergamon, New York.

Fraser, M. and Hawkins, J. (1984). The social networks of opioid users. *International Journal of the Addictions* **19**, 903–17.

Freedman, R. and Czertko, G. (1981). A comparison of thrice weekly LAAM and daily methadone in employed heroin addicts. *Drug and Alcohol Dependence* **8**, 215–22.

Friedman, S., Horvat, G., and Levinson, R. (1982). The Narcotic Addict Rehabilitation Act: its impact upon federal prisons. *Contemporary Drug Problems* **82**, 101–11.

Friedman, S., Jose, B., DesJarlais, D., and Neaigus, A. (1995). Risk factors for human immunodeficiency virus seroconversion among out-of-treatment drug injectors in high and low seroprevalence cities. The National AIDS Research Consortium. *American Journal of Epidemiology* **142**, 864–74.

Frischer, M., Bloor, M., Goldberg, D., Clark, J., Green, S., and McKeganey, N. (1993). Mortality among injecting drug users: a critical reappraisal. *Journal of Epidemiology and Community Health* **47**, 59–63.

Fuchs, D., Unterweger, B., Hausen, A., Reibnegger, G., Werner, E., Hengster, P., Hinterhuber, H., Dierich, M., and Wachter, H. (1988). Anti-HIV-1 antibodies, anti-HTLV-I antibodies and neopterin levels in parenteral drug addicts in the Austrian Tyrol. *AIDS* **1**, 65–6.

Fugelstad, A., Annell, A., Rajs, J., and Agren, G. (1997). Mortality and causes and manner of death among drug addicts in Stockholm during the period 1981–1992. *Acta Psychiatrica Scandinavica* **96**, 169–75.

Galaif, E., Nyamathi, A., and Stein, J. (1999). Psychosocial predictors of current drug use, drug problems, and physical drug dependence in homeless women. *Addictive Behaviors* **24**, 801–14.

Galanter, M., Egelko, S., and Edwards, H. (1993). Rational recovery: alternative to AA for addiction? *American Journal of Drug and Alcohol Abuse* **19**, 499–510.

Gambert, S. (1997). The elderly. In *Substance abuse: a comprehensive textbook* (ed. J. Lowinson, P. Ruiz, R. Millman, and J. Langrod). Williams and Wilkins, Baltimore.

Gardner, R. and Connell, P.H. (1971). Opioid users attending a special drug dependence clinic 1968–1969. *Bulletin on Narcotics* **XXIII**, 915.

Gardner, R. and Connell, P.H. (1972). Amphetamine and other non-opioid drug users attending a special drug dependence clinic. *British Medical Journal* **2**, 322–5.

Garfein, R., Vlahov, D., Galai, N., Doherty, M., and Nelson, K. (1996). Viral infections in short term injecting drug users: the prevalence of hepatitis C, hepatitis B, human immunodeficiency and human T-lymphotropic viruses. *American Journal of Public Health* **86**, 655–61.

Gaston, L. (1990). The concept of the alliance and its role in psychotherapy. *Psychotherapy* **27**, 143–53.

Gawin, F. and Kleber, H. (1984). Cocaine abuse treatment: open trial with desipramine and lithium carbanoate. *Archives of General Psychiatry* **42**, 903–10.

Gawin, F. and Kleber, H. (1986). Abstinence symptomatology and psychiatric diagnosis in cocaine abusers. Clinical observations. *Archives of General Psychiatry* **43**, 107–13.

Gerlach, R. (2000). Substitution treatment in the European Union: Germany. In *Insights: reviewing current practice in drug-substitution treatment in the European Union*. EMCDDA, Belgium.

Gersema, L., Alexander, B., and Kunze, K. (1987). Major withdrawal symptoms after abrupt discontinuation of phenobarbital. *Clinical Pharmacology* **6**, 420–2.

Ghodse A.H. (1977). Drug dependent individuals dealt with by London casualty departments *British Journal of Psychiatry* **131**, 273–80.

Ghodse, A.H. (1978). The attitudes of casualty staff and ambulance personnel towards patients who take drug overdoses. *Social Science and Medicine* **12**, 341–6.

Ghodse, A.H. (1995). *Drugs and addictive behaviour: a guide to treatment.* Blackwells, Oxford.

Ghodse, A.H. and Howse, K. (1994). Substance use of medical students: a nationwide survey. *Health Trends* **26**, 85–8.

Ghodse, A.H. and Rawson, N. (1978). Distribution of drug-related problems among London casualty departments. *British Journal of Psychiatry* **132**, 467–72.

Ghodse, A.H., Sheehan, M., Stevens, B., Taylor, C., and Edwards, G. (1978). Mortality among drug addicts in Greater London. *British Medical Journal* **2**, 1742–4.

Ghodse, A.H., Sheehan, M., Taylor, C., and Edwards, G. (1985). Deaths of drug addicts in the United Kingdom 1967–81. *British Medical Journal* **290**, 425–8.

Ghodse, A.H., Oyefeso, A., and Kilpatrick, B. (1998). Mortality of drug addicts in the United Kingdom 1967–1993. *International Journal of Epidemiology* **27**, 473–8.

Gibson, D.R., Flynn, N.M., and McCarthy, J.J. (1999). Effectiveness of methadone treatment in reducing HIV risk behaviour and HIV seroconversion among injecting drug users. *AIDS* **13**, 1807–18.

Gilbody, S., Wahlbeck, K., and Adams, C. (2002). Randomised controlled trials in schizophrenia: a critical perspective on the literature. *Acta Psychiatrica Scandinavica* **105**, 243–51.

Glanz, M., Klawansky, S., McAuliffe, S., and Chalmers, T. (1997). Methadone vs l-alpha-acetylmethadol in the treatment of opiate addiction. A meta-analysis of the randomized controlled trials. *American Journal on Addictions* **6**, 339–49.

Glaser, F. (1999). The unsinkable Project MATCH. *Addiction* **94**, 34–6.

Glasscote, R., Sussex, J., and Jaffe, J. (1972). *The treatment of drug abuse: programs, problems, prospects.* Joint Information Service, Washington, DC.

Glassroth, J., *et al.* (1986). The impact of substance abuse treatment on the respiratory system. *Chest* **91**, 596–602.

Godfrey, C. and Sutton, M. (1996). Costs and benefits of treating drug problems. In *Welfare and policy: research agenda and issues* (ed. N. Lunt and D. Coyle). Taylor and Francis, London.

Godfrey, C., Stewart, D., and Gossop, M. (2001). *National Treatment Outcome Research Study: economic analysis of the two year outcome data.* Department of Health, London.

Gold, M., Redmond, D., and Kleber, H. (1978a). Clonidine in opiate withdrawal *Lancet* **i**, 929.

Gold, M., Redmond, D., and Kleber, H. (1978b). Clonidine blocks acute opiate withdrawl symptoms *Lancet* **ii**, 599.

Gold, M., Redmond, D., and Kleber, H. (1979). Noradrenergic hyperactivity in opiate withdrawal supported by clonidine reversal of opiate withdrawl. *American Joural of Psychiatry* **136**, 100.

Gold, M. and Miller, N. (1992). Cocaine (and crack) neurobiology. In *Substance abuse: a comprehensive textbook* (ed. J. Lowinson, p. Ruiz, R. Millman, and J. Langrod). Williams and Wilkins, Baltimore.

Goldfried, M.R. (1988). Application of rational restructuring to anxiety disorders. *The Counseling Psychologist* **16**, 50–68.

Goldstein, P. (1979). *Prostitution and drugs.* Lexington Books, Lexington.

Goodwin, D. and Guze, S. (1988). *Psychiatric diagnosis.* Oxford University Press, Oxford.

Gossop, M. (1987). Beware cocaine. *British Medical Journal* **295**, 945.

Gossop, M. (1988). (Clonidine and the treatment of the opiate withdrawal syndrome. *Drug and Alcohol Dependence,* **21**, 253–9.

Gossop, M. (1989a). *Relapse and addictive behaviour.* Routledge, London.

Gossop, M. (1989b). The detoxification of high dose heroin addicts in Pakistan. *Drug and Alcohol Dependence* **24**, 143–50.

Gossop, M. (1993). Volatile substances and the law. *Addiction* **88**, 311–14.

Gossop, M. (1994). Prescribing heroin and other injectable drugs to addicts: a British perspective. *Sucht* **5**, 325–33.

Gossop, M. (2001). A web of dependence. *Addiction* **96**, 677–8.

Gossop, M. and Connell, P. (1975). Attitudes of oral and intravenous multiple drug users toward drugs of abuse. *International Journal of the Addictions* **10**, 453–66.

Gossop, M. and Connell, P. (1983). Drug dependence, who gets treated? *International Journal of the Addictions* **18**, 99–109.

Gossop, M. and Bradley, B. (1984). Insomnia among addicts during supervised withdrawal from opiates: a comparison of oral methadone and electro-stimulation. *Drug and Alcohol Dependence* **13**, 191–8.

Gossop, M. and Grant, M. (1990). *The content and structure of methadone treatment programmes: a study in six countries,* WHO/PSA/90.3. World Health Organization, Geneva.

Gossop, M. and Strang, J. (1991). A comparison of the withdrawal responses of heroin and methadone addicts during detoxification. *British Journal of Psychiatry* **158**, 697–9.

Gossop, M. and Strang, J. (2000). Price, cost and value of opiate detoxification treatments. Reanalysis of data from two randomised trials. *British Journal of Psychiatry* **177**, 262–6.

Gossop, M., Bradley, B., and Brewis, R. (1982*a*). Amphetamine withdrawal and sleep disturbance. *Drug and Alcohol Dependence* **10**, 177–83.

Gossop, M., Strang, J., and Connell, P. (1982*b*). The response of outpatient opiate addicts to the provision of a temporary increase in their prescribed drugs. *British Journal of Psychiatry* **141**, 338–43.

Gossop, M., Bradley, B., Strang, J., and Connell, P. (1984). A comparison of the clinical effectiveness of electro-stimulation and a graduated oral methadone withdrawal schedule in the management of the opiate withdrawal syndrome. *British Journal of Psychiatry* **144**, 203–8.

Gossop, M., Johns, A., and Green, L. (1986). Opiate withdrawal: inpatient versus outpatient programmes and preferred versus random assignment to treatment. *British Medical Journal* **293**, 103–4.

Gossop, M., Bradley, B., and Phillips, G. (1987). An investigation of withdrawal symptoms shown by opiate addicts during and subsequent to a 21-day inpatient methadone detoxification procedure. *Addictive Behaviors* **12**, 1–6.

Gossop, M., Griffiths, P., and Strang, J. (1988). Chasing the dragon: a comparison of heroin chasers and injectors seen by a London community drug team. *British Journal of Addiction* **83**, 1159–62.

Gossop, M., Green, L., Phillips, G., and Bradley, B. (1989*a*). Lapse, relapse and survival among opiate addicts after treatment: a prospective follow-up study. *British Journal of Psychiatry* **154**, 348–53.

Gossop, M., Bradley, B., Phillips, G., and Green, L. (1989*b*). Circumstances surrounding the initial lapse to opiate use following detoxification. *British Journal of Psychiatry* **154**, 354–9.

Gossop, M., Grant, M., and Wodak, A. (1989*c*). *The uses of methadone in the treatment and management of opioid dependence*, WHO/MNH/DAT/89.1. World Health Organization, Geneva.

Gossop, M., Griffiths, P., Bradley, B., and Strang, J. (1989*d*). Opiate withdrawal symptoms in response to 10-day and 21-day methadone withdrawal programmes. *British Journal of Psychiatry* **154**, 360–3.

Gossop, M., Green L., Phillips, G., and Bradley, B. (1990). Factors predicting outcome among opiate addicts after treatment. *British Journal of Clinical Psychology* **29**, 209–16.

Gossop, M., Griffiths, P., and Strang, J. (1991*a*). Chasing the dragon. *Journal of Substance Abuse Treatment* **8**, 89–91.

Gossop, M., Battersby, M., and Strang, J. (1991*b*). Self-detoxification by opiate addicts: a preliminary investigation. *British Journal of Psychiatry* **159**, 208–12.

Gossop, M., Kirsch, A., and Goos, C. (1993). *AIDS among Drug Users in Europe*. World Health Organisation, Copenhagen.

Gossop, M., Griffiths, P., Powis, B., and Strang, J. (1993*a*). Severity of heroin dependence and HIV risk: I. Sexual behaviour. *AIDS Care* **5**, 149–57.

Gossop, M., Griffiths, P., Powis, B., and Strang, J. (1993*b*). Severity of heroin dependence and HIV risk: II. Sharing injecting equipment. *AIDS Care* **5**, 159–68.

Gossop, M., Griffiths, P., Powis, B., and Strang, J. (1994*a*). Cocaine: patterns of use, route of administration, and severity of dependence. *British Journal of Psychiatry* **164**, 660–4.

Gossop, M., Powis, B., Griffiths, P., and Strang, J (1994*b*). Sexual behaviour and its relationship to drug-taking among prostitutes in south London. *Addiction* **89**, 961–70.

Gossop, M., Powis, B., Griffiths, P., and Strang, J (1994c). Multiple risks for HIV and hepatitis B infection among heroin users. *Drug and Alcohol Review* **13**, 293–300.

Gossop, M., Darke, S., Griffiths, P., Hando, J., Powis, B., Hall, W., and Strang, J. (1995). The Severity of Dependence Scale (SDS): psychometric properties of the SDS in English and Australian samples of heroin, cocaine and amphetamine users. *Addiction* **90**, 607–14.

Gossop, M., Griffiths, P., Powis, B., Williamson, S., and Strang, J. (1996). Frequency of non-fatal heroin overdose: survey of heroin users recruited in non-clinical settings. *British Medical Journal* **313**, 402.

Gossop, M. and Strang, J. (1997). Rapid anaesthetic-antagonist detoxification of heroin addicts. What origins, evidence base and clinical justification? *British Journal of Intensive Care* **7**, 66–9.

Gossop, M., Best, D., and Marsden, J. (1997a). Abus de temazepam en Grande-Bretagne. *Psychotropes* **3**, 7–18.

Gossop, M., Griffiths, P., Powis, B., Williamson, S., Fountain, J., and Strang, J. (1997b). Continuing drug risk behaviour: shared use of injecting paraphernalia among London heroin injectors. *AIDS Care* **9**, 651–60.

Gossop, M., Marsden, J., and Stewart, D. (1998a). *NTORS at one year: changes in substance use, health and criminal behaviour one year after intake*. Department of Health, London.

Gossop, M., Marsden, J., Stewart, D., Lehmann, P., Edwards, C., Wilson, A., and Segar, G. (1998b). Substance use, health and social problems of clients at 54 drug treatment agencies: intake data from the National Treatment Outcome Research Study (NTORS). *British Journal of Psychiatry* **173**, 166–71.

Gossop, M., Marsden, J., Stewart, D., Lehmann, P., and Strang, J. (1999a). Methadone treatment practices and outcome for opiate addicts treated in drug clinics and in general practice: results from the National Treatment Outcome Research Study. *British Journal of General Practice* **49**, 31–4.

Gossop, M., Marsden, J., Stewart, D., and Rolfe, A. (1999b). Treatment retention and one year outcomes for residential programmes in England. *Drug and Alcohol Dependence* **57**, 89–98.

Gossop, M., Marsden, J., Stewart, D., and Rolfe, A. (2000a). Patterns of improvement after methadone treatment: one year follow-up results from the National Treatment Outcome Research Study (NTORS). *Drug and Alcohol Dependence* **60**, 275–86.

Gossop, M., Marsden, J., Stewart, D., and Rolfe, A. (2000b). Patterns of drinking and drinking outcomes among drug misusers: 1-year follow-up results. *Journal of Substance Abuse Treatment* **19**, 45–50.

Gossop, M., Marsden, J., Stewart, D., and Rolfe, A. (2000c). Reductions in acquisitive crime and drug use after treatment of addiction problems: one year follow-up outcomes. *Drug and Alcohol Dependence* **58**, 165–172.

Gossop, M., Marsden, J., Stewart, D., and Treacy, S. (2000d). Routes of drug administration and multiple drug misuse: regional variations among clients seeking treatment at programmes throughout England. *Addiction* **95**, 1197–206.

Gossop, M., Marsden, J., Stewart, D., and Treacy, S. (2001a). Outcomes after methadone maintenance and methadone reduction treatments: two-year follow-up results from the National Treatment Outcome Research Study. *Drug and Alcohol Dependence* **62**, 255–64.

Gossop, M., Stephens, S., Stewart, D., Marshall, J., Bearn, J., and Strang, J. (2001*b*). Healthcare professionals referred for treatment of alcohol and drug problems. *Alcohol and Alcoholism* **36**, 160–4.

Gossop, M., Marsden, J., Stewart, D., and Treacy, S. (2002*a*). Reduced injection risk and sexual risk behaviours after drug misuse treatment: results from the National Treatment Outcome Research Study. *AIDS Care* **14**, 77–93.

Gossop, M., Marsden, J., Stewart, D., and Treacy, S. (2002*b*). A prospective study of mortality among drug misusers during a four year period after seeking treatment. *Addiction* **97**, 39–47.

Gossop, M., Marsden, J., and Stewart, D. (2002*c*). Dual dependence: assessment of dependence upon alcohol and illicit drugs, and the relationship of alcohol dependence among drug misusers to patterns of drinking, illicit drug use, and health problems. *Addiction* **97**, 169–78.

Gossop, M., Stewart, D., Browne, N., and Marsden, J. (2002*d*). Factors associated with abstinence, lapse or relapse to heroin use after residential treatment: protective effect of coping responses. *Addiction* **97**, 1259–67.

Gowing, L., Ali, R., and White, J. (2000). *The management of opioid withdrawal: an overview of the research literature*, DASC Monograph no. 9. University of Adelaide, Adelaide.

Graber, A., Davidson, P., Brown, A., McRae, J., and Woolridge, K. (1992). Dropout and relapse during diabetes care. *Diabetes Care* **15**, 1477–83.

Grabowski, J., O'Brien, C., Greenstein, R., Ternes, J., Long, M., and Steinberg-Donato, S. (1979). Effects of contingent payment on compliance with a naltrexone regimen. *American Journal of Drug and Alcohol Abuse* **6**, 355–65.

Green, L. and Gossop, M. (1988). The management of pregnancy in opiate addicts. *Journal of Reproduction and Infant Psychology* **6**, 51–7.

Greenstein, R.A., O'Brien, C.P., McLellan, A.T., Woody, G.E., Grabowski, J., Long, M., Coyle-Perkins, G., and Vittor, A. (1981). Naltrexone: a short-term treatment for opiate dependence. *American Journal of Drug and Alcohol Abuse* **8**, 291–300.

Greenstein, R.A., Arndt, J.C., McLellan, A.T., O'Brien, C.P., and Evans, B. (1984). Naltrexone: a clinical perspective. *Journal of Clinical Psychiatry* **45**, 25–8.

Greenwood, J. (1992). Persuading general practitioners to prescribe-good husbandry or a recipe for chaos? *British Journal of Addiction* **87**, 567–75.

Grella, C.E., Anglin, M.D., and Wugaalter, S.E. (1995). Cocaine and crack use and HIV risk behaviours among high risk methadone maintenance clients. *Drug and Alcohol Dependence* **37**, 15–21.

Grella, C., Hser, Y., Joshi, V., and Anglin, D. (1999). Patient histories, retention, and outcome models for younger and older adults in DATOS. *Drug and Alcohol Dependence* **57**, 151–66.

Griffin, M., Weiss, R., Mirin, S., and Lange, U. (1989). A comparison of male and female cocaine abusers. *Archives of General Psychiatry* **46**, 122–6.

Griffith, J., Rowan-Szal, G., Roark, R., and Simpson, D. (2000). Contingency management in outpatient methadone treatment: a meta-analysis, *Drug and Alcohol Dependence* **58**, 55–66.

Griffiths, P., Gossop, M, Powis, B., and Strang, J. (1994). Transitions in patterns of heroin administration: a study of heroin chasers and heroin injectors. *Addiction* **89**, 301–9.

Groves, P., Heuston, J., Durand, M.A., Albery, I., Gossop, M., and Strang, J. (1996). The identification and management of substance misuse problems by general practitioners. *Journal of Mental Health* **5**, 183–93.

Groves, P., Heuston, J., Albery, I., Gerada, C., Gossop, M., and Strang, J. (2002). Evaluation of a service to strengthen primary care responses to substance-misusing patients: welcomed, but little impact. *Drugs: Education, Prevention and Policy* **9**, 21–33.

Gruer, L., Wilson, P., Scott, R., Elliott, L., Macleod, J., Harden, K., Forrester, E., Hinshelwood, S., McNulty, H., and Silk, P. (1997). General practitioner centred scheme for treatment of opiate dependent drug injectors in Glasgow. *British Medical Journal* **314**, 1730–5.

Grund, J-P. and Blanken, P. (1993). *From chasing the dragon to Chinezen: the diffusion of heroin smoking in The Netherlands*, Institut voor Verslavingson der Zoek (IVO Series 3). Erasmus University, Rotterdam.

Hagan, H. (1998). Hepatitis C virus transmission dynamics in injection drug users. *Substance Use and Misuse* **33**, 1197–212.

Hagan, T., Finnegan, L., and Nelson-Zlupko, L. (1994). Impediments to comprehensive treatment models for substance-dependent women: treatment and research questions. *Journal of Psychoactive Drugs* **26**, 163–71.

Halikas, J., Nugent, S., Crosby, R., and Carlson, G. (1993). 1990–1991 survey of pharmacotherapies used in the treatment of cocaine abuse. *Journal of Addictive Diseases* **12**, 129–39.

Hall, J. and Baker, R. (1986). Token economies and schizophrenia: a review. In *Contemporary issues in schizophrenia* (ed. A. Kerr and R. Snaith). Gaskell, London.

Hall, S., Bass, A., Hargreaves, W., and Loeb, P. (1979). Contingency management and information feedback in outpatient heroin detoxification. *Behaviour Therapy* **10**, 443–51.

Hall, W. (1999). Reducing the toll of opioid overdose deaths in Australia. *Drug and Alcohol Review* **18** (2), 213–20.

Hall, W. and Darke, S. (1998). Trends in opiate overdose deaths in Australia 1979–1995. *Drug and Alcohol Dependence* **52**, 71–7.

Hall, W. and Farrell, M. (1997). Comorbidity of mental disorders with substance misuse. *British Journal of Psychiatry* **171**, 4–5.

Hall, W., Bell, J., and Carless, J. (1993a). Crime and drug use among applicants for methadone maintenance. *Drug and Alcohol Dependence* **31**, 123–9.

Hall, W., Darke, S., Ross, M., and Wodak, A. (1993b). Patterns of drug use and risk taking behaviour among injecting amphetamine and opioid users in Sydney, Australia. *Addiction* **88**, 509–16.

Hall, W., Solowji, N., and Lemon, J. (1994). *The health and psychological consequences of cannabis use*. Australian Government Publishing Services, Canberra.

Hallstrom, C. and Lader, M. (1981). Benzodiazepine withdrawal phenomena. *International Pharmacopsychiatry* **16**, 235–44.

Hamid, R., Deren, S., Beardsley, M., and Tortu, S. (1999). Agreement between urinalysis and self-reported drug use. *Substance Use and Misuse* **34**, 1585–92.

Hammersley, R., Forsyth, A., Morrison, V., and Davies, J. (1989). The relationship between crime and opioid use. *British Journal of Addiction* **84**, 1029–43.

Hammersley, R., Forsyth, A., and Lavelle, T. (1990). The criminality of new drug users in Glasgow. *British Journal of Addiction* **85**, 1583–94.

Hammersley, R., Cassidy, M., and Oliver, J. (1995). Drugs associated with drug-related deaths in Edinburgh and Glasgow, November 1990 to October 1992. *Addiction* **90**, 959–65.

Hando, J., Topp, L., and Hall, W. (1997). Amphetamine-related harms and treatment preferences of regular amphetamine users in Sydney, Australia. *Drug and Alcohol Dependence* **46**, 105–13.

Hartel, D.M. and Schoenbaum, E.E. (1998). Methadone treatment protects against HIV infection: two decades of experience in the Bronx, New York City. *Public Health Reports* **113**, 107–15.

Hartgers, C. (1990). AIDS in the nineties: from science to policy. Drug user interventions. *AIDS Care* **2**, 399–402.

Hartnoll, R., Mitcheson, M., Battersby, A., Brown, G., Ellis, M., Flemming, P., and Hedley, N. (1980). Evaluation of heroin maintenance in controlled trial. *Archives of General Psychiatry* **37**, 877–84.

Harwood, H., Hubbard, R., Collins, J., and Rachal, J. (1988). *The costs of crime and the benefits of drug abuse treatment: a cost–benefit analysis using TOPS data*, NIDA Research Monograph no. 86, pp. 209–35. NIDA, Rockville, Maryland.

Havassy, B., Wasserman, D., and Hall, S. (1995). Social relationships and abstinence from cocaine in an American treatment sample. *Addiction* **90**, 699–710.

Hawkins, J., Catalano, R., and Miller, J. (1992). Risk and protective factors for alcohol and other drug problems in adolescence and early adulthood: implications for substance abuse prevention. *Psychological Bulletin* **112**, 64–105.

Hawton, K., Salkovskis, P., Kirk, J., and Clark, D. (2000). The development and principles of cognitive–behavioural treatments. In *Cognitive behaviour therapy for psychiatric problems* (ed. K. Hawton, P. Salkovskis, J. Kirk, and D. Clark). Oxford Medical Publications, Oxford.

Haynes, R. (1979). Strategies to improve compliance with referrals, appointments and prescribed medical regimens. In *Compliance in healthcare* (R. Haynes, D. Taylor, and D. Sackett). Johns Hopkins University Press, Baltimore.

Heather, N. (1998). Using brief opportunities for change in medical settings. In *Treating addictive behaviors* (ed. W. Miller and N. Heather). Plenum, New York.

Heather, N. (2002). Effectiveness of brief interventions proved beyond reasonable doubt. *Addiction* **97**, 293–4.

Heather, N. and Bradley, B. (1990). Cue exposure as a practical treatment for addictive disorders: why are we waiting? *Addictive Behaviors* **15**, 335–7.

Heather, N. and Robertson, I. (1989). *Problem drinking*. Oxford University Press, Oxford.

Heather, N. and Stallard, A. (1989). Does the Marlatt model underestimate the importance of conditioned craving in the relapse process? In *Relapse and addictive behaviour* (ed. M. Gossop). Routledge, London.

Hedberg, A. and Campbell, L. (1974). A comparison of four behavioural treatment approaches to alcoholism. *Journal of Behaviour Therapy and Experimental Psychiatry* **5**, 251–6.

Heimer, R., Khoshnood, K., Jariwala-Freeman, B., Duncan, B., and Harima, Y. (1996). Hepatitis in used syringes: the limits of sensitivity techniques to detect hepatitis B virus (HBV) DNA, hepatitis C virus (HCV) RNA, and antibodies to HBV core and HCV antigens. *Journal of Infectious Diseases* **173**, 997–1000.

Henderson, G. (1993). Mechanisms of drug incorporation into hair. *Forensic Science International* **63**, 19–29.

Henman, J.O. and Henman, S. (1990). Cognitive–perceptual reconstruction in the treatment of alcoholism. In *Neuro-linguistic programming in alcoholism treatment* (ed. C.M. Sterman), pp. 105–24. Haworth Press, New York.

Henretig, F. (1996). Inhalant abuse in children and adolescents. *Pediatric Annals* **25**, 47–52.

Henry, W., Strupp, H., Schacht, T., and Gaston, L. (1994). Psychodynamic approaches. In *Handbook of psychotherapy and behavior change* (ed. A. Bergin and S. Garfield). Wiley, New York.

Hersh, D. and Modesto-Lowe, V. (1998). Drug abuse and mood disorders. In *Dual diagnosis and treatment* (ed. H. Kranzler and B. Rounsaville). Marcel Dekker, New York.

Hickman, M., Drummond, N., and Grimshaw, A. (1994). The operation of shared care for chronic disease. *Health Bulletin* **52**, 118–26.

Higgins, S., Delaney, D., Budney, A., Bickel, W., Hughes, J., Foerg, F., and Fenwick, J. (1991). A behavioral approach to achieving initial cocaine abstinence. *American Journal of Psychiatry* **148**, 1218–24.

Higgins, S.T., Budney, A.J., Bickel, W.K., and Badger, G.J. (1993). Participation of significant others in outpatient behavioral treatment predicts greater cocaine abstinence. *American Journal of Drug and Alcohol Abuse* **20**, 47–56.

Higgins, S.T., Budney, A.J., Bickel, W.K., Foerg, F.E., Donham, R., and Badger, G.J. (1994). Incentives improve outcome in outpatient behavioral treatment of cocaine dependence. *Archives of General Psychiatry* **51**, 568–76.

Hill, S. (1985). The disease concept of alcoholism: a review. *Drug and Alcohol Dependence* **16**, 193–214.

Hodgson, R. (1972). Behaviour therapy. In *Alcoholism-new knowledge and new responses* (ed. G. Edwards and M. Grant). Croom Helm, Beckenham.

Hodgson, T. and Meiners, M. (1982). Cost-of-illness methodology: a guide to current practices and procedures. *Milbank Memorial Fund Quarterly. Health and Society* **60**, 429–62.

Holland, S. (1982). *Residential drug free programs for substance abusers: the effect of planned duration on treatment.* Gateway Foundation, Chicago.

Holland, S. (1986). Measuring process in drug abuse treatment research. In *Therapeutic communities for addictions: readings in theory, research and practice* (ed. G. De Leon and J.T. Ziegenfuss), pp. 169–81. Charles C. Thomas, Springfield, Illinois.

Hollister, L., Johnson, K., Boukhabza, D., and Gillespie, H. (1981). Aversive effects of naltrexone in subjects not dependent on opiates. *Drug and Alcohol Dependence* **8**, 37–41.

Holroyd, S. and Duryee, J. (1997). Substance use disorders in a geriatric psychiatry outpatient clinic: prevalence and epidemiologic characteristics. *Journal of Nervous and Mental Diseases* **185**, 627–32.

Horgan, C. (1997). Need and access to drug abuse treatment. In *Treating drug abusers effectively* (ed. J.A. Egerton, D.M. Fox, and A.I. Leshner). Blackwells, Oxford.

Horvath, A. and Symonds, B. (1991). Relation between working alliance and outcome in psychotherapy. A meta-analysis. *Journal of Counseling Psychology* **38**, 139–49.

Howard, M. and Jenson, J. (1999). Inhalant use among antisocial youth: prevalence and correlates. *Addictive Behaviors* **24**, 59–74.

Hser, Y-I., Anglin, M.D., and Booth, M. (1987). Sex differences in addict careers. *American Journal of Drug and Alcohol Abuse* **13**, 231–51.

Hser, Y.I., Anglin, D., and Powers, K. (1993). A 24-year follow-up of California narcotics addicts. *Archives of General Psychiatry* **50**, 577–84.

Hubbard, R.L., Marsden, M.E., Rachal, J.V., Harwood, H.J., Cavanaugh, E.R., and Ginzberg, H.M. (1989). *Drug abuse treatment: a national study of effectiveness*. Chapel Hill, London.

Hubbard, R.L., Craddock, S.G., Flynn, P., Anderson, J., and Etheridge, R. (1997). Overview of 1-year outcomes in the Drug Abuse Treatment Outcome Study (DATOS). *Psychology of Addictive Behaviors* **11**, 279–93.

Hughes, J. (1987). Craving as a psychological concept. *British Journal of Addiction* **82**, 38–9.

Hughes, S. and Calverley, P.M. (1988). Heroin inhalation and asthma. *British Medical Journal* **297**, 1511–12.

Hulse, G.K., English, D.R., Milne, E., and Holman, C.D.J. (1999). The quantification of mortality resulting from the regular use of illicit opiates. *Addiction* **94**, 221–9.

Hunt, D.E., Lipton, D.S., and Spunt, B. (1984). Patterns of criminal activity among methadone clients and current narcotic users in treatment. *Journal of Drug Issues* **14**, 687–702.

Hunt, D., Lipton, D., Goldsmith, D., *et al.* (1986). 'It takes your heart': the image of methadone maintenance in the addict world and its effect on recruitment to treatment. *International Journal of the Addictions* **20**, 1751–71.

Hunt, L. and Chambers, C. (1976). *Heroin epidemics: a study of heroin use in the United States 1965–1975*. Spectrum, New York.

Hunt, N., Griffiths, P., Southwell, M., Stillwell, G., and Strang, J. (1999). Preventing and curtailing injecting drug use: a review of opportunities for developing and delivering 'route transition interventions'. *Drug and Alcohol Review* **18**, 441–51.

Hunt, W. A., Barnett, L. W., and Branch, L. G. (1971). Relapse rates in addiction programs. *Journal of Clinical Psychology* **27** (4), 455–6.

Hunter, G.M., Donoghoe, M.C., and Stimson, G.V. (1995). Crack use and injection on the increase among injecting drug users in London. *Addiction* **90**, 1397–400.

Hunter, G.M., Stimson, J., Judd, A., Jones, S., and Hickman, M. (2000). Measuring injecting risk behaviour in the second decade of harm reduction: a survey of injecting drug users in England. *Addiction* **95**, 1351–61.

Hurt, R., Finlayson, R., Morse, R., and Davis, L. (1988). Alcoholism in elderly persons: medical aspects and prognosis of 216 inpatients. *Mayo Clinic Proceedings* **63**, 753–60.

Hutchinson, S., Taylor, A., Gruer, L., Barr, C., Mills, C., Elliott, L., Goldberg, D., Scott, R., and Gilchrist, G. (2000). One-year follow-up of opiate injectors treated with oral methadone in a GP-centred programme. *Addiction* **95**, 1055–68.

ICD-10 (1992). *The ICD-10 classification of mental and behavioural disorders*. World Health Organization, Geneva.

Iguchi, M.Y. and Stitzer, M.L. (1991). Predictors of opiate drug abuse during a 90-day methadone detoxification. *American Journal of Drug and Alcohol Abuse* **17** (3), 279–94.

Iguchi, M., Stitzer, M., Bigelow, G., and Liebson, I. (1988). Contingency management in methadone maintenance: effects of reinforcing and aversive consequences on illicit polydrug use. *Drug and Alcohol Dependence* **22**, 1–7.

Iguchi, M., Handelsman, L., Bickel, W., and Griffiths, R. (1993). Benzodiazepine and sedative use/abuse by methadone maintenance clients. *Drug and Alcohol Dependence* **32**, 257–66.

Iguchi, M., Lamb, R., Belding, M., Platt, J., Husband, S., and Morral, A. (1996). Contingent reinforcement of group participation versus abstinence in a methadone maintenance program. *Experimental and Clinical Psychopharmacology* **4**, 315–21.

Imperato, A., Mele, A., Scrocco, M.G., and Puglisi-Allegra, S. (1992). Chronic cocaine alters limbic extracellular dopamine. Neurochemical basis for addiction. *European Journal of Pharmacology* **212**, 299–300.

Inciardi J.A. (1979). Heroin use and street crime. *Crime and Delinquency* **25**, 332–46.

Institute of Medicine (1990*a*). *Treating drug problems*, Vol.1 (ed. D. Gerstein and H. Harwood). National Academy Press, Washington, DC.

Institute of Medicine (1990*b*). *Broadening the base of treatment for alcohol problems*. National Academy Press, Washington, DC.

Isbell, H. (1955). Craving for alcohol. *Quarterly Journal of Studies on Alcohol* **16**, 38–42.

Isbell, H., Wikler, A., Eisenman, A., Daingerfield, M., and Frank K. (1948). Liability of addiction to 6-dimethylamino-4-4-diphenyl-3-heptanone (methadone, 'amidone' or '10820') in man. *Archives of Internal Medicine* **82**, 362–92.

Jaffe, J. (1985). Drug addiction and drug abuse. In *The phamacological basis of therapeutics* (ed. A. Goodman, L. Gilman, and T. Rall). Macmillan, New York.

Jaffe, J., Senay, E., Schuster, C., Renault, P., Smith, B., and DiMenza, S. (1972). Methadyl acetate vs methadone. *Journal of the American Medical Association* **222**, 437–42.

Jamieson, A., Glanz, A., and MacGregor, S. (1984). *Dealing with drug misuse*. Tavistock, London.

Janis, I. and Mann, L. (1977). *Decision making*. Free Press, New York.

Jansson, L., Svikis, D., Lee, J., Paluzzi, P., Rutigliano, P., and Hackerman, F. (1996). Pregnancy and addiction: a comprehensive care model. *Journal of Substance Abuse Treatment* **13**, 321–9.

Jarvis, G. and Parker, H. (1989). Young heroin users and crime. *British Journal of Criminology* **29**, 175–85.

Jessor, R., Donovan, J., and Costa, F. (1991). *Beyond adolescence: problem behavior and young adult development*. Cambridge University Press, Cambridge.

Joe, G.W. and Simpson, D.D. (1975). Retention in treatment of drug users: 1971–1972 DARP admissions. *American Journal of Drug and Alcohol Abuse* **2**, 63–71.

Joe, G. W. and Friend, H. (1989). Treatment process factors and satisfaction with drug abuse treatment. *Psychology of Addictive Behaviors* **3**, 53–64.

Joe, G.W. and Simpson, D.D. (1990). Death rates and risk factors. In *Opioid addiction and treatment: a 12-year follow-up* (ed. D.D. Simpson and S.B. Sells). Krieger, Malabar, Florida.

Joe, G.W., Lehman, W., and Simpson, D.D. (1982). Addict death rates during a four-year post-treatment follow-up. *American Journal of Public Health* **72**, 703–9.

Joe, G.W., Chastain, R., and Simpson, D.D. (1990). Reasons for addiction stages. In *Opioid addiction and treatment: a 12-year follow-up* (ed. D.D. Simpson and S.B. Sells). Krieger, Malabar, Florida.

Joe, G.W., Simpson, D.D., and Hubbard, R.L. (1991). Treatment predictors of tenure in methadone maintenance. *Journal of Substance Abuse* **3**, 73–84.

Joe, G.W., Simpson, D.D., and Broome, K.M. (1999). Retention and patient engagement models for different treatment modalities in DATOS. *Drug and Alcohol Dependence* **57**, 113–25.

Johnsen, E. and Herringer, L. (1993). A note on the utilisation of common support activities and relapse following substance abuse treatment. *Journal of Psychology* **127**, 73–8.

Johnson, B., Goldstein, P., Preble, E., Schmeidler, J., Lipton, D., Spunt, B., and Miller, T. (1985). *Taking care of business: the economics of crime by heroin abusers.* Lexington Books, Lexington, Maine.

Johnson, J. (1973). Effects of accurate expectations about sensations on the sensory and distress components of pain. *Journal of Personality and Social Psychology* **27**, 261–75.

Johnson, R., Chutuape, M., Strain, E., Walsh, S., Stitzer, M., and Bigelow, G. (2000). A comparison of levomethadyl acetate, buprenorphine, and methadone for opioid dependence. *New England Journal of Medicine* **343**, 1290–7.

Johnson, S. (1997). Dual diagnosis of severe mental illness and substance misuse: a case for specialist services? *British Journal of Psychiatry* **171**, 205–8.

Jones, H. and Jones, H. (1977). *Sensual drugs.* Cambridge University Press, London.

Jones, H., Strain, E., Bigelow, G., Walsh, S., Stitzer, M., Eissenberg, T., and Johnson, R. (1998). Induction with levomethadyl acetate: safety and efficacy. *Archives of General Psychiatry* **55**, 729–36.

Jones, H., Haug, N., Silverman, K., Stitzer, M., and Svikis, D. (2001). The effectiveness of incentives in enhancing treatment attendance and drug abstinence in methadone-maintained pregnant women. *Drug and Alcohol Dependence* **61**, 297–306.

Joseph, H. and Paone, D. (1997). The homeless. In *Substance abuse: a comprehensive textbook* (ed. J. Lowinson, P. Ruiz, R. Millman, and J. Langrod). Williams and Wilkins, Baltimore.

Joseph, J., Breslin, C., and Skinner, H. (1999). Critical perspectives on the transtheoretical model and stages of change. In *Changing addictive behaviour* (ed. J. Tucker, D. Donovan, and G.A. Marlatt). Guilford, New York.

Kall, K. (1997). Amphetamine abuse in Sweden. In *Amphetamine misuse* (ed. H. Klee). Harwood, Amsterdam.

Kandall, S., Albin, S., Lowinson, J., Berle, B., Eidelman, A., and Gartner, L. (1976). Differential effects of maternal heroin and methadone use on birth-weight. *Paediatrics* **58**, 681–5.

Kashner, T., Rodell, D., Ogden, S., Guggenheim, F., and Karson, C. (1992). Outcomes and costs of two VA inpatient treatment programs for older alcoholic patients. *Hospital and Community Psychiatry* **43**, 985–9.

Katz, J. (1989). Drugs as reinforcers: pharmacological and behavioural factors. In *The neuropharmacological basis of reward* (ed. J. Liebman and S. Cooper). Oxford University Press, Oxford.

Kaufman, M., Levin, J., Ross, M., Lange, N., Rose, S., Kukes, T., Mendelson, J., Lukas, S., Cohen, B., and Renshaw, P. (1998). Cocaine-induced cerebral vasoconstriction detected in humans with magnetic resonance angiography. *Journal of the American Medical Association* **279**, 376–80.

Kazdin, A. (1978). *History of behavior medification.* University Park Press, Baltimore.

Keaney, F., Crimlisk, H., and Bearn, J. (2002). Lofexidine and desiprimine: interaction results in breakthrough opioid withdrawal symptoms. *International Journal of Psychiatry in Clinical Practice* **6**, 179–81.

Kendall, P., Vitousek, K., and Kane, M. (1991). Thought and action in psychotherapy: cognitive–behavioral approaches. In *Clinical psychology handbook* (ed. M. Hersen, A. Kazdin, and A. Bellack). Pergamon, New York.

Kennard, D. (1998). *An introduction to therapeutic communities.* Jessica Kingsley, London.

Kessler, R., McGonagle, K., and Zhao, S. (1994). Lifetime and 12 month prevalence of DSM-IIIR psychiatric disorders in the United States: results from the National Comorbidity Study. *Archives of General Psychiatry* **51**, 8–19.

Khantzian, E.J. and Mack, J.E. (1994). Alcoholics Anonymous and contemporary psychodynamic theory. In *Recent developments in alcoholism*, Vol. 7 (ed. M. Galanter), pp. 67–89. Plenum Press, New York.

Khantzian, E.J. and Treece, C. (1985). DSM-III psychiatric diagnosis of narcotic addicts. *Archives of General Psychiatry* **42**, 1067–71.

Kidorf, M. and Stitzer, M. (1993). Descriptive analysis of cocaine use of methadone patients. *Drug and Alcohol Dependence* **32**, 267–75.

Kidorf, M., Stitzer, M.L., Brooner, R.K., and Goldberg, J. (1994). Contingent methadone take-home doses reinforce adjunct therapy attendance of methadone maintenance patients. *Drug and Alcohol Dependence* **36**, 221–6.

King, D., Griffiths, K., and Hall, C. (1980). Effect of the CURB campaign on barbiturate prescribing in Northern Ireland. *Royal College of General Practitioners* **30**, 614–18.

King, G.R. and Ellinwood, E.H. (1997). Amphetamines and other stimulants. In *Substance abuse: a comprehensive textbook* (ed. J.Lowinson, P.Ruiz, R.Millman, and J.Langrod). Williams and Wilkins, Baltimore.

King, V., Stoller, K., Hayes, M., Umbricht, A., Currens, M., Kidorf, M., Carter, J., Schwarz, R., and Brooner, R. (2002). A multicenter randomized evaluation of methadone medical maintenance. *Drug and Alcohol Dependence* **65**, 137–48.

Kintz, P. (2001). Deaths involving buprenorphine: a compendium of French cases. *Forensic Science International* **121**, 65–9.

Kirk, J. (2000). Cognitive behavioural assessment. In *Cognitive behaviour therapy for psychiatric problems* (ed. K. Hawton, P. Salkovskis, J. Kirk, and D. Clark). Oxford Medical Publications, Oxford.

Kleber, H. (1981). Detoxification from narcotics. In *Substance abuse* (ed. J. Lowinson and P. Ruiz). Williams and Wilkins, Baltimore.

Kleber, H. (1988). Epidemic cocaine abuse: America's present, Britain's future? *British Journal of Addiction* **83**, 1359–71.

Kleber, H. (1993). The US anti-drug prevention strategy: science and policy connections. In *Drugs, alcohol and tobacco: making the science and policy connections* (ed. G. Edwards, J. Strang, and J. Jaffe). Oxford University Press, Oxford.

Kleber, H., Gold, M., and Riordan, C. (1980). The use of clonidine in detoxification from opiates. *United Nations Bulletin on Narcotics* **32**, 1–10.

Kleber, H., Kosten, T., Gaspari, J., and Topazian, M. (1985). Nontolerance to the opioid antagonism of naltrexone. *Biological Psychiatry* **20**, 66–72.

Kleber, H., Topazian, M., Gaspari, J., Riordan, C., and Kosten, T. (1987). Clonidine and naltrexone in the outpatient treatment of heroin withdrawal. *American Journal of Drug and Alcohol Abuse* **13**, 1–17.

Klee, H. (1997). Amphetamine misusers in contemporary Britain: the emergence of a hidden population. In *Amphetamine misuse* (ed. H. Klee). Harwood, Amsterdam.

Klee, H., Faugier, J., Hayes, C., and Morris, J. (1991). Risk reduction among injecting drug users: changes in the sharing of injecting equipment and in condom use. *AIDS Care* **3**, 63–73.

Kleinman, P., Goldsmith, D., Friedman, S., Hopkins, W., and DesJarlais, D. (1990*a*). Knowledge about and behaviours affecting the spread of AIDS: a street survey of intravenous drug users and their associates in New York. *International Journal of the Addictions* **24**, 345–61.

Kleinman, P., Miller, A., Millman, R., Woody, G., Todd, T., Kemp, J., and Lipton, D.S. (1990*b*). Psychopathology among cocaine abusers entering treatment. *Journal of Nervous and Mental Diseases* **178**, 442–7.

Klonoff, D., Andrews, B., and Obana, W. (1989). Stroke associated with cocaine use. *Archives of Neurology* **46**, 989–93.

Knight, K., Simpson, D., Chatham, L., and Camacho, L. (1997). An assessment of prison-based drug treatment: Texas' in-prison therapeutic community program. *Journal of Offender Rehabilitation* **24**, 75–100.

Knight, K., Simpson, D., and Hiller, M. (1999). Three-year reincarceration outcomes for in-prison therapeutic community treatment in Texas. *The Prison Journal* **79**, 337–51.

Knupfer, G. (1972). Ex-problem drinkers. In *Life history research in psychopathology* (ed. M. Roff, L. Robins, and H. Pollack). University of Minneapolis Press, Minneapolis.

Koester, S. (1994). Copping, running, and paraphernalia laws: contextual variables and needle risk behavior among injection drug users in Denver. *Human Organization* **53**, 287–95.

Kolar, A., Brown, B., Hertzen, C., and Michaelson, B. (1994). Children of substance abusers: the life experiences of children of opiate addicts in methadone maintenance. *American Journal of Drug Abuse* **20**, 159–71.

Kosten, T. (1992). Pharmacotherapies. In *A Clinician's Guide to Cocaine Addiction* (ed. T. Kosten and H. Kleber). Guilford Press, New York.

Kosten, T.R., Morgan, C., and Kosten, T.A. (1990). Depressive symptoms during buprenorphine treatment of opioid abusers. *Journal of Substance Abuse Treatment* **7**, 51–4.

Kosten, T.R., Morgan, C., and Kleber, H. (1992). Phase II clinical trials of buprenorphine: detoxification and induction onto naltrexone. In *Buprenorphine, an alternative treatment for opioid dependence* (ed. J. Blaine), pp. 101–119, NIDA Research Monograph. NIDA, Rockville, Maryland.

Kothari, G., Marsden, J., and Strang, J. (2002). Opportunities and obstacles for effective treatment of drug misusers in the criminal justice system in England and Wales. *British Journal of Criminology* **42**, 412–32.

Kozlowski, L. and Wilkinson, A. (1987). Use and misuse of the concept of craving by alcohol, tobacco, and drug researchers. *British Journal of Addiction* **82**, 31–6.

Kreek, M.J. (1981). Medical management of methadone-maintained patients. In *Substance abuse: clinical problems and perspectives* (ed. J. Lowinson and P. Ruiz). Williams and Wilkins, Baltimore.

Kreek, M.J. (1996). Long-term pharmacotherapy for opiate (primarily heroin) addiction: opioid agonists. In *Pharmacological aspects of drug dependence* (ed. C. Schuster and M. Kuhar). Springer, Berlin.

Kreek, M.J. (1997*a*). Clinical update of opioid agonist and partial agonist medications for the maintenance treatment of opioid addiction. *Seminars in Neuroscience* **9**, 140–57.

Kreek, M.J. (1997b). Opiate and cocaine addictions: challenge for pharmacotherapies. *Pharmacology Biochemistry and Behavior* **57**, 551–69.

Kreek, M.J. (2000). Methadone-related opioid agonist pharmacotherapy for heroin addiction. History, recent molecular and neurochemical research and future in mainstream medicine. *Annals of the New York Academy of Sciences* **909**, 186–216.

Kreek, M.J. and Vocci, F. (2002). History and current status of opioid maintenance treatments. *Journal of Substance Abuse Treatment* **23**, 93–105.

Krupka, L. and Blume, E. (1980). Alcoholics Anonymous in a therapeutic community. *Journal of Drugs Education* **10**, 145–51.

Kuehnle, J. and Spitzer, R. (1981). DSM-III classification of substance use disorders. In *Substance abuse: clinical problems and perspectives* (ed. J. Lowinson and P. Ruiz). Williams and Wilkins, Baltimore.

Kumar, R. and Stolerman, I.P. (1977). Experimental and clinical aspects of drug dependence. In *Handbook of psychopharmacology* (ed. L.I. Iverson and S.D. Iverson). Plenum Press, New York.

Kurtzman, T.L., Otsuka, K.N., and Wahl, R.A. (2001). Inhalant abuse by adolescents. *Journal of Adolescent Health* **28**, 170–80.

Lacoste Marin, J. (1992). Esta cambiando la via de administracion de la heroina? [Is the administration route of heroin changing?] *Medicina Clinica* (*Barcelona*) **99**, 517.

Lader, M. and Marks, I. (1971). *Clinical anxiety*. Heineman, London.

Lambert, M. and Bergin, A. (1994). The effectiveness of psychotherapy. In *Handbook of psychotherapy and behavior change* (ed. A. Bergin and S. Garfield). Wiley, New York.

Lehman, A., Myers, C., Corty, E., and Thompson, J. (1994). Prevalence and patterns of 'dual diagnosis' among psychiatric inpatients. *Comprehensive Psychiatry* **35**, 106–12.

Lehman, W.E.R. and Simpson, D.D. (1990). Alcohol use. In *Opioid addiction and treatment: a 12 year follow-up* (ed. D.D. Simpson and S.B. Sells), pp. 177–92. Kreiger, Melbourne, Florida.

Leshner, A. (1997). Introduction to the special issue: the National Institute on Drug Abuse's Drug Abuse Treatment Outcome Study (DATOS). *Psychology of Addictive Behaviors* **11**, 211–15.

Levine, D.P. (1991). Skin and soft tissue infection in intravenous drug users. In *Infections in intravenous drug abusers* (ed. D.P. Levine and J.D. Sobel), pp. 3–26. Oxford University Press, New York.

Lewis, R. (1994). Flexible hierarchies and dynamic disorder: the trading and distribution of illicit heroin in Britain and Europe, 1970–1990. In *Heroin addiction and public policy: the British system* (ed. J. Strang and M. Gossop). Oxford University Press, Oxford.

Liese, B. and Najavits, L. (1997). Cognitive and behavioral therapies. In *Substance abuse: a comprehensive textbook* (ed. J. Lowinson, P. Ruiz, R. Millman, and J. Langrod). Williams and Wilkins, Baltimore.

Lincourt, P., Kuettel, T., and Bombardier, C. (2002). Motivational interviewing in a group setting with mandated clients: a pilot study. *Addictive Behaviors* **27**, 381–91.

Linden, C. (1990). Volatile substances of abuse. *Emergency Medicine Clinics in North America* **8**, 559–78.

Lindsay, S. (1983). The fear of dental treatment: a critical and theoretical analysis. In *Contributions to medical psychology*, Vol.III (ed. S. Rachman). Pergamon, Oxford.

Ling, W. and Wesson, D. (1984). Naltrexone treatment for addicted healthcare professionals: a collaborative private practice experience. *Journal of Clinical Psychiatry* **49**, 46–8.

Ling, W., Charuvastra, C., Kaim, S., and Klett, C. (1976). Methadyl acetate and methadone as maintenance treatments for heroin addicts. *Archives of General Psychiatry* 33, 709–20.

Lipton, D. and Appel, P. (1984). The state perspective. In *Strategies, progress and prospects* (ed. F. Tims and J. Ludford), NIDA Research Monograph no. 51. NIDA, Rockville, Maryland.

Lipton, D. and Maranda, M. (1983). Detoxification from heroin dependency: an overview of method and effectiveness. In *Evaluation of drug treatment programmes* (ed. B. Stimmel), pp. 31–55. Hawarth, New York.

Lipton, D., Brewington, V., and Smith, M. (1994). Acupuncture for crack-cocaine detoxification: experimental evaluation of efficacy. *Journal of Substance Abuse Treatment* 11, 205–15.

Litman, G.K., Eiser, J.R., Rawson, N., and Oppenheim, A.N. (1979). Differences in relapse precipitants and coping behaviours between alcohol relapsers and survivors. *Behaviour Research and Therapy* 17, 89–94.

Litt, M., Cooney, N., Kadden, R., and Gaupp, L. (1990). Reactivity to alcohol cues and induced moods in alcoholics. *Addictive Behaviors* 15, 137–46.

Loimer, N., Schmid, R, Presslich, O., and Lenz, K. (1989). Continuous naloxone administration suppresses opiate withdrawal symptoms in human opiate addicts during detoxification treatment. *Journal of Psychiatric Research* 23, 81–6.

Loimer, N., Lenz, K., Schmid, R., and Presslich, O. (1991). Technique for greatly shortening the transition from methadone to naltrexone maintenance of patients addicted to opiates. *American Journal of Psychiatry* 148, 933–5.

Loimer, N., Hoffman, P., and Chaudry, H. (1992). Nasal administration of naloxone for detection of opiate dependence. *Journal of Psychiatric Research* 26, 39–43.

Longshore, D., Hsieh, S.C., Danila, B., and Anglin, M.D. (1993). Methadone maintenance and needle/syringe sharing. *International Journal of the Addictions* 28, 983–96.

Louie, A.K., Lannon, R.A., and Ketter, T.A. (1989). Treatment of cocaine-induced panic. *American Journal of Psychiatry* 146, 40–4.

Love, J. and Gossop, M. (1985). The processes of referral and disposal within a London drug dependence clinic. *British Journal of Addiction* 80, 435–40.

Lowenstein, D., Massa, S., Rowbotham, M., Collins, S., McKinney, H., and Simon, P. (1987). Acute neurologic and psychiatric complications associated with cocaine abuse. *American Journal of Medicine* 83, 841–6.

Loxley, W., Phillips, M., Carruthers, S., and Bevan, J. (1997). The Australian study of HIV and injecting drug use: Part I: prevalence for HIV, hepatitis B and hepatitis C among injecting drug users in four Australian cities. *Drug and Alcohol Review* 16, 207–14.

Luborsky, L., McLellan, A.T., Woody, G., O'Brien, C., and Auerbach, A. (1985). Therapist success and its determinants. *Archives of General Psychiatry* 42, 602–11.

Maddux, J. (1988). Clinical experience with civil commitment. *Journal of Drug Issues* 18, 575–94.

Maddux, J., Desmond, D., and Esquivel, M. (1980). Outpatient methadone withdrawal for heroin dependence. *American Journal of Drug and Alcohol Abuse* 7, 323–33.

Maggio, C.A., Presta, E., and Bracco, E.F. (1985). Naltrexone and human eating behavior: a dose-ranging inpatient trial in moderately obese men. *Brain Research Bulletin* 14, 657–61.

Makela, K. (1993). International comparisons of Alcoholics Anonymous. *Alcohol, Health, and Research World* **17**, 228–34.

Mansour, A., Fox, C., Burke, S., and Watson, S. (1994). Immunohistochemical localization of the kappa1 opioid receptors. *Regulatory Peptides*, **54**, 177–8.

Mardones, J. (1955). Craving for alcohol. *Quarterly Journal of Studies on Alcohol* **16**, 51–3.

Margison, F., McGrath, G., Barkham, M., Mellor-Clark, J., Audin, K., and Connell, J. (2000). Measurement and psychotherapy. *British Journal of Psychiatry* **177**, 123–30.

Mark, T., Woody, G., Juday, T., and Kleber, H. (2001). The economic costs of heroin addiction in the United States. *Drug and Alcohol Dependence* **61**, 195–206.

Marks, J. (1985*a*). *The benzodiazepines: use, overuse, misuse, abuse*. MTP Press, Lancaster.

Marks, J. (1985*b*). Opium, the religion of the people. *Lancet* **1**, 1439–40.

Marlatt, G.A. (1985). Relapse prevention: theoretical rationale and overview of the model. In *Relapse prevention: maintenance strategies in the treatment of addictive behavior* (ed. G. A. Marlatt and J.R. Gordon). Guilford Press, New York.

Marlatt, G.A. (1987). Craving notes. *British Journal of Addiction* **82**, 42–4.

Marlatt, G.A. (1999). From hindsight to foresight: a commentary on Project MATCH. In *Changing addictive behavior* (ed. J. Tucker, D. Donovan, and G.A. Marlatt). Guilford Press, New York.

Marlatt, G.A. and Gordon, J.R. (1985). *Relapse prevention: maintenance strategies in the treatment of addictive behavior*. Guildford Press, New York.

Marlowe, D., Merikle, E., Kirby, K., Festinger, D., and McLellan, A.T. (2001). Multidimensional assessment of perceived treatment—entry pressures among substance abusers. *Psychology of Addictive Behaviors* **15**, 97–108.

Marrazzi, M., Wroblewski, J., Kinzie, J., and Lubie, E. (1997). High dose naltrexone and liver function safety. *American Journal on Addictions* **6**, 21–9.

Marsch, L.A. (1998). The efficacy of methadone maintenance interventions in reducing illicit opiate use, HIV risk behaviour and criminality: a meta-analysis. *Addiction* **93**, 515–32.

Marsden, J., Gossop, M., Stewart, D., Best, D., Farrell, M., Lehmann, P., Edwards, C., and Strang, J. (1998*a*). The Maudsley Addiction Profile (MAP): a brief instrument for assessing treatment outcome. *Addiction* **93**, 1857–67.

Marsden, J., Griffiths, P., Farrell, M., Gossop, M., and Strang, J. (1998*b*). Cocaine in Britain: prevalence, problems and treatment responses. *Journal of Drug Issues* **28**, 225–41.

Marsden, J., Gossop, M., Stewart, D., Rolfe, A., and Farrell, M. (2000*a*). Psychiatric symptoms amongst clients seeking treatment for drug dependence: intake data from the National Treatment Outcome Research Study. *British Journal of Psychiatry* **176**, 285–9.

Marsden, J., Stewart, D., Gossop, M., Rolfe, A., Bacchus, L., Griffiths, P., Clarke, K., and Strang, J. (2000*b*). Assessing client satisfaction with treatment for substance use problems and the development of the Treatment Perceptions Questionnaire (TPQ). *Addiction Research* **8**, 455–70.

Marsh, A. (1997). Hair analysis for drugs of abuse. *Syva Drug Monitor* **2**, 1–4.

Marsh, J., D'Aunno, T., and Smith, B. (2000). Increasing access and providing social services to improve drug abuse treatment for women with children. *Addiction* **95**, 1237–47.

Marsh, K. and Simpson, D.D. (1986). Sex differences in opioid addiction careers. *American Journal of Drug and Alcohol Abuse* **12**, 309–29.

Martin, D., Garske, J., and Davis, M. (2000). Relation of the therapeutic alliance with outcome and other variables: a meta-analytic review. *Journal of Consulting and Clinical Psychology* **68**, 438–50.

Martin, E. (1987). Managing drug addiction in general practice—the reality behind the guidelines. *Journal of the Royal Society of Medicine* **80**, 305–7.

Martin, S., Butzin, C., Saum, C., and Inciardi, J. (1999). Three-year outcomes of therapeutic community treatment for drug-involved offenders in Delaware: from prison to work release to aftercare. *The Prison Journal* **79**, 294–320.

Martin, W., Jasinski, D., and Mansky, P. (1973). Naltrexone: an antagonist for the treatment of heroin dependence. *Archives of General Psychiatry* **28**, 784–91.

Masek, B. (1982). Compliance and medicine. In *Behavioral medicine: assessment and treatment strategies* (ed. D. Doleys, R. Meredith, and A. Ciminero). Plenum, New York.

Matthai, S.M., Sills, J.A., Davidson, D.C., and Alexandrou, D. (1996). Cerebral oedema after ingestion of MDMA ('ecstasy') and unrestricted intake of water. *British Medical Journal* **312**, 1359.

Mattick, R. and Hall, W. (1996). Are detoxification programmes effective? *Lancet* **347**, 97–100.

Mattick, R., Oliphant, D., Ward, J., and Hall, W. (1998). The effectiveness of other opioid replacement therapies: LAAM, heroin, buprenorphine, naltrexone and injectable maintenance. In *Methadone maintenance treatment and other replacement therapies* (ed. J. Ward, R. Mattick, and W. Hall). Harwood, Amsterdam.

McBride, A.J., Sullivan, G., Blewitt, A.E., and Morgan, S. (1997). Amphetamine prescribing as a harm reduction measure: a preliminary study. *Addiction Research* **5**, 95–112.

McCann, U., Szabo, Z., Scheffel, U., Dannals, R., and Ricaurte, G. (1998). Positron emission tomographic evidence of toxic effect of MDMA ('Ecstasy') on brain serotonin neurones in human beings. *Lancet* **352**, 1433–7.

McCusker, J., Vickers-Lahti, M., Stoddard, A., Hindin, R., Bigelow, C., Zorn, M., Garfield, F., Frost, R., Love, C., and Lewis, B. (1995). The effectiveness of alternative planned durations of residential drug abuse treatment. *American Journal of Public Health* **85**, 1426–9.

McCusker, J., Bigelow, C., Vickers-Lahti, M., Spotts, D., Garfield, F., and Frost, R. (1997). Planned duration of residential drug abuse treatment: efficacy versus effectiveness. *Addiction* **92**, 1467–78.

McDowell, D. and Kleber, H. (1994). MDMA: its history and pharmacology. *Psychiatric Annals* **24**, 127–30.

McGarvey, E., Canterbury, R., and Waite, D. (1996). Delinquency and family problems in incarcerated adolescents with and without a history of inhalant use. *Addictive Behaviors* **21**, 537–42.

McInnes, E. and Powell, J. (1994). Drug and alcohol referrals: are elderly substance abuse diagnoses and referrals being missed? *British Medical Journal* **308**, 444–6.

McKay, J., Alterman, A., McLellan, A.T., and Snider, E. (1994). Treatment goals, continuity of care, and outcome in a day hospital substance abuse rehabilitation program. *American Journal of Psychiatry* **151**, 254–9.

McKay, J.R., Alterman, A.I., Rutherford, M.J., Cacciola, J.S., and McLellan, A.T. (1999). The relationship of alcohol use to cocaine relapse in cocaine dependent patients in an aftercare study. *Journal of Studies on Alcohol* **60**, 176–80.

McKeganey, N. (1988). Shadowland: general practitioners and the treatment of opiate-abusing patients. *British Journal of Addiction* **83**, 373–86.

McKeganey, N., Barnard, M., and Bloor, M. (1990). A comparison of HIV-related risk behaviour and risk reduction between female street working prostitutes and male rent boys in Glasgow. *Sociology of Health and Illness* **12**, 275–92.

McKim, W. (2000). *Drugs and behaviour*. Prentice Hall, New Jersey.

McLatchie, B. and Lomp, K. (1988). Alcoholics Anonymous affiliation and treatment outcome among a clinical sample of problem drinkers. *American Journal of Alcohol Abuse* **14**, 309–24.

McLellan, A.T. (2002). Have we evaluated addiction treatment correctly? Implications from a chronic care perspective. *Addiction* **97**, 249–52.

McLellan, A.T., Luborsky, L., O'Brien, C.P., and Woody, G.E. (1980). An improved evaluation instrument for substance abuse patients: the Addiction Severity Index. *Journal of Nervous and Mental Disease* **168**, 26–33.

McLellan A.T., Luborsky, L., Woody, G., Druley, K., and O'Brien, C. (1983). Predicting response to alcohol and drug abuse treatments: role of psychiatric severity. *Archives of General Psychiatry* **40**, 620–5.

McLellan, A.T., Luborsky, L., Cacciola, J., and Griffith, J.E. (1985). New data from the Addiction Severity Index: reliability and validity in three centers. *Journal of Nervous and Mental Disorders* **173**, 412–23.

McLellan, A.T., Childress, A., Ehrman, A., O'Brien, C., and Pasko, S. (1986). Extinguishing conditioned responses during opiate dependence treatment: turning laboratory findings into clinical procedures. *Journal of Substance Abuse Treatment* **3**, 33–40.

McLellan, A.T., Cacciola, J., Kushner, H., Peters, F., Smith, I., and Pettinati, H. (1992). The fifth edition of the Addiction Severity Index: cautions, additions and normative data. *Journal of Substance Abuse Treatment* **5**, 312–16.

McLellan, A.T., Arndt, I., Metzger, D., Woody, G., and O'Brien, C. (1993). The effects of psychosocial services in substance abuse treatment. *Journal of the American Medical Association* **269**, 1953–9.

McLellan A.T., Alterman, A., Metzger, D., Grissom, G., Woody, G., Luborsky, L., and O'Brien, C. (1994). Similarity of outcome predictors across opiate, cocaine, and alcohol treatments: role of treatment services. *Journal of Consulting and Clinical Psychology* **62**, 1141–58.

McLellan, A.T., Grissom, G.R., Zanis, D., Randall, M., Brill, P., and O'Brien, C. (1997*a*). Problem-service 'matching' in addiction treatment: a prospective study in 4 programs. *Archives of General Psychiatry* **54**, 730–5.

McLellan, A.T., Wood, G.E., Metzger, D.S., McKay, J., and Alterman, A.I. (1997*b*). Evaluating the effectiveness of addiction treatments: reasonable expectations, appropriate comparisons. In *Treating drug abusers effectively* (ed. J.A. Egerton, D.M. Fox, and A.I. Leshner). Blackwells, Oxford.

McLellan, A.T., Hagan, T., Levine, M., Gould, F., Meyers, K., Bencivengo, M., and Durrell, J. (1998). Supplemental social services improve outcomes in public addiction treatment. *Addiction* **93**, 1489–99.

McLellan, A.T., Lewis, D., O'Brien, C., and Kleber, H. (2000). Drug dependence, a chronic medical illness: implications for treatment, insurance, and outcome evaluation. *Journal of the American Medical Association* **284**, 1689–95.

McLellan, D.L. (1997). Introduction to rehabilitation. In *Rehabilitation studies handbook* (ed. B. Wilson and D.L. McLellan). Cambridge University Press, Cambridge.

McPherson, T. and Hersch, R. (2000). Brief substance use screening instruments for primary care settings: a review. *Journal of Substance Abuse Treatment* **18**, 193–202.

Meichenbaum, D. (1977). *Cognitive–behavior modification: an integrative approach*. Plenum Press, New York.

Meichenbaum, D. and Turk, D. (1987). *Facilitating treatment adherence*. Plenum, New York.

Mello, N., Mendelson, J., Kuehnle, J., and Sellers, M. (1981). Operant analysis of human heroin self-administration and the effects of naltrexone. *Journal of Pharmacology and Experimental Therapeutics* **216**, 45–54.

Messina, N., Wish, E., and Nemes, S. (2000). Predictors of treatment outcomes in men and women admitted to a therapeutic community. *American Journal of Drug and Alcohol Abuse* **26**, 207–27.

Metrebian, N., Shanahan, W., Wells, B., and Stimson, G. (1998). Feasibility of prescribing injectable heroin and methadone to opiate-dependent drug users: associated health gains and harm reductions. *Medical Journal of Australia* **168**, 596–600.

Metzger, D.S., Woody, G.E., McLellan A.T., O'Brien, C.P., Druley, P., Navaline, H., DePhilippis, D., Stolley, P., and Abrutyn, E. (1993). Human immunodeficiency virus seroconversion among intravenous drug users in-and out of treatment: an 18 month prospective follow up. *AIDS* **6**, 1049–56.

Meyer, R. and Mirin, S. (1979). *The heroin stimulus*. Plenum, New York.

Meyers, K., Hagan, T., Zanis, D., Webb, A., Frantz, J, Ring-Kurtz, S., Rutherford, M., and McLellan, A.T. (1999). Critical issues in adolescent substance use assessment. *Drug and Alcohol Dependence* **55**, 235–46.

Miller, N., Belkin, B., and Gold, M. (1991). Alcohol and drug dependence among the elderly. *Comprehensive Psychiatry* **32**, 153–65.

Miller, W.R. (1978). Behavioural treatment of problem drinkers: a comparative outcome study of three controlled drinking therapies. *Journal of Consulting and Clinical Psychology* **46**, 74–86.

Miller, W.R. (1983). Motivational interviewing with problem drinkers. *Behavioural Psychotherapy* **1**, 147–72.

Miller, W.R. and McCrady, B.S. (1993). The importance of research on Alcoholics Anonymous. In *Research on Alcoholics Anonymous* (ed. B.S. McCrady and W.R. Miller), pp. 3–11. Rutgers Center of Alcohol Studies, New Brunswick, New Jersey.

Miller, W.R. and Rollnick, S. (1991). *Motivational interviewing*. Guilford, New York.

Miller, W.R., Leckman, A.L., Delaney, H.D., and Tinkcom, M. (1992). Long-term follow-up of behavioural self-control training. *Journal of Studies on Alcohol* **53**, 249–61.

Mirin, S.M., Meyer, R.E., and McNamee, H.B. (1976). Psychopathology and mood during heroin use: acute vs. chronic effects. *Archives of General Psychiatry* **33**, 1503–8.

Mitcheson, M. (1994). Drug clinics in the 1970s. In *Heroin addiction and drug policy: the British system* (ed. J. Strang and M. Gossop). Oxford University Press, London.

Mitcheson, M., Edwards, G., Hawks, D., and Ogborne, A. (1976). Treatment of methylamphetamine users during the 1968 epidemic. In *Drugs and drug dependence* (ed. G. Edwards, M. Russell, D. Hawks, and M. MacCafferty). Saxon House, Westmead.

Mo, B. and Way, E. (1966). Assessment of inhalation as a mode of administration of heroin by addicts. *Journal of Pharmacology and Experimental Therapeutics* **154**, 142–51.

Modesto-Lowe, V. and Kranzler, H. (1999). Using cue reactivity to evaluate medications for treatment of cocaine dependence: a critical review. *Addiction* **94**, 1639–51.

Moggi, F., Ouimette, P., Moos, R., and Finney, J. (1999). Dual diagnosis patients in substance abuse treatment: relationship of general coping and substance specific coping to 1 year outcomes. *Addiction* **94**, 1805–16.

Moise, R., Reed, B., and Ryan, V. (1982). Issues in the treatment of heroin-addicted women: a comparison of men and women entering two types of drug abuse programs. *International Journal of the Addictions* **17**, 109–39.

Montgomery, H.A., Miller, W.R., and Tonigan, J.S. (1995). Does Alcoholics Anonymous involvement predict treatment outcome? *Journal of Substance Abuse Treatment* **12**, 241–6.

Moos, R.H. (1997). *Evaluating treatment environments.* Transaction, New Brunswick.

Moos, R.H., Finney, J.W., and Cronkite, R.C. (1990). *Alcoholism treatment: context, process and outcome.* Oxford University Press, New York.

Moos, R.H., Mertens, J., and Brennan, P. (1993). Patterns of diagnosis and treatment among late middle-aged and older substance abuse patients. *Journal of Studies on Alcohol* **54**, 479–87.

Moos, R.H., Finney, J.W., Ouimette, P.C., and Suchinsky, R. (1999). A comparative evaluation of substance abuse treatment: I. Treatment orientation, amount of care, and 1-year outcomes. *Alcoholism, Clinical and Experimental Research* **23**, 529–36.

Moos, R.H., Finney, J. W., Federman, E., and Suchinsky, R. (2000). Speciality mental health care improves patients' outcomes: findings from a nationwide program to monitor the quality of care for patients with substance use disorders. *Journal of Studies on Alcohol* **61**, 704–13.

Morgan, J. (1981). Amphetamine. In *Substance abuse: clinical problems and perspectives* (ed. J. Lowinson and P. Ruiz). Williams and Wilkins, Baltimore.

Morgenstern, J., Labouvie, E., McCrady, B.S., Kahler, C.W., and Frey, R.M. (1997). Affiliation with Alcoholics Anonymous after treatment: a study of its therapeutic effects and mechanisms of action. *Journal of Consulting and Clinical Psychology* **65** (5), 768–77.

Morral, A., Iguchi, M., Belding, M., and Lamb, R. (1997). Natural classes of treatment response. *Journal of Consulting and Clinical Psychology* **65**, 673–85.

Morral, A.R., McCaffrey, D., and Iguchi, M. (2000). Hardcore drug users claim to be occasional users: frequency underreporting. *Drug and Alcohol Dependence* **57**, 193–202.

Moss, A. and Chaisson, R. (1988). AIDS and intravenous drug use in San Francisco. *AIDS and Public Policy* **3**, 37–41.

Moss, A.R., Vranizan, K., Gorter, R., and Bacchetti, P. (1994). HIV seroconversion in intravenous drug users in San Francisco, 1985–1990. *AIDS* **8**, 223–31.

Mueser, K., Drake, R., and Miles, K. (1997). The course and treatment of substance use disorders in persons with severe mental illness. In NIDA Research Monograph no.172. NIDA, Rockville, Maryland.

Mulvaney, F., Brown, L., Alterman, A., Sage, R., Cnaan, A., Cacciola, J., and Rutherford, M. (1999). Methadone maintenance outcomes for Hispanic and African-American men and women. *Drug and Alcohol Dependence* **54**, 11–18.

Myers, T., Cocherill, R., Worthington, C., Millson, M., and Rankin, J. (1998). Community pharmacist perspectives on HIV/AIDS and interventions for injection drug users in Canada. *AIDS Care* **10**, 689–700.

Myles, J. (1997). Treatment for amphetamine misuse in the United Kingdom. In *Amphetamine misuse* (ed. H. Klee). Harwood, Amsterdam.

Narcotics Anonymous (1988). *The NA big book*. World Service Office, Van Nuys, California.

National Research Council Committee on Clinical Evaluation of Narcotic Antagonists. (1978). Clinical evaluation of naltrexone treatment of opiate-dependent individuals. *Archives of General Psychiatry* **35**, 335–40.

Negrete, J. (1992). Cocaine problems in the coca-growing countries of South America. In *Cocaine: scientific and social dimensions* (ed. G. Bock and J. Whelan). Wiley, Chichester.

Negrete, J. (1999). A contrast in treatment philosophies. *Addiction* **94**, 59–62.

Neeleman, J. and Farrell, M. (1997). Fatal methadone and heroin overdoses: time trends in England and Wales. *Journal of Epidemiology and Community Health* **51**, 435–7.

Nemoto, T., Aoki, B., Huang, K., Morris, A., Nguyen, H., and Wong, W. (1999). Drug use behaviors among Asian drug users in San Francisco. *Addictive Behaviors* **24**, 823–38.

Newcomb, M. (1995). Identifying high risk youth: prevalence and patterns of adolescent drug abuse. In *Adolescent drug abuse: clinical assessment and therapeutic interventions* (ed. E. Rahdert and D. Czechowicz), NIDA Research Monograph no. 156. US Government Printing Office, Washington, DC.

Nictern, S. (1973). The children of drug users. *Journal of the Academy of Child Psychiatry* **12**, 24–31.

Nir, I. (1980). Central nervous system stimulants. In *Meyler's side effects of drugs* (ed. M. Dukes). Excerpta Medica, Amsterdam.

Nirenberg, T., Cellucci, T., Liepman, L., Swift, R., and Sirota, A. (1996). Cannabis versus other illicit drug use among methadone maintenance patients. *Psychology of Addictive Behaviours* **10**, 222–7.

Noble, A., Best, B., Finch, E., Gossop, M., Sidwell, C., and Strang, J. (2000). Injecting risk behaviour and year of first injection as predictors of hepatitis B and C status among methadone maintenance patients in south London. *Journal of Substance Use* **5**, 131–5.

Nunes, E.V., Quitkin, F.M., Brady, R., and Stewart, J.W. (1991). Imipramine treatment of methadone maintenance patients with affective disorder and illicit drug use. *American Journal of Psychiatry* **148**, 667–9.

Nurco, D. and Makofsky, A. (1981). The self-help movement and Narcotics Anonymous. *American Journal of Drug and Alcohol Abuse* **8**, 139–51.

Nurco, D., Wegner, N., Stephenson, P., Makofsky, A., and Shaffer, J. (1983). *Ex-addicts' self-help groups*. Praeger, New York.

Nurco, D., Shaffer, J., and Cisin, I.H. (1984). An ecological analysis of the interrelationships among drug abuse and other indices of social pathology. *International Journal of the Addictions* **19**, 441–51.

Nurco, D.N., Hanlon, T.E., Kinlock, T.W., and Duszynski, K.R. (1989). The consistency of types of criminal behaviour over preaddiction, addiction, non-addiction status periods. *Comprehensive Psychiatry* **30**, 391–402.

Nurco, D., Kinlock, T., and Balter, M. (1993). The severity of pre-addiction criminal behaviour among urban, male narcotic addicts and two non addicted control groups. *Journal of Research in Crime and Delinquency* **30** (3), 293–316.

Obadia, Y., Perrin, V., Feroni, I., Vlahov, D., and Moatti, J.P. (2001). Injecting misuse of buprenorphine among French drug users. *Addiction* **96**, 267–72.

O'Brien, C. (1994). Opioids: antagonists and partial antagonists. In *Textbook of substance abuse treatment* (ed. M. Galanter and H. Kleber). American Psychiatric Press, Washington, DC.

O'Brien, C. and Childress, A.R. (1991). Behaviour therapy of drug dependence. In *Addiction behaviour* (ed. I. Glass). Routledge, London.

O'Brien, C. and Cornish, J. (1999). Opioids: antagonists and partial antagonists. In *Textbook of substance abuse treatment*, 2nd edn (ed. M. Galanter and H. Kleber). American Psychiatric Press, Washington, DC.

O'Brien, C., Chaddock, B., Woody, G., and Greenstein, R. (1974). Systematic extinction of addiction-associated rituals using narcotic antagonists. *Psychosomatic Medicine* **36**, 458.

O'Brien, C., Greenstein, R., Mintz, J., and Woody, G. (1975). Clinical experience with naltrexone. *American Journal of Drug and Alcohol Abuse* **2**, 365–77.

O'Brien, C., Childress, A., McLellan, A., and Ehrman, R. (1990). Integrating systematic cue exposure with standard treatment in recovering drug dependent patients. *Addictive Behaviors* **15**, 355–65.

O'Donnell, J. (1969). *Narcotic addicts in Kentucky*. US Government Printing Office, Washington, DC.

Office of National Drug Control Policy (1998). *Pulse check trends in drug abuse January–June 1998*. Office of National Drug Control Policy, Rockville, Maryland.

O'Leary, K. and Wilson, G. (1975). *Behavior therapy: application and outcome*. Prentice Hall, Englewood Cliffs, New Jersey.

Oleske, J. (1977). Experiences with 118 infants born to narcotic-using mothers. *Clinical Pediatrics* **16**, 418–23.

O'Neil, J., Baker, P., and Gough, T. (1984). Illicitly imported heroin products: some physical and chemical features indicative of their origin. *Journal of Forensic Science* **29**, 885–902.

Onken, L.S., Blaine, J.D., and Boren, J.J. (1997). *Treatment for drug addiction: it won't work if they don't receive it*, NIDA Research Monograph no. 165. NIDA, Rockville, Maryland.

Oppenheimer, E., Tobutt, C., Taylor, C., and Andrew, T. (1994). Death and survival in a cohort of heroin addicts from London clinics: a 22-year follow-up. *Addiction* **89**, 1299–308.

Orford, J. (1985). *Excessive appetites*. Wiley, New York.

Orford, J. (1999). Future directions: a commentary on Project MATCH. *Addiction* **94**, 62–6.

Orford, J. (2001). *Excessive appetites: a psychological view of addictions*. Wiley, Chichester.

Ouimette, P.C., Finney, J.W., and Moos, R.H. (1997). Twelve-step and cognitive–behavioral treatment for substance abuse: a comparison of treatment effectiveness. *Journal of Consulting and Clinical Psychology* **65**, 230–40.

Ouimette, P.C., Moos, R.H., and Finney, J.W. (1998). Influence of outpatient treatment and 12-step group involvement on one-year substance abuse treatment outcomes. *Journal of Studies on Alcohol* **59**, 513–22.

Ouimette, P., Humphreys, K., Moos, R.H., Finney, J.W., Cronkite, R., and Federman, B. (2001). Self-help group participation among substance use disorder patients with posttraumatic stress disorder. *Journal of Substance Abuse Treatment* **20**, 25–32.

Parker, H., Newcombe, R., and Bakx, K. (1987). The new heroin users: prevalence and characteristics in the Wirral, Merseyside. *British Journal of Addiction* **82**, 147–58.

Parrott, A. (2002). Recreational Ecstasy/MDMA, the serotonin syndrome, and serotonergic neurotoxicity. *Pharmacology, Biochemistry and Behavior* **71**, 837–44.

Pascal, C. (1988). *Intravenous drug abuse and AIDS transmission: federal and state laws regulating needle availability*, NIDA Research Monograph no. 80. NIDA,Rockville, Maryland.

Patterson, L. and Welfel, E.R. (1994). *The counseling process*. Brooks/Cole Publishing, Pacific Grove, California.

Pearson, G. (1991). The local nature of drug problems. In *Drug misuse in local communities: perspectives across Europe* (ed. T. Bennett). The Police Foundation, London.

Pearson, G. and Gilman, M. (1994). Local and regional variations in drug misuse: the British heroin epidemic of the 1980s. In *Heroin addiction and drug policy: the British system* (ed. J. Strang and M. Gossop). Oxford University Press, Oxford.

Pechnick, R. and Ungerleider, J.T. (1997). Hallucinogens. In *Substance abuse: a comprehensive textbook* (ed. J. Lowinson, P. Ruiz, R. Millman, and J. Langrod). Williams and Wilkins, Baltimore.

Pederson, L. and Lefcoe, N. (1976). A psychological and behavioural comparison of ex-smokers and smokers. *Journal of Chronic Diseases* **29**, 431–4.

Perez-Reyes, M., White, R., McDonald, S., Hill, J., Jeffcoat, R., and Cook, C. (1991). Phamacologic effects of methamphetamine vapor inhalation (smoking). in man. In *CPDD, problems of drug dependence*, NIDA Research Monograph no. 105. Government Printing Office, Washington, DC.

Perneger, T., Giner, F., del Rio, M., and Mino, A. (1998). Randomised trial of heroin maintenance programme for addicts who fail in conventional drug treatments. *British Medical Journal* **317**, 13–18.

Pessione, F., Degos, F., Marcellin, P., Duchatelle, V., Njapoum, C., Martinot-Peignoux, M., Degott, C., Valla, D., Erlinger, S., and Rueff, B. (1998). Effect of alcohol consumption on serum hepatitis C virus RNA and histological lesions in chronic hepatitis C. *Hepatology* **27**, 1717–22.

Peterson, K., Swindle, R., Phibbs, C., Recine, B., and Moos, R. (1994). Determinants of readmission following inpatient substance abuse treatment. *Medical Care* **32**, 535–50.

Petrakis, I., Carroll, K., Gordon, L., Cushing, G., and Rounsaville, B. (1994). Fluoxetine treatment for dually diagnosed methadone maintained opioid addicts: a pilot study. In *Experimental therapeutics in addiction medicine*, pp. 25–33. Haworth Press, New York.

Petursson, H. and Lader, M. (1984). *Dependence on tranquillizers*. Oxford University Press, Oxford.

Pfohl, D., Allen, J., Atkinson, R., Knopman, D., Malcolm, R., Mitchell, J., and Morley, J. (1986). *Naltrexone hydrochloride (Trexan): a review of serum transaminase elevations at high dosage*, NIDA Research Monograph no. 67, pp. 66–72. Rockville, Maryland.

Phillips, G., Gossop, M., and Bradley, B. (1986). The influence of psychological factors on the opiate withdrawal syndrome. *British Journal of Psychiatry* **149**, 235–8.

Philpot, C., Harcourt, C., and Edwards, J. (1989). Drug use in Sydney. *British Journal of Addiction* **84**, 499–505.

Platt, J.J. (1995). *Heroin addiction: theory, research, and treatment*. Krieger, Malabar, Florida.

Podell, R. and Gary, L. (1976). Compliance: a problem in medical management. *American Family Physician* **13**, 74–80.

Polcin, D. and Weisner, C. (1999). Factors associated with coercion in entering treatment for alcohol problems. *Drug and Alcohol Dependence* **54**, 63–8.

Pottier, A., Taylor, J., Norman, C., Meyer, L., Anderson, H., and Ramsey, J. (1992). *Trends in deaths associated with abuse of volatile substances 1971–1990*, Department of Public Health Sciences, report no.5. Department of Public Health Sciences, London.

Powell, J., Dawe, S., Richards, D., Gossop, M., Marks, I., Strang, J., and Gray, J. (1993). Can opiate addicts tell us about their relapse risk? Subjective predictors of clinical prognosis. *Addictive Behaviors* **18**, 473–90.

Powis, B., Griffiths, P., Gossop, M., and Strang, J. (1996). The differences between male and female drug users: community samples of heroin and cocaine users compared. *Substance Use and Misuse* **31**, 529–43.

Powis, B., Strang, J., Griffiths, P., Taylor, C., Williamson, S., Fountain, J., and Gossop, M. (1999). Self-reported overdose among injecting drug users in London: extent and nature of the problem. *Addiction* **94**, 471–8.

Powis, B., Gossop, M., Bury, C., Payne, K. and Griffiths, P. (2000). Drug using mothers: social, psychological and substance use problems of women opiate users with children. *Drug and Alcohol Review* **19**, 171–80.

Prescott, L. (1983). Safety of the benzodiazepines. In *The benzodiazepines* (ed. E. Costa). Raven Press, New York.

Prochaska, J. and DiClemente, C. (1982). Transtheoretical therapy: towards a more integrative model of change. *Psychotherapy: Theory, Research and Practice* **19**, 276–88.

Prochaska, J., Velicer, W., Guadagnoli, E., Rossi, J., and DiClemente, C. (1991). Patterns of change: dynamic typology applied to smoking cessation. *Multivariate Behavioral Research* **26**, 83–107.

Prochaska, J., DiClemente, C., and Norcross, J. (1992). In search of how people change: applications to the addictive behaviors. *American Psychologist* **47**, 1102–14.

Project MATCH Research Group (1997). Matching alcoholism treatment to client heterogeneity: project MATCH posttreatment drinking outcomes. *Journal of Studies on Alcohol* **58**, 7–29.

Project MATCH Research Group (1998). Matching alcoholism treatment to client heterogeneity: project MATCH three year drinking outcomes. *Alcoholism: Clinical and Experimental Research* **22**, 1300–11.

Rachman, S. and Teasdale, J. (1969). *Aversion therapy and behaviour disorders*. University of Miami Press, Florida.

Rapaport, R.N. (1960). *Community as doctor*. Tavistock Publications, London.

Ravndal, E. and Vaglum, P. (1994). Treatment of female addicts: the importance of relationships to parents, partners, and peers for the outcome. *International Journal of the Addictions* **29**, 115–25.

Rawson, R., Washton, A., Resnick, R., and Tennant, F. (1981). Clonidine hydrochloride detoxification from methadone treatment: the value of naltrexone aftercare. In *Problem of drug dependence 1980* (ed. L. Harris), Research Monograph no. 34. NIDA, Rockville, Maryland.

Rawson, R., Hasson, A., Huber, A., McCann, M., and Ling, W. (1998). A 3-year progress report on the implementation of LAAM in the United States. *Addiction* **93**, 533–40.

Rawson, R., McCann, M., Hasson, A., and Ling, W. (2000). Addiction pharmacology 2000: new options, new challenges. *Journal of Psychoactive Drugs* **32**, 371–8.

Rawson, R., Gonzales, R., and Brethen, P. (2002). Treatment of methamphetamine use disorders: an update. *Journal of Substance Abuse Treatment* **23**, 145–50.

Reddy, D., Smith, R., Elliott, J., Haddad, G., and Wanek, E. (1986). Infected femoral artery false aneurysms in drug addicts: evolution of selective vascular reconstruction. *Journal of Vascular Surgery* **3**, 718–24.

Redliner, I. (1994). Healthcare for the homeless: lessons from the front line. *New England Journal of Medicine* **331**, 327–8.

Reed, B. (1987). Developing women-sensitive drug dependence treatment services: why so difficult? *Journal of Psychoactive Drugs* **19**, 151–64.

Regan, D., Ehrlich, S., and Finnegan, L. (1987). Infants of drug addicts: at risk for child abuse, neglect, and placement in foster care. *Neurotoxicology and Teratology* **9**, 315–19.

Regier, D.A., Farmer, M.E., Rae, D.S., Locke, B.Z., Keith, S.J., Judd, L.L., and Goodwin, F.K., (1990). Comorbidity of mental disorders with alcohol and other drug abuse: results from the Epidemiological Catchment Area (ECA). Study. *Journal of the American Medical Association* **21**, 2511–18.

Rehm, J., Gschwend, P., Steffen, T., Gutzwiller, F., Dobler-Mikola, A., and Uchtenhagen, A. (2001). Feasibility, safety, and efficacy of injectable heroin prescription for refractory opioid addicts: a follow-up study. *The Lancet* **358**, 1417–23.

Reilly, P. M., Sees, K.L., Hall, S.M., Shropshire, M.S., Delucchi, K.L., Tusel, D.J., Banys, P., Clark, H.W., and Piotrowski, N.A. (1995). Self efficacy and illicit opioid use in a 180-day methadone detoxification treatment. *Journal of Consulting and Clinical Psychology* **63** (1), 158–62.

Rementaria, J. and Nunag, N. (1973). Narcotic withdrawal in pregnancy: stillbirth incidence with a case report. *American Journal of Obstetrics and Gynecology* **116**, 1152.

Resnick, R. (1983). Methadone detoxification from illicit opiates and methadone maintenance. In *Research on the treatment of narcotic addiction* (ed. J. Cooper, F. Altman, B. Brown, and D. Czechowicz). NIDA, US Dept of Human Sciences, Rockville, Maryland.

Resnick, R., Kestenbaum, R., Washton, A., and Poole, D. (1977). Naloxone-precipitated withdrawal: a method for rapid induction onto naltrexone. *Clinical Pharmacology and Therapeutics* **21**, 409–13.

Resnick, R., Schuyten-Resnick, E., and Washton, A. (1979). Narcotic antagonists in the treatment of opioid dependence: review and commentary. *Comprehensive Psychiatry* **20**, 116–25.

Reuter, P. (1997). Why can't we make prohibition work better? Some consequences of ignoring the unattractive. *Proceedings of the American Philosophical Society* **141**, 262–75.

Reuter, P., MacCoun, R., and Murphy, P. (1990). *Money from crime: a study of the economics of drug dealing in Washington, D.C.* RAND, Santa Monica.

Reynaud, M., Petit, G., Potard, D., and Courty, P. (1998). Six deaths linked to concomitant use of buprenorphine and benzodiazepines. *Addiction* **93**, 1385–92.

Ricaurte, G., Yuan, J., and McCann, U. (2000). 3, 4-Methylenedioxymethamphetamine (MDMA, 'Ecstasy')-induced serotonin neurotoxicity: studies in animals. *Neuropsychobiology* **42**, 5–10.

Richardson, H. (1989). Volatile substance abuse: evaluation and treatment. *Human Toxicology* **8**, 319–22.

Ridgely, M., Goldman, H., and Willenbring, M. (1990). Barriers to the care of persons with dual diagnoses: organisational and financing issues. *Schizophrenia Bulletin* **16**, 123–32.

Risser, D. and Schneider, B. (1994). Drug-related deaths between 1985 and 1992 examined at the Institute of Forensic Medicine in Vienna, Austria. *Addiction* **89**, 851–7.

Risser, D., Uhl, A., Stichenwirth, M., Honigschabl, S., Hirz, W., Schneider, B., Stellag-Carion, C., Klupp, N., Vycudilik, W., and Bauer, G. (2000). Quality of heroin and heroin-related deaths from 1987–1995 in Vienna, Austria. *Addiction* **95**, 375–82.

Rivara, F.P., Mueller, B.A., Somes, G., Mendoza, C.T., Rushforth, N.B., and Kellerman, A.L. (1997). Alcohol and illicit drug abuse and the risk of violent death in the home. *Journal of the American Medical Association* **278**, 569–75.

Roberts, K., McNulty, H., Gruer, L., Scott, R., and Bryson, S. (1997). The role of Glasgow pharmacists in the management of drug misuse. *International Journal of Drug Policy* **9**, 187–94.

Robles, E., Silverman, K., and Stitzer, M. (1999). Contingency management therapies. In *Methadone treatment for opioid dependence* (ed. E. Strain and M. Stitzer). Johns Hopkins University Press, Baltimore.

Robles, E., Silverman, K., Preston, K, Cone, E., Katz, E., Bigelow, G., and Stitzer, M. (2000). The brief abstinence test: voucher-based reinforcement of cocaine abstinence. *Drug and Alcohol Dependence* **58**, 205–12.

Roche, A., Guray, C., and Saunders, J. (1991). General practitioners' experiences of patients with drug and alcohol problems. *British Journal of Addiction* **86**, 263–75.

Rohsenow, D., Monti, P., Abrams, D., Rubonis, A., Niaura, R., Sirota, A., and Colby, S. (1992). Cue elicited urge to drink and salivation in alcoholics: relationship to individual differences. *Advances in Behavior Research and Therapy* **14**, 195–210.

Rollnick, S. (2001). Enthusiasm, quick fixes and premature controlled trials. Addiction **96**, 1769–75.

Rosenbaum, M. and Murphy, S. (1981). Getting the treatment: recycling women addicts. *Journal of Psychoactive Drugs* **13**, 1–13.

Rossetti, Z.L., Hmaidan, Y., and Gessa, G.L. (1992). Marked inhibition of mesolimbic dopamine release: a common feature of ethanol, morphine, cocaine and amphetamine abstinence in rats. *European Journal of Pharmacology* **221**, 227–34.

Rossow, I. and Lauritzen, G. (1999). Balancing on the edge of death: suicide attempts and life-threatening overdoses among drug addicts. *Addiction* **94**, 209–19.

Roszell, D.K., Calsyn, D.A., and Chaney, E.F. (1986). Alcohol use and psychopathology in opioid addicts on methdone maintenance. *American Journal of Drug and Alcohol Abuse* **12**, 269–78.

Rotgers, F. (1992). Coercion in addictions treatment. *Annual Review of Addiction Research and Treatment* **2**, 403–16.

Rounsaville, B.J. (1995). Can psychotherapy rescue naltrexone treatment of opioid addiction? In *Integrating behavioral therapies with medications in the treatment of drug dependence* (ed. L. Onken, J. Blaine, and J. Boren), NIDA Monograph no.150. NIDA, Rockville, Maryland.

Rounsaville, B.J. and Kleber, H. (1985). Psychotherapy/counseling for opiate addicts: strategies for use in different treatment settings. *International Journal of the Addictions* **20**, 869–96.

Rounsaville, B.J., Weissman, M.M., Crits-Christoph, K., Wilber, C., and Kleber, H. (1982). Diagnosis and symptoms of depression in opiate addicts. *Archives of General Psychiatry* **39**, 151–6.

Rounsaville, B.J., Kosten, T., Weissman, M., and Kleber, H. (1986). Prognostic significance of psychopathology in treated opiate addicts. *Comprehensive Psychiatry* **27**, 480–98.

Rounsaville, B.J., Kosten, T., and Kleber, H. (1987). The antecedents and benefits of achieving abstinence in opioid addicts: a 2.5 year follow-up study. *American Journal of Drug and Alcohol Abuse* **13**, 213–29.

Rounsaville, B.J., Bryant, K., Babor, T., Kranzler, H., and Kadden, R. (1993). Cross system agreement for substance use disorders. DSM-III-R, DSM-IV, and ICD10. *Addiction* **88**, 337–48.

Royal College of Physicians. (1987). *The medical consequences of alcohol abuse.* Tavistock, London.

Royal College of Psychiatrists (1986). *Alcohol: our favourite drug.* Royal College of Psychiatrists, Tavistock, London.

Royal College of Psychiatrists and Royal College of Physicians (2000). *Drugs: dilemmas and choices.* Gaskell, London.

Ruben, S. and Morrison, C. (1992). Temazepam misuse in a group of injecting drug users. *British Journal of Addiction* **87**, 1387–92.

Russo, J. (1968). *Amphetamine abuse.* Charles C. Thomas, Springfield, Illinois.

Ruttenber, A. and Luke, J. (1984). Heroin-related deaths: new epidemiological insights. *Science* **226**, 14–20.

Ryan, L., Ehrlich, S., and Finnegan, L. (1987). Cocaine abuse in pregnancy: effects on the fetus and newborn. *Neurotoxicology and Teratology* **9**, 295–9.

Sackett, D. and Snow, J. (1979). The magnitude of compliance and noncompliance. In *Compliance in healthcare* (ed. R. Haynes, D. Taylor, and D. Sackett). Johns Hopkins University Press, Baltimore.

SAMHSA (Substance Abuse and Mental Health Services Administration). (1996). *National Drug and Alcoholism Treatment Unit Survey (NDATUS): data for 1994 and 1980–1994.* US Department of Health and Human Services, Public Health Service, Rockville, Maryland.

SAMHSA (2001). *Summary of findings from the 2000 National Household Survey on Drug Abuse.* Substance Abuse and Mental Health Services Administration, Rockville, Maryland.

San, L., Puig, M., Bulbena, A., and Farre, M. (1995). High risk of ultra-short noninvasive opiate detoxification. *American Journal of Psychiatry* **152**, 956.

Saunders, B., Wilkinson, C., and Phillips, M. (1995). The impact of a brief motivational intervention with opiate users attending a methadone programme. *Addiction* **90**, 415–24.

Saunders, W. and Kershaw, P. (1979). Spontaneous remission from alcoholism—a community study. *British Journal of Addiction* **74**, 251–6.

Sax, D., Kornetsky, C., and Kim, A. (1994). Lack of hepatotoxicity with naltrexone treatment. *Journal of Clinical Pharmacology* **34**, 898–901.

Saxon, A., Caslyn, D., Greenberg, D., Blaes, P., Haver, V., and Stanton, V. (1993). Urine screening for marijuana among methadone-maintained patients. *American Journal on Addictions* **2**, 207–11.

Saxon, A., Wells, E., Fleming, C., Jackson, R., and Calsyn, D. (1996). Pre-treatment characteristics, program philosophy and level of ancillary services as predictors of methadone maintenance treatment outcome. *Addiction* **91**, 1197–209.

Schachter, S. (1982). Recidivism and self-cure of smoking and obesity. *American Psychologist* **37**, 436–44.

Schlomer, G. (1955). Morphine withdrawal in addicts by the method of prolonged sleep. In *Management of addictions* (ed. E. Podolsky). Philosophical Library, New York.

Schoenbaum, E., Hartel, D., Selwyn, P., *et al.* (1989). Risk factors for human imm unodeficiency virus infection in intravenous drug users. *New England Journal of Medicine* **321**, 874–9.

Schuckit, M.A. (1983*a*). Alcoholism and other psychiatric disorders. *Hospital and Community Psychiatry* **34**, 1022–6.

Schuckit, M.A. (1983*b*). A clinical review of alcohol, alcoholism, and the elderly patient. *Journal of Clinical Psychiatry* **43**, 396–9.

Schuckit, M.A. (1985). The clinical implications of primary diagnostic groups among alcoholics. *Archives of General Psychiatry* **42**, 1043–9.

Schuckit, M.A. (1989). *Drug and alcohol abuse: a clinical guide to diagnosis and treatment.* Plenum, New York.

Schuckit, M.A. and Hesselbrock, V. (1994). Alcohol dependence and anxiety disorders: what is the relationship? *American Journal of Psychiatry* **151**, 1723–34.

Schut, J., Wohlmuth, T., and File, K. (1973). Low dosage maintenance: a reexamination. *International Journal of Clinical Pharmacology and Toxicology* **7**, 48–53.

Scott, J., Kennedy, A.J., Winfield, J., and Bond, C. (1997). Investigation into the effectiveness of filters for use by intravenous drug users. *International Journal of Drug Policy* **9**, 181–6.

Scott, J., Gilvarry, E., and Farrell, M. (1998). Managing anxiety and depression in alcohol and drug dependence. *Addictive Behaviors* **23**, 919–31.

Scott, R., Gruer, L., Wilson, P., and Hinshelwood, S. (1995). Glasgow has an innovative scheme for encouraging GPs to manage drug misusers. *British Medical Journal* **310**, 464–5.

Sees, K., Delucchi, K., Masson, C., Rosen, A., Westley Clark, H., Robillard, H., Banys, P., and Hall, S. (2000). Methadone maintenance vs 180-day psychosocially enriched detoxification for treatment of opioid dependence: a randomized controlled trial. *Journal of the American Medical Association* **283**, 1303–10.

Seivewright, N. (2000). *Community treatment of drug misuse: more than methadone.* Cambridge University Press, Cambridge.

Seivewright, N. and Dougal, W. (1993). Withdrawal symptoms from high dose benzodiazepines in polydrug users. *Drug and Alcohol Dependence* **32**, 15–23.

Seligman, M.E.P. (1995). The effectiveness of psychotherapy. *American Psychologist* **50**, 965–74.

Sell, L., Farrell, M., and Robson, P. (1997). Prescription of diamorphine, dipipanone and cocaine in England and Wales. *Drug and Alcohol Review* **16**, 221–6.

Sell, L., Segar, G., and Merrill, J. (2001). One hundred and twenty five patients prescribed injectable opiates in the north west of England. *Drug and Alcohol Review* **20**, 57–66.

Selwyn, P., Feiner, C., Cox, C., Lipshutz, C., and Cohen, R. (1987). Knowledge about AIDS and high-risk behavior among intravenous drug users in New York City. *AIDS* **1**, 247–54.

Senay, E.C., Dorus, W., Goldberg, F., and Thornton, W. (1977). Withdrawal from methadone maintenance: rate of withdrawal and expectation. *Archives of General Psychiatry* **34**, 361–7.

Shaner, A., Khalsa, M., Roberts, L., Wilkins, J., Anglin, D., and Hsieh, S. (1993). Unrecognized cocaine use among schizophrenic patients. *American Journal of Psychiatry* **150**, 758–62.

Sharp, C. and Rosenberg, N. (1992). Volatile substances In *Substance abuse: a comprehensive textbook* (ed. J. Lowinson, P. Ruiz, R. Millman, and J. Langrod). Williams and Wilkins, Baltimore.

Sharples, A. (1975). *The scorpion's tail.* Elek, London.

Shearer, J., Wodak, A., Mattick, R., van Beek, I., Lewis, J., Hall, W., and Dolan, K. (2001). Pilot randomized controlled study of dexamphetamine substitution for amphetamine dependence. *Addiction* **96**, 1289–96.

Sheeren, M. (1988). The relationship between relapse and involvement in Alcoholics Anonymous. *Journal of Studies in Alcoholism* **49**, 104–6.

Shepherd, R. (1989). Mechanism of sudden death associated with volatile substance abuse. *Human Toxicology* **8**, 287–91.

Sheridan, J., Lovell, S., Turnbull, P., Parsons, J., Stimson, G., and Strang, J. (2000). Pharmacy-based needle exchange (PBNX). schemes in south east England: a survey of service providers. *Addiction* **95**, 1551–60.

Sherman, M. and Bigelow, G. (1992). Validity of patients' self-reported drug use as a function of treatment status. *Drug and Alcohol Dependence* **30**, 1–11.

Shiffman, S. (1989). Conceptual issues in the study of relapse. In *Relapse and addictive behaviour* (ed. M. Gossop). Routledge, London.

Siegel, R. (1978). Cocaine hallucinations. *American Journal of Psychiatry* **135**, 309–14.

Siegel, S. (1979). The role of conditioning in drug tolerance and addiction. In *Psychopathology in animals: research and treatment implications* (ed. J. Keehn). Academic Press, New York. .

Siegel, S. (1983). Classical conditioning, drug tolerance and drug dependence. In *Research advances in alcohol and drug problems*, Vol.7 (ed. Y. Israel, F. Glaser, H. Kalant, R. Popham, W. Schmidt, and R. Smart). Plenum, New York.

Silverman, K., Chutuape, M., Bigelow, G., and Stitzer, M. (1996*a*). Voucher-based reinforcement of attendance by unemployed methadone patients in a job skills training program. *Drug and Alcohol Dependence* **41**, 197–207.

Silverman, K., Higgins, S.T., Brooner, R.K., Montoya, I.D., Cone, E.J., Schuster, C.R., and Preston, K.L. (1996*b*). Sustained cocaine abstinence in methadone patients through voucher-based reinforcement therapy. *Archives of General Psychiatry* **53**, 409–15.

Simpson, D.D. (1981). Treatment for drug use: follow-up outcomes and length of time spent. *Archives of General Psychiatry* **38**, 875–80.

Simpson, D.D. (1997). Effectiveness of drug-abuse treatment: a review of research from field settings. In *Treating drug abusers effectively* (ed. J.A. Egerton, D.M. Fox, and A.I. Leshner). Blackwells, Oxford.

Simpson, D.D. and Friend, J. (1986). Legal status and long-term outcomes for addicts in the DARP follow-up project. In *Compulsory treatment of drug abuse: research and clinical practice* (ed. C. Leukefeld and F.Tims), NIDA Research Monograph no.86. NIDA, Rockville, Maryland.

Simpson, D.D. and Joe, G. (1993). Motivation as a predictor of early dropout from drug abuse treatment. *Psychotherapy* **30**, 357–68.

Simpson, D.D. and Lloyd, M.R. (1977). *Alcohol and illicit drug use: national follow-up study of admissions to drug abuse treatments in the DARP during 1969–1971*, Services Research Report. National Institute on Drug Abuse, Rockville, Maryland.

Simpson, D.D. and Lloyd, M.R. (1981). Alcohol use following treatment for drug addiction: a four year follow-up. *Journal of Studies on Alcohol* **42**, 323–35.

Simpson, D. and Savage, L. (1980). Drug abuse treatment readmissions and outcomes. *Archives of General Psychiatry* **37**, 896–901.

Simpson, D. and Sells, S. (1983). Effectiveness for treatment of drug abuse: an overview of the DARP research programme. *Advances in Alcohol and Substance Abuse* **2** (1), 7–29.

Simpson, D.and Sells, S. (1990). *Opioid addiction and treatment.* Krieger, Malabar, Florida.

Simpson, D., Savage, L., and Lloyd, M. (1979). Follow-up evaluation of treatment of drug abuse during 1969–1972. *Archives of General Psychiatry* **36**, 772–80.

Simpson, D., Crandall, R., Savage, L., and Pavia-Kreuger, E. (1981). Leisure of addicts at post-treatment follow-up. *Journal of Counseling Psychology* **28**, 36–9.

Simpson, D.D., Joe, G., Rowan-Szal, G., and Greener, J. (1995). Client engagement and change during drug abuse treatment. *Journal of Substance Abuse* **7**, 117–34.

Simpson, D.D., Joe, G., Broome, K., Hiller, M., Knight, K., Rowan-Szal, G. (1997*a*). Program diversity and treatment retention rates in the Drug Abuse Treatment Outcome Study (DATOS). *Psychology of Addictive Behaviors* **11**, 279–93.

Simpson, D.D., Joe, G., Rowan-Szal, G., and Greener, J. (1997*b*). Drug abuse treatment process components that improve retention. *Journal of Substance Abuse Treatment* **14**, 565–72.

Sklar, S., Annis, H., and Turner, N. (1997). Development and validation of the Drug Taking Confidence Questionnaire: a measure of coping self-efficacy. *Addictive Behaviors* **22**, 655–70.

Sleight, P. (1996). Myocardial infarction. In *Oxford textbook of medicine*, Vol 2 (ed. D. Weatherall, J. Ledingham, and D. Warrell). Oxford University Press, Oxford.

Smith, D. (1969). "Speed kills": a review of amphetamine abuse. *Journal of Psychodelic Drugs* **2**, 2.

Smith, D. and Wesson, D. (1999). Benzodiazepines and other sedative-hypnotics. In *Textbook of Substance Abuse Treatment* (ed. M. Galanter and H. Kleber). American Psychiatric Press, Washington.

Sobell, L. and Sobell, M. (1978). Validity of self-reports in three populations of alcoholics. *Journal of Consulting and Clinical Psychology* **46**, 901–7.

Sobell, M. and Sobell, L. (1998). Guiding self-change. In *Treating addictive behaviors* (ed. W. Miller and N. Heather). Plenum, New York.

Sobell, M. and Sobell, L. (1999). Stepped care for alcohol problems: an efficient method for planning and delivering clinical services. In *Changing addictive behavior* (ed. J. Tucker, D. Donovan, and G.A. Marlatt). Guilford, New York.

Sorensen, J.L. and Copeland, A.L. (2000). Drug abuse treatment as an HIV preventative strategy: a review. *Drug and Alcohol Dependence* **59**, 17–31.

Spanagel, R., Kirschke, C., Tretter, F., and Holsboer, F. (1998). Forced opiate withdrawal under anaesthesia augments and prolongs the occurrence of withdrawal signs in rats. *Drug and Alcohol Dependence* **52**, 251–6.

Spear, H.B. and Mott, J. (1993). Cocaine and crack within the British system: a history of control. In *Cocaine and crack: supply and use* (ed. P. Bean). St Martin's Press, New York.

Speckart, G. and Anglin, M.D. (1985). Narcotics use and crime. An analysis of existing evidence for a causal relationship. *Behavioural Science and Law* **3**, 259–83.

Sperry, L., Brill, P., Howard, K., and Grissom, G. (1996). *Treatment outcomes in psychotherapy and psychiatric interventions*. Brunner/Mazel, New York.

Stark, M. (1994). Management of drug addicts in police custody. *Journal of the Royal Society of Medicine* **87**, 584–7.

Steigerwald, F. and Stone, D. (1999). Cognitive restructuring and the 12-step program of Alcoholics Anonymous. *Journal of Substance Abuse Treatment* **16**, 321–7.

Stephens, R., Roffman, R., and Curtin, L. (2000). Comparison of extended versus brief treatments for marihuana use. *Journal of Consulting and Clinical Psychology* **68**, 898–908.

Sterling, R., Gottheil, E., Weinstein, S., and Serota, R. (2001). The effect of therapist/patient race- and sex-matching in individual treatment. *Addiction* **96**, 1015–22.

Stevens, A. and Raftery, J. (1994). Introduction. In *Health care needs assessment: the epidemiologically based needs assessment reviews* (ed. A. Stevens and J. Raftery), p. 1. Radcliffe Medical, Oxford.

Stewart, D., Gossop, M., Marsden, J., and Rolfe, A. (2000*a*). Drug misuse and acquisitive crime among clients recruited to the National Treatment Outcome Research Study (NTORS). *Criminal Behaviour and Mental Health* **10**, 10–20.

Stewart, D., Gossop, M., Marsden, J., and Strang, J. (2000*b*). Variation between and within drug treatment modalities: data from the National Treatment Outcome Research Study (UK). *European Addiction Research* **6**, 106–14.

Stewart, D., Gossop, M., and Marsden, J. (2002). Reductions in non-fatal overdose after drug misuse treatment: results from the National Treatment Outcome Research Study (NTORS). *Journal of Substance Abuse Treatment* **22**, 1–9.

Stewart, D., Gossop, M., Marsden, J., Kidd, T., and Treacy, S. (2003). Similarities in outcomes for men and women after drug misuse treatment: results from the National Treatment Outcome Research Study (NTORS). *Drug and Alcohol Review* **22**, 35–41.

Stewart, J., de Wit, H., and Eikelboom, R. (1984). Role of unconditioned and conditioned drug effects in the self-administration of opiates and stimulants. *Psychological Review* **91**, 251–68.

Stiles, W., Shapiro, D., and Elliot, R. (1986). Are all psychotherapies equivalent? *American Psychologist* **41**, 165–80.

Stimson, G. (1973). *Heroin and behaviour*. Irish University Press, Shannon.

Stimson, G. (1974). Obeying doctor's orders. A view from the other side. *Social Science and Medicine* **8**, 97–104.

Stimson, G. (1995). AIDS and injecting drug use in the United Kingdom, 1987–1993: The policy response and the prevention of the epidemic. *Social Science and Medicine* **41**, 699–716.

Stimson, G.V. (1996). Has the United Kingdom averted an epidemic of HIV-1 infection among drug injectors? *Addiction* **91**, 1085–8.

Stimson, G. (1998). Harm reduction in action: putting theory into practice. *International Journal of Drug Policy* **9**, 401–9.

Stimson, G., Oppenheimer, E., and Stimson, C. (1984). Drug abuse in the medical profession: addict doctors and the Home Office. *British Journal of Addiction* **79**, 395–402.

Stimson, G., Alldritt, L., Dolan, K., and Donoghoe, M. (1988). Syringe exchange schemes for drug users in England and Scotland. *British Medical Journal* **296**, 1717.

Stimson, G., Donoghoe, M., Lart, R., and Dolan, K. (1990). Distributing sterile needles and syringes to people who inject drugs: the syringe-exchange experiment. In *AIDS and drug misuse* (ed. J. Strang and G. Stimson). Routledge, London.

Stitzer, M., Bigelow, G., Lawrence, C., Cohen, J., D'Lugoff, B., and Hawthorne, J. (1977). Medication take-home as a reinforcer in a methadone maintenance program. *Addictive Behaviors* **2**, 9–14.

Stitzer, M., Bigelow, G., Liebson, I., and Hawthorne, J. (1982). Contingent reinforcement of benzodiazepine-free urines. *Journal of Applied Analysis of Behavior* **15**, 493–503.

Stitzer, M., Bickel, W., Bigelow, G., and Liebson, I. (1986). Effect of methadone dose contingencies on urinalysis test results of polydrug-abusing methadone-maintenance patients. *Drug and Alcohol Dependence* **18**, 341–8.

Stitzer, M., Bigelow, G., and Gross, J. (1989). Behavioral treatment of drug abuse. In *Treatments of psychiatric disorders: a task force* (ed. T.B. Karasu), Report of the American Psychiatric Association, Vol. 2. American Psychiatric Association, Washington, DC.

Stitzer, M.L. and Chutape, M.A. (1999). Other substance use disorders in methadone treatment: Prevalence, consequences, detection, and management. In *Methadone treatment for opioid dependence* (ed. E.C. Strain and M.L. Stitzer). Johns Hopkins University Press, Baltimore.

Stockwell, T. (1987). Is there a better word than 'craving'? *British Journal of Addiction* **82**, 44–5.

Stone, A.M., Greenstein, R.A., Gamble, G., and McLellan, A.T. (1993). Cocaine use by schizophrenic outpatients who receive depot neuroleptic medication. *Hospital and Community Psychiatry* **44**, 176–7.

Strain, E.C. (1998). Useful predictors of outcome in methadone-treated patients: results from a controlled clinical trial with three doses of methadone. *Journal of Maintenance in the Addictions* **1**, 15–28.

Strain, E.C. (1999). Methadone dose during maintenance treatment. In *Methadone treatment for opioid dependence* (ed. E. C. Strain and M. Stitzer). Johns Hopkins, Baltimore.

Strain, E.C. and Stoller, K.B. (1999). Introduction and historical overview. In *Methadone treatment for opioid dependence* (ed. E. C. Strain and M. Stitzer). Johns Hopkins, Baltimore.

Strain, E.C., Brooner, R.K., and Bigelow, G.E. (1991*a*). Clustering of multiple substance use and psychiatric diagnoses in opiate addicts. *Drug and Alcohol Dependence* **27**, 127–34.

Strain, E.C., Stitzer, M.L., and Bigelow, G.E. (1991*b*). Early treatment time course of depressive symptoms in opiate addicts. *Journal of Nervous and Mental Disease* **179**, 215–21.

Strain, E.C., Preston, K., Liebson, I., and Bigelow, G. (1995). Buprenorphine effects in methadone-maintained volunteers: effects at two hours after methadone. *Journal of Pharmacology and Experimental Therapeutics* **272**, 628–38.

Strain, E.C., Bigelow, G., Liebson, I., and Stitzer, M. (1999). Moderate- versus high-dose methadone in the treatment of opioid dependence. *Journal of the American Medical Association* **281**, 1000–5.

Strang, J. (1990). Intermediate goals and the process of change. In *AIDS and drug misuse* (ed. J. Strang and G. Stimson). Routledge, London.

Strang, J. (1993). Drug use and harm reduction: responding to the challenge. In *Psychoactive drugs and harm reduction: from faith to science* (ed. N. Heather, A. Wodak, E. Nadelmann, and P. O'Hare). Whurr, London.

Strang, J. and Edwards, G. (1989). Cocaine and crack. *British Medical Journal* **299**, 337–8.

Strang, J. and Gossop, M. (1990). Comparison of linear versus inverse exponential methadone reduction curves in the detoxification of opiate addicts. *Addictive Behavior* **15**, 541–7.

Strang, J. and King, L. (1996). Heroin is more than just diamorphine. *Addiction Research* **5**, iii–vii.

Strang, J. and Sheridan, J. (1997). Prescribing amphetamines to drug misusers: data from the 1995 national survey of community pharmacies in England and Wales. *Addiction* **92**, 833–8.

Strang, J. and Sheridan, J. (1998). National and regional characteristics of methadone prescribing in England and Wales: local analyses of data from the 1995 national survey of community pharmacies. *Journal of Substance Misuse* **3**, 240–6.

Strang, J., Griffiths, P., and Gossop, M. (1992a). First use of heroin: changes in route of administration over time. *British Medical Journal* **304**, 1222–3.

Strang, J., Seivewright, N., and Farrell, M. (1992b). Intravenous and other novel abuses of benzodiazepines: the opening of Pandora's box? *British Journal of Addiction* **87**, 1373–5.

Strang, J., Griffiths, P., Abbey, J., Gossop, M. (1994a). Survey of use of injected benzodiazepines among drug users in Britain. *British Medical Journal* **308**, 1082.

Strang, J., Ruben, S., Farrell, M., and Gossop, M. (1994b). Prescribing heroin and other injectable drugs. In *The British system* (ed. J. Strang and M. Gossop). Oxford University Press, London.

Strang, J., Sheridan, J., and Barber, N. (1996a). Prescribing injectable and oral methadone to opiate addicts: results from the 1995 national postal survey of community pharmacies. *British Medical Journal* **313**, 270–2.

Strang, J., Powis, B., Griffiths, P., and Gossop, M. (1996b). The better-travelled treatment tourist: service overlap among heroin and cocaine users. *Druglink* **11**, 10–13.

Strang, J., Bearn, J., and Gossop, M. (1997a). Opiate detoxification under anaesthesia. *British Medical Journal* **315**, 1249–50.

Strang, J., Finch, E., Hankinson, L., Farell, M., Taylor, C., and Gossop, M. (1997b). Methadone treatment for opiate addiction: benefits in the first month. *Addiction Research* **5**, 71–6.

Strang, J., Griffiths, P., and Gossop, M. (1997c). Heroin in the United Kingdom: different forms, different origins, and the relationship to different routes of administration. *Drug and Alcohol Review* **16**, 329–37.

Strang, J., Marks, I., Dawe, S., Powell, J., Gossop, M., Richards, D., and Grey, J. (1997d). Type of hospital setting and treatment outcome with heroin addicts. Results from a randomised trial. *British Journal of Psychiatry* **171**, 335–9.

Strang, J., Griffiths, P., Powis, B., Fountain, J., Williamson, S., and Gossop, M. (1999a). Which drugs cause overdose among opiate misusers? Study of personal and witnessed overdoses. *Drug and Alcohol Review* **18**, 253–61.

Strang, J., Powis, B., Best, D., Vingoe, L., Griffiths, P., Taylor, C., Welsh, S., and Gossop, M. (1999b). Preventing opiate overdose fatalities with take-home naloxone: pre-launch study of possible impact and acceptability. *Addiction* **94**, 199–204.

Strang, J., Bearn, J., and Gossop, M. (1999c). Lofexidine for opiate detoxification: review of recent randomised and open trials. *American Journal on Addictions* **8**, 337–48.

Strang, J., Best, D., Man, L-H., Noble, A., and Gossop, M. (2000a). Peer-initiated overdose resuscitation: fellow drug users could be mobilised to implement resuscitation. *International Journal of Drug Policy* **11**, 437–45.

Strang, J. Marsden, J. Cummins, M. Farrell, M., Finch, E., Gossop, M., Stewart, D., and Welch, S. (2000b). Randomised trial of supervised injectable versus oral methadone maintenance: report of feasibility and 6-month outcomes. *Addiction* **95**, 1631–45.

Sutton, S. (1996). Can 'stages of change' provide guidance in the treatment of addictions? In *Psychotherapy, psychological treatments and the addictions* (ed. G. Edwards and C. Dare). Cambridge University Press, Cambridge.

Svikis, D., Golden, A., Huggins, G., and Pickens, R. (1997). Cost-effectiveness of treatment for drug-abusing women. *Drug and Alcohol Dependence* **45**, 105–13.

Swift, R. and Miller, N. (1997). Integration of health care economics for addiction treatment in clinic care. *Journal of Psychoactive Drugs* **29**, 255–62.

Swift,W., Copeland, J., and Hall, W. (1996). Characteristics of women with alcohol and other drug problems: findings of an Australian national survey. *Addiction* **91**, 1141–50.

Swift, W., Maher, L., and Sunjic, S. (1999). Transitions between routes of heroin administration: a study of Caucasian and Indochinese heroin users in south-western Sydney, Australia. *Addiction* **94**, 71–82.

Talbott, G., Gallegos, K., Wilson, P., and Porter, T. (1987). The Medical Association of Georgia's impaired physician program—review of the first 1000 physicians: analysis of specialty. *Journal of the American Medical Association* **257**, 2927–30.

Tashkin, D.P., Simmons, M.S., Caulson, A.H., Clark, V.A., and Gong, H. (1987). Respiratory effects of cocaine freebasing among habitual users of marijuana with or without tobacco. *Chest* **92**, 638–44.

Task Force to Review Services for Drug Misusers (1996). *Report of an independent review of drug treatment services in England*. Department of Health, London.

Taylor, A. (1993). *An ethnography of a female injecting community*. Clarendon, Oxford.

Taylor, D., Poulton, R., Moffitt, T., Ramankutty, P., and Sears, M. (2000). The respiratory effects of cannabis dependence in young adults. *Addiction* **95**, 1669–77.

Teasdale, J. (1973). Conditioned abstinence in narcotic addicts. *International Journal of the Addictions* **8**, 273–92.

Telch, M., Hannon, R., and Telch, C. (1984). A comparison of cessation strategies for the outpatient alcoholic. *Addictive Behaviors* **9**, 103–9.

Tennant, F.S. (1987). Inadequate plasma concentrations in some high dose methadone maintenance patients. *American Journal of Psychiatry* **144**, 1349–50.

Tennant, F.S. and Sagherian, A. (1987). Double blind comparison of amantidine and bromocriptine for ambulatory withdrawal from cocaine dependence. *Archives of Internal Medicine* **147**, 109–12.

Tennant, F.S., Rawson, R.A., Cohen, A.J., and Mann, A. (1984). Clinical experience with naltrexone in suburban opioid addicts. *Journal of Clinical Psychiatry* **45**, 41–5.

Thirion, X., Lapierre, V., Micallef, J., Ronflé, E. Masutb, A., Pradela, V., Coudertb, C., Mabriez, J., and Sanmarco, J. (2002). Buprenorphine prescription by general practitioners in a French region. *Drug and Alcohol Dependence* **65**, 197–204.

Thomas, R., Plant, M.A., Plant, M.L., and Sales, D. (1989). Risks of AIDS among workers in the 'sex industry': some initial results from a Scottish study. *British Medical Journal* **299**, 148–9.

Tinetti, M., Speechley, M., and Ginter, S. (1988). Risk factors for falls among elderly persons living in the community. *New England Journal of Medicine* **319**, 1701–7.

Tracqui, A., Kintz, P., and Ludes, B. (1998). Buprenorphine-related deaths among drug addicts in France: a report on 20 fatalities. *Journal of Analytic Toxicology* **22**, 430–4.

Trinkoff, A. and Storr, C. (1994). Relationship of speciality and access to substance use among registered nurses: an exploratory analysis. *Drug and Alcohol Dependence* **36**, 215–19.

Tuchfeld, B. (1981). Spontaneous remission in alcoholics: empirical observations and theoretical implications. *Journal of Studies on Alcohol* **42**, 626–41.

Turnbull, P., McSweeney, T., and Hough, M. (2000). *Drug treatment and testing orders: the 18 months evaluation*, Home Office paper no.128. Home Office, London.

Tyrer, P., Rutherford, D., and Huggett, T. (1981). Benzodiazepine withdrawal symptoms and propranolol. *Lancet* i, 520–2.

Uchtenhagen, A., Dobler-Mikola, A., Steffan, T., Gutzwiller, F., Blattler, R., and Pfeifer, S. (1999). *Prescription of narcotics for heroin addicts*. Karger, Basel.

Unnithan, S., Gossop, M., and Strang, J. (1992). Factors associated with relapse among opiate addicts in an outpatient detoxification programme. *British Journal of Psychiatry* **161**, 654–7.

US Surgeon General's Report (1988). *The health consequences of smoking*. US Dept of Health and Human Services, Rockville, Maryland.

Utting, J. (1989). Major catastrophes in anaesthesia. In *General anaesthesia* (ed. J.F. Nunn, J.E. Utting, and B.R. Brown). Butterworths, London.

Vaillant, G. (1966). A twelve-year follow-up of New York addicts: II. The natural history of a chronic disease. *New England Journal of Medicine* **275**, 1282–8.

Vaillant, G. (1973). A 20 year follow-up of New York narcotic addicts. *Archives of General Psychiatry* **29**, 237–41.

van den Brink, W., Hendriks, V., Blanken, P., Huijsman, I., and van Ree, J. (2002). *Medical co-prescription of heroin: two randomized controlled trials*. CCBH, Utrecht.

Verkes, R., Gigsman, H., Pieters, M., Schoemaker, R., de Visser, S., and Kuijpers, M. (2001). Cognitive performance and serotonergic function in users of ecstasy. *Psychopharmacology* **153**, 196–202.

Vermeulen, E. and Walburg, J. (1997). What happens if a criminal can choose between detention and treatment: results of a 4-year experiment in the Netherlands. *Alcohol and Alcoholism* **33**, 33–6.

Vetter, H., Ramsey, L., Luscher, T., Schrey, A., and Vetter, W. (1985). Symposium on compliance—improving strategies in hypertension. *Journal of Hypertension* **3**, 1–99.

Vignau., J., Duhamel, A., Catteau, J, Legal, G., Huynh Pho, A., Grailles, I., Beauvillain, J., Petit, P., Beauvillain, P., and Parquet, P. (2001). Practice-based buprenorphine maintenance treatment (BMT): how do French healthcare providers manage the opiate-addicted patients? *Journal of Substance Abuse Treatment* **21**, 135–44.

Vincent, P. (1971). Factors influencing patient noncompliance. *Nursing Research* **20**, 509–16.

Vingoe, L., Finch, E., and Griffiths, P. (1997). *Improving the quality and comparability of data related to hepatitis B/C and delta virus infection in drug users.* European Monitoring Centre for Drugs and Drug Addiction, National Addiction Centre, London.

Voegtlin, W. (1940). The treatment of alcoholism by establishing a conditioned reflex. *American Journal of the Medical Sciences* **199**, 802–10.

Vogel, V., Isbell, H., and Chapman, K. (1948). Present status of narcotic addiction. *Journal of the American Medical Association* **138**, 1019–26.

Vogler, R., Compton, J., and Weissbach, T. (1975). Integrated behaviour change techniques for alcoholism. *Journal of Consulting and Clinical Psychology* **43**, 233–43.

Volkow, N., Chang, L., Wang, G., Fowler, J., Franceschi, D., Sedler, M., Gatley, J., Miller, E., Hitzemann, R., Ding, Y., and Logan, J., (2001). Loss of dopamine transporters in methamphetamine abusers recovers with protracted abstinence *Journal of Neuroscience* **21**, 9414–18.

Wahren, C., Allebeck, P., and Rajs, J. (1997). Unnatural causes of death among drug addicts in Stockholm: an analyis of health care and autopsy records. *Substance Use and Misuse* **32**, 2163–83.

Waldorf, D., Reinarman, D., and Murphy, S. (1991). *Cocaine changes: the experience of using and quitting.* Temple University Press, Philadelphia.

Wallerstein, R.S. (1956). Comparative study of treatment methods for chronic alcoholism. *American Journal of Psychiatry* **113**, 228–33.

Walsh, S., Johnson, R., Cone, E., and Bigelow, G. (1998). Intravenous and oral l-alpha-acetylmethadol: pharmacodynamics and pharmacokinetics in humans. *Journal of Pharmacology and Experimental Therapeutics* **285**, 71–82.

Ward, J., Mattick, R., and Hall, W. (1992). *Key issues in methadone maintenance treatment.* New South Wales Press, Sydney.

Ward, J., Mattick, R., and Hall, W. (1998). *Methadone maintenance treatment and other opioid replacement therapies.* Harwood, Australia.

Washton, A. (1987). Outpatient treatment techniques. In *Cocaine: a clinician's handbook* (ed. A. Washton and M. Gold). Wiley, Chichester.

Washton, A. (1989). *Cocaine addiction: treatment, recovery and relapse.* Norton, New York.

Washton, A., Pottash, A., and Gold, M. (1984). Naltrexone in addicted business executives and physicians. *Journal of Clinical Psychiatry* **49**, 39–41.

Weisberg, D. (1985). *Children of the night.* Lexington Books, Lexington, Maine.

Weiss, F., Markou, A., Lorang, M.T., and Koob, G.F. (1992). Basal extracellular dopamine levels in the nucleus accumbens are decreased during cocaine withdrawal after unlimited-access self-administration. *Brain Research* **593**, 314–18.

Weiss, R.D. (1999). Inpatient treatment. In *The American Psychiatric Press textbook of substance abuse treatment,* 2nd edn (ed. M. Galanter and H.D. Kleber). American Psychiatric Press Inc, Washington, DC.

Weiss, R.D., Griffin, M.S., and Mirin, S.M. (1992). Drug abuse as self medication for depression: an empirical study. *American Journal of Drug and Alcohol Abuse* **18**, 121–30.

Weiss, R., Martinez-Raga, J., Griffen, M., Greenfield, S., and Hufford, C. (1997). Gender differences in cocaine dependent patients: a 6 month follow up study. *Drug and Alcohol Dependence* **44**, 35–40.

Weiss, R.D., Najavits, L.M., Greenfield, S.F., Soto, J.A., Shaw, S.R., and Wyner, D. (1998). Validity of substance use self-reports in dually diagnosed outpatients. *American Journal of Psychiatry* **155**, 127–8.

Weiss, R.D., Greenfield, S.F., Griffin, M.L., Najavits, L.M., and Fucinto, L. (2000). The use of collateral reports for patients with bipolar and substance use disorders. *American Journal of Drug and Alcohol Abuse* **26**, 369–78.

Weissman, M. and Merikangas, K. (1986). The epidemiology of anxiety and panic disorders. *Journal of Clinical Psychiatry* **46**, 11–17.

Welch, M., Sniegoski, L., Allgood, C., and Habram, M. (1993). Hair analysis for drugs of abuse: evaluation of analytical methods, environmental issues, and development of reference materials. *Journal of Analytical Toxicology* **17**, 389–98.

Wells, B. (1994). Narcotics Anonymous (NA) in Britain. In *Heroin addiction and drug policy: the British system* (ed. J. Strang and M. Gossop), pp. 240–7. Oxford University Press, Oxford.

Wells, E.A., Hawkins, J.D., and Catalano, R.F. (1988). Choosing drug use measures for treatment outcome studies. I. The influence of measurement approach on treatment results. *International Journal of the Addictions* **23**, 851–73.

West, R. and Gossop, M. (1994). A comparison of withdrawal symptoms from different drug classes. *Addiction* **89**, 1483–9.

Wexler, H., Falkin, G., and Lipton, D. (1990). Outcome evaluation of a prison therapeutic community for substance abuse treatment. *Criminal Justice and Behavior* **17**, 71–92.

Wexler, H., Melnick, G., Lowe, L., and Peters, J. (1999). Three-year revicarceration outcomes for Amity in-prison therapeutic community and aftercare in California. *The Prison Journal* **79**, 321–36.

White, B. and Madara, E. (1992). *The self-help sourcebook*. American Self-help Clearinghouse, Denville, New Jersey.

White, J.M. and Irvine, R.J. (1999). Mechanisms of fatal opioid overdose. *Addiction* **94**, 961–72.

White, R., Alcorn, R., and Feinmann, C. (2001). Two methods of community detoxification from opiates: an open-label comparison of lofexidine and buprenorphine. *Drug and Alcohol Dependence* **65**, 77–83.

Wiens, A., Montague, J., Manaugh, T., and English, C. (1976). Pharmacological aversive counter-conditioning to alcohol in a private hospital: one year follow-up. *Journal of Studies on Alcoholism* **37**, 1320–4.

Wiesbeck, G., Schuckit, M., Kalmijn, J., Tipp, J., Bucholz, K., and Smith, T. (1996). An evaluation of the history of a marijuana withdrawal syndrome in a large population. *Addiction* **91**, 1469–78.

Wikler, A. (1948). Recent progress in research on the neurophysiologic basis of morphine addiction. *American Journal of Psychiatry* **105**, 329–38.

Wikler, A. (1980). *Opioid dependence*. Plenum, New York.

Williams, A.B., McNelly, E.A., Willaims, A.E., and D'Aquila, R.T. (1992). Methadone maintenance treatment and HIV type 1 seroconversion among injecting drug users. *AIDS Care* **4**, 35–41.

Williams, B., Chang, K., Van Truong, M., and Saad, F. (1992). *Canadian profile: alcohol and other drugs*. Addiction Research Foundation, Toronto.

Williams, H. (1971). Low and high dose methadone maintenance in the outpatient treatment of the hard core heroin addict. In *Methadone maintenance* (ed. S. Einstein). Marcel Dekker, New York.

Williams, R.J. and Chang, S.Y. (2000). A comprehensive and comparative review of adolescent substance abuse treatment outcome. *Clinical Psychology: Science and Practice* **7**, 138–66.

Williamson, S., Gossop, M., Powis, B., Griffiths, P., Fountain, J., and Strang, J. (1997). Adverse effects of stimulant drugs in a community sample of drug users. *Drug and Alcohol Dependence* **44**, 87–94.

Wilson, B., Elms, R., and Tompson, C. (1975). Outpatient vs hospital methadone detoxification: experimental comparison. *International Journal of the Addictions* **10**, 13–21.

Wilson, G.T. (1980). Toward specifying the 'nonspecific' factors in behavior therapy. In *Psychotherapy process* (ed. M. Mahoney). Plenum, New York.

Wilson, G.T. (1996). Treatment manuals in clinical practice. *Behaviour Research and Therapy* **34**, 295–314.

Winick, C. (1990–91). The counselor in drug abuse treatment. *International Journal of the Addictions* **25**, 1479–502.

Withers, N.W., Pulvirenti, L., Koob, G.F., and Gillin, J.C. (1995). Cocaine abuse and dependence. *Journal of Clinical Psychopharmacology* **15**, 63–78.

Wolfe, B. and Goldfried, M. (1988). Research on psychotherapy integration. *Journal of Consulting and Clinical Psychology* **56**, 448–51.

Wolff, K. and Strang, J. (1999). Therapeutic drug monitoring for methadone: scanning the horizon. *European Addiction Research* **5**, 36–42.

Wolff, K., Hay, A., Raistrick, D., Calvert, R., and Feely, M. (1991). Measuring compliance in methadone maintenance patients: use of a pharmacological indicator to 'estimate' methadone plasma levels. *Clinical Pharmacological Therapies* **50**, 199–207.

Wolff, K., Rostami-Hodjegan, A., Shires, S., Hay, A., Feely, M., Calvert, R., Raistrick, D., and Tucker, G. (1997). The pharmacokinetics of methadone in healthy subjects and opiate users. *British Journal of Clinical Pharmacology* **44**, 325–34.

Wolff, K. Farrell, .M., Marsden, J., Monteiro, M., All, R., Welch, S., and Strang, J. (1999). A review of biological indicators of illicit drug use, practical considerations and clinical usefulness. *Addiction* **94**, 1279–98.

Wolk, J., Wodak, A., Morlet, A., Guinan, J., Wilson, E., Gold, J., and Cooper, D. (1988). Syringe HIV seroprevalence and behavioural and demographic characteristics of intravenous drug users in Sydney, Australia, 1987. *AIDS* **2**, 373–7.

Wolpe, J. (1969). *The practice of behavior therapy*. Pergamon, New York.

Woods, J., Katz, J., and Winger, G. (1987). Abuse liability of benzodiazepines. *Pharmacological Reviews* **39**, 251–413.

Woody, G., O'Hare, K., Mintz, J., and O'Brien, C. (1975). Rapid intake: a method for increasing retention rate of heroin addicts seeking methadone treatment. *Comprehensive Psychiatry* **16**, 165–9.

Woody, G., McLellan, A.T., and Luborsky, L. (1984). Psychiatric severity as a predictor of benefits from psychotherapy. *American Journal of Psychiatry* **141**, 1171–7.

Woody, G., McLellan, A.T., Luborsky, L., and O'Brien, C. (1987). 12 month follow-up of psychotherapy for opiate dependence. *American Journal of Psychiatry* **144**, 38–46.

World Health Organisation (1993). *AIDS among drug users in Europe* (ed. M. Gossop, A. Kirsch, and C. Goos). World Health Organisation, Copenhagen.

Wray, I. and Dickerson, M. (1981). Cessation of high frequency gambling and 'withdrawal symptoms'. *British Journal of Addiction* **76**, 401–5.

Wutzke, S., Conigrave, K., Saunders, J., and Hall, W. (2002). The long-term effectiveness of brief interventions for unsafe alcohol consumption: a 10-year follow-up. *Addiction* **97**, 665–75.

Yablonsky, L. (1965). *Synanon: the tunnel back.* Macmillan, New York.

Yancovitz, S., DesJarlais, D., and Peyser, N. (1991). A randomized trial of an interim methadone clinic. *American Journal of Public Health* **81**, 1185–91.

Zanis, D., McLellan, A.T., and Randall, M. (1994). Can you trust patients' self-reports of drug use during treatment? *Drug and Alcohol Dependence* **35**, 127–32.

Zanis, D., McLellan, A.T., Alterman, A., and Cnaan, R. (1996). Efficacy of enhanced outreach counseling to reenroll high-risk drug users 1 year after discharge from treatment. *American Journal of Psychiatry* **153**, 1095–6.

Ziedonis, D. and Kosten, T. (1991). Depression as a prognostic factor for pharmacological treatment of cocaine dependence. *Psychopharmacology Bulletin* **27**, 337–43.

Index